Hong Kong Notable Doctors

Hong Kong Notable Doctors

Individuals Who Shaped the Medical Services 1842–2015

By

Wong Tai-wai

Moira M. W. Chan-Yeung

The Chinese University of Hong Kong Press

Hong Kong Notable Doctors:
Individuals Who Shaped the Medical Services, 1842–2015
By Wong Tai-wai & Moira M. W. Chan-Yeung

ISBN: 978-988-237-354-9 (hardcover)
978-988-237-902-2 (ebook)

The Chinese University of Hong Kong Press
The Chinese University of Hong Kong
Sha Tin, N.T., Hong Kong
Fax: +852 2603 7355
Email: cup@cuhk.edu.hk
Website: cup.cuhk.edu.hk

This book is dedicated to all men and women of science and humanity in the art of healing, through the inspiration of God.

Contents

Foreword

When the Hong Kong Museum of Medical Sciences Society was inaugurated in 1995, the first main objective was to collect and preserve materials of historical interest relating to the development of medical sciences in Hong Kong for exhibition in the Museum. The second objective was to promote research and public interest in the development of medicine in Hong Kong. To this end, the Museum has organized guided tours of heritage trails and published articles, pamphlets, and books on local medical history. In addition, the Society has organized regular talks of medical history and medical topics to the public not only to arouse the public's interest in the history of medicine, but also to alert them on the importance of health and prevention of diseases.

Both authors of the present book have been regular contributors to the Museum's column in the *Hong Kong Medical Journal*—"Reminiscence: Artefacts from The Hong Kong Museum of Medical Sciences." Dr. T. W. Wong was the editor of the Museum's publication for the 20th anniversary—*Footprints of Medicine: From the Collections of Hong Kong Museum of Medical Sciences* and other medical history books. Professor Moira Chan-Yeung has published three well-researched books on the medical history of Hong Kong covering the period of 1842 to 2015. When I learned of their new project on writing about notable doctors of the past, I eagerly awaited the results of their labour.

This is probably the first book dedicated to the life and times of the doctors who have shaped the medical development of Hong Kong. It is a fascinating story of how the pioneers transformed a city with primitive medical services into what it is today—a city with advanced medical facilities as in any major Western city. As a pathologist, I am naturally drawn to the stories of trailblazers such as Dr. William Hunter, Professors Wang Chung-yik, Hou Pao-chang, and James Gibson, who built a strong foundation for modern pathology in Hong Kong. Hunter, in particular, was the one who oversaw the building of the Bacteriological Institute, which stands today as the Museum. In addition to the intriguing stories, the sequence of narration of these exceptional doctors over more than a century and a half guides us through the development of local medicine in areas of public health, public medical services, medical education, and private practice. The book also provides a great source of reference materials for any researcher in this field.

The Museum has been using different artefacts to arouse public interests in medical history. Telling history through the stories of these architects of our medical and health services is also a good way to engage the general public. This new book by Wong Tai-wai and Moira Chan-Yeung, both members of the Society, is therefore a welcomed addition to the scholarly works of local medical history.

Dr. Mak Wai-ping
Chairman (Executive Committee) and Board of Directors
Hong Kong Museum of Medical Sciences Society

Preface

The development of Western medicine in Hong Kong to its current sophisticated state over more than 150 years is a fascinating story, which has been described by Moira Chan-Yeung in her three books on local medical history (*A Medical History of Hong Kong: 1842–1941*; *A Medical History of Hong Kong: 1942–2015*; and *A Medical History of Hong Kong: The Development and Contributions of Outpatient Services*). These books, covering the period from 1842 to 2015, present an account of the major medical events in the context of the socio-political and economic situations of the time.[1] The publication of the Hong Kong Museum of Medical Sciences Society, *Plague, SARS and the Story of Medicine in Hong Kong*, also takes a similar thematic approach to the medical history of Hong Kong.[2] It includes chapters on the control of infectious diseases and tuberculosis and on the development of hospitals and medical education.

Historical events are often driven by many forces—political, economic, and social changes—acting within a certain time frame. However, we believe that human factors are equally important in shaping the events. This book, *Hong Kong Notable Doctors: Individuals Who Shaped the Medical Services, 1842–2015*, gives the history of development of sanitation and medical and health services in Hong Kong from a perspective different from the above books—the personalities responsible for these remarkable achievements during this period, adding another dimension and color to the remarkable medical history of Hong Kong. The personalities include doctors, nurses, paramedics, and also patients who should not be considered as passive recipients of medical service. In view of the limitation of space in this book, we will only discuss the doctors who are no longer with us but have pioneered and engineered the development and growth of medical and health services in Hong Kong.

While these doctors from diverse backgrounds lived in different eras and engaged in different branches of medicine, they were strikingly similar in several aspects: their dedication to serving the community and their tireless labor to achieve their aim at times under adverse conditions, leaving their mark in the history of medicine in Hong Kong. These individuals, spanning over a period of over 150 years, comprised doctors in government public medical and health services who advocated new initiatives and laid the infrastructure; those who established health policies, and moved the health system forward; the medical educators who trained the medical workforce and generated new medical knowledge through their research; and practising doctors, who not only delivered medical care but also offered their free services in education and social welfare. The story of each doctor in this book is narrated in the context of the complex political, social, and economic backdrop of his/her time. We have also identified the few pioneer female doctors before and after World War II, and described their struggle to enter medical school and the achievements in their life-time.

This book is intended for medical students, medical practitioners, other healthcare professionals, and even general readers. We hope that the stories of these medical pioneers will stimulate their interest in local medical history and to learn from them. We also hope that the general readers who are taking a first dip into the world of medical history will find it fascinating. These doctors built the medical services of Hong Kong from scratch to its current state with an advanced infrastructure similar to any developed nation in the world and as a testimony to their work, the men and women in Hong Kong led the world in life expectancy.[3] We wish to remember and honor them, celebrate their lives here, and to give thanks for their inspirations and selflessness.

The Hong Kong public medical and health services were called by different names over its existence, e.g. Medical Department, Medical and Health Services, or Medical and Health Department. We have used the name according to how it was called during the period in question. The appendix has the name of the public medical and health services according to the period for clarification. In addition, the medical profession is notoriously confusing for its numerous professional titles, especially when given in abbreviations. A listing of these titles and their abbreviations can be found in the section on abbreviation in the front matter of the book. Finally, the information of this book came from a number of primary and secondary sources which can be found under bibliography at the back of the book.

Acknowledgements

Throughout the process of researching and writing this book, we have received assistance, and encouragement from a number of friends and colleagues. When the idea of writing about the prominent doctors who contributed significantly to the medical development as a sequel to the series of books on medical history of Hong Kong was first conceived, we sought advice from members of the Hong Kong Museum of Medical Sciences (HKMMS). Both Dr. Mak Wai-ping (Chairman of Executive Committee) and Dr. Betty Young (Chair of Education and Research Committee) showed their enthusiastic support for the project and shared with us their ideas on candidates for notable doctors. The HKMMS also gave us permission to reproduce many valuable photographs from the Museum's archive of historical photographs.

We are also fortunate to be able to contact some of the friends and relatives of these notable doctors. Dr. A. E. Rodrigues, son of Sir Albert Rodrigues, kindly shared his private collection of photographs and anecdotes of his father. Ms. Christine Fang allowed us to use the pictures of Dr. Harry Fang and gave us information and photographs of his father's efforts to promote rehabilitation in mainland China. Dr. Peter Ho spent his valuable time searching for old photographs of his father Dr. Ho Hung-chiu, John, and kindly allowed us to use some of them. Dr. C. T. Hung, past president of the Hong Kong College of Anesthesiologists, contributed photographs of Dr. Zoltan Lett and his achievements in building the discipline in anesthesia in Hong Kong, and Dr. Arthur van Langenberg for information on the history of development of surgery in Hong Kong. We wish also to express our gratitude to the Centre for Research Collections of the Main Research Library of the University of Edinburgh and the University of Glasgow for information on the student record of Professor James Gibson and on his PhD thesis.

The following clinical departments of the University of Hong Kong have kindly allowed us to use pictures of notable educators from their departments: Departments of Medicine, Obstetrics and Gynecology, Orthopaedics and Traumatology, Pediatrics and Adolescent Medicine, Pathology, and Surgery. We are also grateful to the following organizations that have given their consents for reproducing their photographs: Alice Ho Miu Ling Nethersole Charity Foundation, the Chinese University of Hong Kong, Hong Kong College of Family Physicians, Hong Kong Sanatorium & Hospital, Hong Kong Tuberculosis, Chest and Heart Diseases Association, Institute of Mental Health (Castle Peak Hospital), Mental Health Association of Hong Kong, Obstetrical and Gynaecological Society of Hong Kong, Tung Wah Museum Archives, University Archives (the University of Hong Kong) and the Wellcome Collection.

Wong Tai-wai and Moira Chan-Yeung
September 2022

Abbreviations

AFOM	Associateship of the Faculty of Occupational Medicine
AMMH	Alice Memorial Maternity Hospital
BAAG	British Army Aid Group
Bar-at-Law	Barrister-at-Law
BSc	Bachelor of Science
CBE	Commander of the British Empire
CPD	Chinese Public Dispensary
CStJ	Commander of the Order of the Most Venerable Order of the Hospital of Saint John of Jerusalem
CUHK	The Chinese University of Hong Kong
DGO	Diploma of Gynecology and Obstetrics
DIH	Diploma of Industrial Health
DMRD	Diploma in Medical Radio-Diagnosis
DPH (Cantab)	Diploma of Public Health (Cambridge)
DPM	Diploma of Psychological Medicine
DSc	Doctor of Science
DSSc	Doctor of Social Science
DTM&H (Cantab)	Diploma of Tropical Medicine and Hygiene (Cambridge)
ED	Efficiency Decoration
FACS	Fellow of the American College of Surgeons
FACR	Fellow of the American College of Radiologists
FAFOM	Fellow of the Australian Faculty of Occupational Medicine
FAMS	Fellow of the Academy of Medicine (Singapore)
FANZCA	Fellow of the Australian and New Zealand College of Anesthetists

FFARACS	Fellow of the Faculty of Anesthetists of the Royal Australasian College of Surgeons
FFARCS	Fellow of the Faculty of Anesthetists of the Royal College of Surgeons
FFOM	Fellow of the Faculty of Occupational Medicine
FFPH	Fellow of the Faculty of Public Health
FHKAM	Fellow of the Hong Kong Academy of Medicine
FHKCA	Fellow of the Hong Kong College of Anesthesiologists
FHKCCM	Fellow of the Hong Kong College of Community Medicine
FHKCFP	Fellow of the Hong Kong College of Family Physicians
FHKCGP	Fellow of the Hong Kong College of General Practitioners
FHKCP	Fellow of the Hong Kong College of Physicians
FHKCR	Fellow of the Hong Kong College of Radiologists
FRCA	Fellow of the Royal College of Anesthetists
FRACMA	Fellow of the Royal Australasian College of Medical Administrators
FRACP	Fellow of the Royal Australasian College of Physicians
FRANZCR	Fellow of the Royal Australian and New Zealand College of Radiologists
FRCOG	Fellow of the Royal College of Obstetricians and Gynecologists
FRCP	Fellow of the Royal College of Physicians
FRCPath	Fellow of the Royal College of Pathologists
FRCPsych	Fellow of the Royal College of Psychiatry
FRCPS	Fellow of the Royal College of Physicians and Surgeons of Canada
FRCR	Fellow of the Royal College of Radiologists
FRCS	Fellow of the Royal College of Surgeons
FRIPH	Fellow of Royal Institute of Public Health
FRS	Fellow of the Royal Society
FRSM	Fellow of the Royal Society of Medicine

FRSTMH	Fellow of the Royal Society of Tropical Medicine and Hygiene
GCMG, KCMG	Knight Grand Cross (GCMG); Knight Commander (KCMG) of the British Most Distinguished Order of Saint Michael and Saint George.
GMC	General Medical Council
HKAR	Hong Kong Administrative Report
HKCGP	Hong Kong College of General Practitioners
HKCFP	Hong Kong College of Family Physicians
HKCM	Hong Kong College of Medicine
HKMA	Hong Kong Medical Association
HKMMS	Hong Kong Museum of Medical Sciences
HKSP	Hong Kong Sessional Papers
Hon. LLD	Honorary Doctor of Laws
HKU	The University of Hong Kong
ICAC	Independent Commission Against Corruption
ICD	International Classification of Diseases
ISO	International Organization for Standardization
JP	Justice of the Peace
KBE	Knight Commander of the British Empire
KCR	Kowloon-Canton Railway
KStJ	Knight of the Order of the Most Venerable Order of the Hospital of Saint John of Jerusalem
LMSH	Licentiate of Medicine and Surgery, College of Medicine, Hong Kong
LRCS	Licentiate of the Royal College of Surgeons
LRCP	Licentiate of the Royal College of Physicians
LRFPS	Licentiate of the Royal Faculty of Physicians & Surgeons
MA	Master of Arts
MBBS, MBCM, MBChB, BMBCh	Bachelor of Medicine and Bachelor of Surgery
MBE	Member of the Order of the British Empire
MBS	Medical Benevolent Society

MC	Military Cross
MCHC	Maternal and Child Health Centers
MD	Doctor of Medicine
MBCM	Bachelor of Medicine and Master of Surgery
MRCP	Member of the Royal College of Physicians
MRCS	Member of the Royal College of Surgeons
NGO	Non-governmental Organization
NPC	Nasopharyngeal carcinoma
OBE	Officer of the Order of British Empire
PCMO	Principal Civil Medical Officer
PRC	People's Republic of China
PSM	The Most Esteemed Order of Loyalty to the Crown of Malaysia
R&D	Research and Development
RCPE	Royal College of Physicians of Edinburgh
SARDA	Society for the Aid and Rehabilitation of Drug Abusers
SBS	Silver Bauhinia Star
TB	Tuberculosis
TCM	traditional Chinese medicine
WMA	World Medical Association
WONCA	World Organization of Family Doctors

Overview

When Hong Kong was ceded to Britain after the Opium War in 1842, it was a very unhealthy place for the foreigners. The garrison was suffering from "Hong Kong Fever" which was likely due to malaria, and few soldiers were fit for duty. A Government Civil Hospital in a rented house was started around 1850 for the colonial surgeon to see all the sick patients in one place. The scant attention the government paid to sanitary services resulted in Hong Kong becoming well known for its insanitary conditions. In 1894, the horrendous plague finally descended on the city killing thousands. This appalling epidemic became the wakeup call for the administrators to overhaul the public health infrastructure. From then on sanitation and medical services gradually improved. Today, Hong Kong residents enjoy a long life, and their life expectancy leads the world. The standards of medical and health services rank similar to those of developed nations.

This book is organized into three periods—before WWII (Chapters 1–6), during the war (Chapter 7) and after the war (Chapters 8–13)—and by different categories of doctors: medical missionaries, doctors in the government medical and health services, medical educators, private practitioners, and female doctors.

Chapter 1 described medical missionaries who introduced Western medicine to Hong Kong shortly after it was ceded to the British. Two medical missionaries, Drs. William Lockhart and Benjamin Hobson of the London Missionary Society (LMS) arrived in Hong Kong in 1842 and 1843 respectively. Lockhart built the Medical Missionary Society Hospital on Morrison Hill, Wan Chai, while Hobson operated the hospital after Lockhart's departure. The hospital was closed in the early 1850s from lack of funds. Medical missionaries would return to Hong Kong 30 years later and play a major role in propagating Western medicine by founding Alice Memorial Hospital and Hong Kong College of Medicine (HKCM) for Chinese. As a result of their efforts, Western medicine was gradually accepted by the Chinese in Hong Kong.

The cornerstone in medical and health development in Hong Kong was the establishment of a public medical and health service. It began with the appointment of a government doctor, known as Colonial Surgeon, who delivered healthcare to the civil servants, police, and prisoners. In those days, the Colonial Surgeon served both as a clinician and an administrator as exemplified by Dr. Philip Ayres in Chapter 2. He fought long and hard to improve the sanitation in Hong Kong, which only materialized after the city had been visited by the atrocious plague epidemic in 1894. In its aftermath, both the government and the people realized the significance of public health and set about to improve it. Ayres's successor, Dr. John Atkinson, with the new title of Principal Civil Medical Officer, and Dr. Francis Clark, the first Medical Officer of Health, had the formidable task of tackling reforms of both medical and sanitary services in Hong Kong. The appointment of Dr. William Hunter, the first bacteriologist in government service in 1902, and the establishment of the Bacteriology Institute to fight plague and other infectious diseases, were other outcomes of plague. In the 1930s, when Dr. Arthur Wellington became the director of Government Medical and Sanitary Services, he reorganized the structure of the services. By the beginning of World War II, the Hong Kong Government Medical and Health Services was relatively well developed as a result of these conscientious and hard-working medical doctors and administrators.

Chapter 3 tells the story of how three groups of people worked together to realize their mutual interest of educating Chinese young men in Western medicine so that they would popularize and disseminate it locally, by founding the Alice Memorial Hospital and the Hong Kong College of Medicine (HKCM) for Chinese in 1887. First, the missionaries from the LMS donated the land for the building of the Alice Memorial Hospital. The LMS also appointed Dr. J. C. Thomson, a medical missionary, to be the medical superintendent of Alice Memorial Hospital. Second, the Chinese elite in the community, including Dr. Ho Kai, who donated funds to build the hospital as a memorial to his wife, and the others who were responsible for raising operating funds for the hospital. Third, the doctors in private practice in Hong Kong who offered free professional services to the patients in the hospital and taught the students of HKCM, including Patrick Manson, James Cantlie, and Gregory Jordan—prominent doctors in the community then. HKCM produced 60 graduates during its existence, but their license was not recognized by the

General Medical Council (GMC) in Britain and they were not allowed to practice medicine in Hong Kong. Eventually they were able to serve Hong Kong by becoming employees of the government. One of them, Dr. Ho Ko-tsun included in this chapter, was a shining example of a *kaifong* (neighborhood) doctor, who devoted many years of his life to serving the residents in Wan Chai, working in one of the Chinese Public Dispensaries (CPD).

The merging of HKCM with the University of Hong Kong (HKU) to become the Faculty of Medicine led to the arrival of another breed of medical educators from the United Kingdom. These full-time professors, as described in Chapter 4: Drs. Kenelm Digby (anatomy, surgery), H. G. Earle (physiology), Wang Chung-yik (pathology), John Anderson (medicine), and Richard Tottenham (obstetrics and gynecology), were appointed by HKU at various times. They laid the foundation of the new faculty. Unlike the graduates of HKCM, the graduates of the Faculty of Medicine, HKU, were recognized by the GMC in Britain and could practice in Hong Kong.

Before the twentieth century, European doctors were the main providers of medical care in the private sector, serving mainly the European population. Graduates of HKCM and HKU only emerged as an important force in the private sector after the 1920s. Two important events revealed the rise in influence of the local practicing Chinese doctors: 1) the establishment of Hong Kong Chinese Medical Association, and 2) the founding of Yeung Wo Home, the first private hospital run by Chinese doctors. Yeung Wo Home was later transformed into Hong Kong Sanatorium and Hospital, which is an ongoing concern today. Among the medical graduates before World War II, three selfless doctors in the private sector contributed greatly to public services in education and social welfare, in addition to providing medical service. They were Dr. Li Shu-fan, Dr. Arthur Woo, and Dr. Tseung Fat-im described in Chapter 5.

Chapter 6 is devoted to female doctors who appeared rather late on the local medical scene. Dr. Alice Hickling (née Sibree), the first female doctor arrived from England in 1904 to work in Alice Memorial Maternity Hospital and introduced Western method of delivery. She also pioneered in maternal and child health services in Hong Kong. The first local female medical student, Lai Po-chuen, was admitted in 1921 to HKU. Eva Ho Tung entered the university the following spring but graduated in 1927 as the first female medical graduate. All three female doctors specialized in obstetrics and gynecology, an area considered socially acceptable for female doctors.

Japanese invasion of Hong Kong began in December 1941. After Hong Kong government surrendered to the Japanese Army, the medical system collapsed. All European doctors, including many government doctors and university educators, were interned in civilian or prison-of-war (POW) camps. Many local doctors fled to Free China. During this difficult period, three exceptional European doctors chose different paths and served Hong Kong in diverse ways as depicted in Chapter 7. Dr. Percy Selwyn-Clarke, prewar Director of Medical Services, chose to stay in the job to maintain basic public health service despite the risk of allegation of collaboration with the enemy by the British. Dr. Lindsay Ride, Professor of Physiology at HKU, escaped from the POW camp to Free China, where he formed the British Army Aid Group (BAAG). Dr. Gordon King left the HKU Relief Hospital for Free China secretly before he was interned and helped students from HKU to further their education in universities in the mainland.

The postwar period witnessed a rapid development of diagnostic technology and proliferation of new drugs. The advent of antibiotics revolutionized the treatment of infectious diseases, including tuberculosis. Drugs effective in the treatment of mental illnesses resulted in a major paradigm shift in the management of mental illnesses. At the same time Hong Kong underwent transformation in many areas: population, demographics, economic status, lifestyle, and disease patterns. The population explosion in the immediate postwar period overwhelmed all social services in Hong Kong. As Hong Kong transformed from an entrepôt to a manufacturing center, its economy improved in the late 1950s, and really took off in the late 1960s. The progressive affluence enriched the standard of living and the diet. This, in turn, brought alterations in disease patterns with noncommunicable diseases replacing infectious diseases as major threats to health at the dawn of the 1970s. The doctors who greatly influenced the development of medical and health services after World War II also discussed under the same categories as they were before the war.

In the Government Medical and Health Department there were Drs. Yeo Kok-cheang (1952–1957), Gerald Choa (1970–1976), and Lee Shiu-hung (1989–1994), as recounted in Chapter 8. Yeo, the first Chinese Director of Medical and Health Service, led the fight to overcome the many prevalent infectious diseases. When Choa took the baton in 1970, he reorganized the hospital services to meet the increasing demand in a rapidly developing Hong Kong. Lee became the first Director of Health after the Medical and Health Department split into two services: the Hospital Services Department and the Department of Health. He promoted the much-needed primary healthcare.

The Government Medical and Health Department also developed specialty services in public hospitals after the war. In addition to the traditional branches of medicine, such as internal medicine, surgery, obstetrics and gynecology, pediatrics and orthopedics, new specialties arose with recent progress in medical knowledge and innovations in technology. Chapter 9 captured the fascinating stories of pioneers in radiology and radiotherapy (Dr. John Ho), mental health (Dr. Yap Pow-meng), and anesthesia (Dr. Zoltan Lett), who developed their respective services from scratch after World War II to modernity, commensurate with those in developed economies.

In Chapter 10, we summarized the achievements of the postwar university professors who rehabilitated the faculty and developed new specialty areas. They included Professor Hou Po-chang (Chair 1947–1960) and Professor James Gibson (1963–1983) in pathology; Professor A. J. S. McFadzean (1949–1974) and Professor David Todd (1975–1994) in medicine; Professor Arthur Hodgson (1961–1975) in orthopedics, and Professor G. B. Ong (1964–1982) in surgery. They expanded their departments to include new subspecialties to provide up-to-date clinical services to patients and training opportunities for postgraduates. Each of them placed Hong Kong on the world map in his research area of interest.

After the war, the number of doctors in private practice grew with an increasing number of graduates from HKU and later also from the Chinese University of Hong Kong. The three distinguished doctors in the private sector narrated in Chapter 11, Drs. Albert Rodrigues, Harry Fang, and Lee Chung-yin, contributed greatly to the advancement of medical services. Rodrigues and Fang were specialists and they contributed by serving on the Legislative Council and Executive Council, advising the government on the development of medical services during the first two decades after the war. Lee founded the College of General Practitioners (later renamed Family Physicians) to raise the standards of general practice.

Today, there may be slightly more female students (female to male, 1.18:1 in 2020) admitted to the medical faculties of the two universities in Hong Kong, and female doctors are represented in traditionally male-dominant specialties such as orthopedics and heart surgery. It was only after World War II that female doctors were appointed to higher academic or professional positions. Professor Elaine Field and Professor Daphne Chun were the two heroines in Chapter 12. Professor Elaine Field organized and inaugurated the Pediatrics Department of HKU. Professor Daphne Chun, born and educated locally, succeeded Professor Gordon King to become the first female professor of obstetrics and gynecology in HKU. Chun raised the standard of maternity service in Tsan Yuk Hospital and in Hong Kong.

Although the missionary doctors introduced Western medicine in Hong Kong, their role gradually waned (see Chapter 13). Dr. Edward Paterson was the last in the long line of medical missionaries of the LMS when he joined Nethersole Hospital after the war. He built his dream hospital, "hospital without walls"—United Christian Hospital in Hong Kong. The Columban Sisters were medical missionaries invited to operate Ruttonjee Sanatorium in Hong Kong in 1949, and they led the fight against tuberculosis in Hong Kong. The departure of Paterson and the Columban Sisters from Hong Kong in 1989 and 2015 respectively closed an important chapter of medical missionaries in Hong Kong as well as our book. Their invaluable selfless devotion and hard work in caring for the people of Hong Kong for over 150 years will long live in our memories and in our medical history books.

This book on notable doctors from the past focuses on one of the important driving forces behind the evolution of medical and healthcare besides socio-political and economic factors. In addition to providing medical care, their other roles in medical education, research, and in formulating healthcare policies have been pivotal in advancing medical and healthcare in Hong Kong.

1. The Medical Missionaries
Introducing Western Medicine to Hong Kong

The introduction of Western medicine to China is a story of faith, charity, and dedication of missionaries, particularly medical missionaries, from Europe and North America. These missionaries attempted to introduce Christianity to China by packaging it with medical services. Even though Christianity arrived in China as early as 635 C. E., and intermittently thereafter, it had never really taken root until the nineteenth century, when a large number of missionaries arrived in China as a result of a combination of three elements in the Western world—university education, personal Christian awakening, and the call to missionary service.[1] In England itself, the evangelical revival coincided with the imperialistic expansion of the British Empire, leading to a proliferation of overseas missionary activities.

During the early part of the nineteenth century, several medical missionaries reached China. Among them was Dr. Peter Parker, a gifted doctor from the United States, who established a hospital in Guangzhou and performed surgeries mostly on the eyes but also on other organs. The aims of the medical missionaries were to heal the sick and at the same time to introduce the Gospel of Christ to China, by cultivating confidence and friendship. After Hong Kong became a colony in 1842, it was a stepping stone for entering China rather than a mission field. This chapter is devoted to the work of the first two medical missionaries in Hong Kong. Dr. William Lockhart, of the London Missionary Society (LMS) arrived in Hong Kong in 1842 and built a hospital, Medical Missionary Society Hospital. He was succeeded by Dr. Benjamin Hobson, who also left for China after a few years. The hospital did not last long and was closed in 1853 because of funding difficulties.

William Lockhart (1811–1896)

MD, MRCS

William Lockhart was the first medical missionary to set foot in Hong Kong. He was born in Liverpool, trained as a physician at Guy's Hospital, London, and Heath Hospital, Dublin. After he became a member of the Royal College of Surgeons of England, he joined the LMS, arriving in Macau in 1839. In Macau, Lockhart reopened the hospital that was closed by Dr. Peter Parker, an American physician and missionary, when Parker returned to Guangzhou. Soon Lockhart, too, had to leave Macau, when British subjects were evacuated because of preparation for the First Opium War. Lockhart spent the next two years studying Chinese in Batavia (present-day Jakarta), Guangzhou, and Chusan (Zhoushan). He returned to Macau in 1841 when Chusan was evacuated. In 1842, he received orders to return to Chusan via Hong Kong, which by then was ceded to the British as a result of the First Opium War. He was detained in Hong Kong, where he supervised the building of Medical Missionary Society Hospital, planned by the LMS. Although Lockhart was the first medical missionary to arrive in Hong Kong, he did not work as a doctor because, after the completion of the hospital, he was told by the LMS to continue his journey to China for a more important assignment. Lockhart subsequently established a number of hospitals in China, including the ones in Shanghai and Beijing.

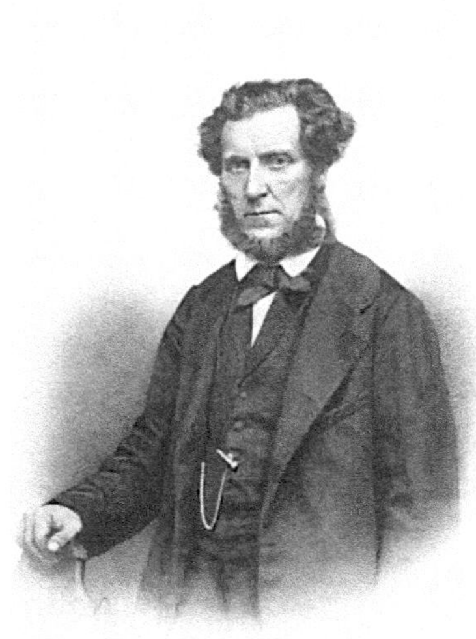

Figure 1.1 Dr. William Lockhart
Source: Wellcome Collection. Attribution 4.0 International (CC BY 4.0)

After 20 years' experience as a medical missionary,[2] he wrote a book, *The Medical Missionary in China: A Narrative of Twenty Years' Experience.*[3] He concluded that the medical and the missionary work should not be carried out by the same individual, as the doctor could hardly find time for "saving the soul."

Benjamin Hobson (1816–1873)
MB, MRCS

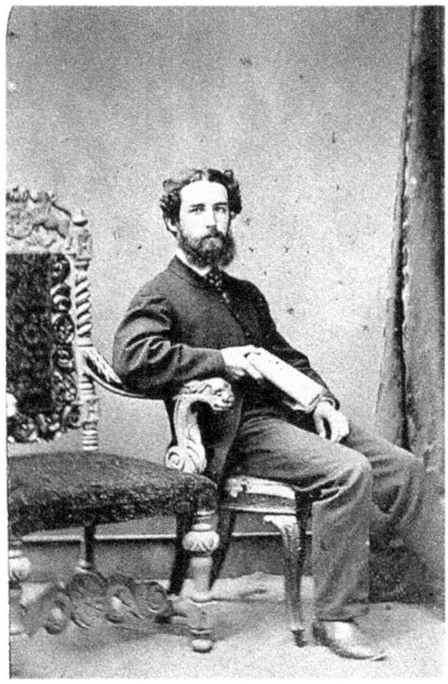

Figure 1.2 Dr. Benjamin Hobson
Source: Wellcome Collection. Attribution 4.0 International (CC BY 4.0)

The next medical missionary to reach Hong Kong was Benjamin Hobson, a distinguished graduate of the University of London with a MB and a Member of the Royal College of Surgeons (MRCS). He arrived in Macau in December 1839 as a LMS medical missionary and was in charge of a missionary hospital there.[4] When Lockhart left Hong Kong in 1843, Hobson was ordered to close the hospital in Macau and move the facilities to the newly completed Medical Missionary Society Hospital in Hong Kong. The 42-bed hospital was situated at Morrison Hill, where a school had been established by the Morrison Education Society. At the end of three years, Hobson returned to England on leave, as his wife developed intermittent fever. While on board, she passed away. Before he returned to Hong Kong in 1847, he married the daughter of Robert Morrison, the first Protestant missionary to Macau. However, shortly after his return to Hong Kong, Hobson was reassigned to Guangzhou, and he left Medical Missionary Society Hospital. In Guangzhou, he opened a hospital in Kam-li-fau, a place where no foreigners had taken up residence. Between 1854 and 1855, Guangzhou was under siege because of fighting between the government troops and the Taiping rebels. Hobson was forced to leave for Shanghai. It was just as well, because the hospital in Kam-li-fau was destroyed by fire in 1856. In Shanghai, Hobson took over the management of a hospital from Lockhart, who was due to go on leave. Hobson did not stay in Shanghai for long. He left China in 1859 and remained in England until he died in 1873.[5]

Hobson achieved a great deal during the time he was in Hong Kong and China and under very unsettling political conditions. He was a highly successful clinician, treating various eye diseases which were incredibly prevalent in Hong Kong. He described eye conditions such as ophthalmia tarsi, chronic ophthalmia, trichiasis (turning in of the eyelash), entropion (inversion of the eyelid), opacity, and vascularity of the cornea. These conditions could be the various manifestations of trachoma, a disease now known to be caused by the highly infectious agent, chlamydia. Hobson rightly pointed out that the infection was transmitted from one person to another during the common practice of "washing the eye" by Chinese barbers who rubbed the everted lower lid with an ivory or bamboo instrument.[6] Hobson treated the chlamydia infection with "nitrate of silver in distilled water, and strong solutions of sub-acetate of lead and sulphate of copper and zinc." Until the advent of antibiotics, the remedy using solutions containing 1% silver nitrate and ¼% copper sulphate remained the standard treatment of trachoma infection. Hobson operated on patients with cataract and had complete success in 11 out of 25 cases, partial success in 12 and failure in 2. As did other medical missionaries, such as Dr. Parker, Hobson operated on patients with hernia, large pedunculated tumors and even cancer of the breast, with remarkable success in some. In his second report to the LMS, Hobson described in detail leprosy patients with marked disfiguration and the lack of effective treatment.[7] He also vaccinated children in Hong Kong with cowpox vaccine which was brought in from England and seldom gave rise to severe reactions.[8] Vaccination using material from active smallpox lesions had long been practiced in China but at times led to virulent smallpox infection.

Hobson's more significant contribution was in medical education, not so much in teaching medical students but by the medical books he wrote in Chinese. Having been trained in a scientific discipline and believing that traditional Chinese medicine had no scientific basis, Hobson wanted to give Hong Kong and China a rational system of medicine. He offered his young assistant, Chan Apun, instructions on physics, chemistry, physiology, treatment of various diseases, and operations on the eye. On 13 May 1845, during the first meeting of the China Medico-Chirurgical Society in Hong Kong, of which Hobson was its first secretary, there was general support from the local medical colleagues to train local Chinese doctors in Western medicine. Some members expressed the hope that one day a proper medical school would be established in Hong Kong.[9] After Apun passed an examination conducted by a group of local doctors,[10]

Hobson asked the Committee of the Medical Missionary Society for permission to recruit boys for a preparatory medical course, and to observe treatment of diseases in the hospital.[11] In 1846, when Hobson went on leave, he raised about £300 for a medical school. His hopes were dashed on returning to Hong Kong because the interested local doctors had either moved away or died, and the principal of the Morrison Education Society School had taken all the bright students to the United States for further education.[12] Unable to realize his dream of opening a medical school in Hong Kong, Hobson used the money he raised to open a hospital in Kam-li-fau in Guangzhou and to further the education of Chan Apun.

Despite his disappointment in Hong Kong, he wrote six medical books in Chinese that helped to advance Western medical education in China. These books were rewritten by Chinese scholars in elegant Chinese, and were easy and interesting to read. One of the scholars, Guan Maocai, was the best-known translator interested in Western medicine.[13] The six medical books were: 1) *Outline of Anatomy and Physiology*, 1851; 2) *Natural Philosophy and Natural History*, 1851; 3) *Practice of Medicine and Materia Medica*, 1858; 4) *First Lines of Practice of Surgery in the West*, 1857; 5) *Treatise on Midwifery and Diseases of Children*, 1858; and 6) *The Medical Vocabulary in English and Chinese*, 1858. The first two books were published in Guangzhou and the rest in Shanghai, where Hobson was relocated around 1855. Hobson's books, with their attractive illustrations and detailed anatomical diagrams, were widely distributed and eventually used more extensively in Japan.[14]

Despite the Chinese mistrust of foreigners and their medicine, Hobson gained the trust of the local people. The Medical Missionary Society Hospital, even though it had 42 beds, had at times up to 85 inpatients. It offered free medical services to the Chinese, along with the gospel. Hobson was succeeded by Dr. Henri Hirschberg in 1848. The Medical Missionary Society Hospital flourished under Hirschberg's management for a while.[15] Around 1853, the hospital closed its doors from lack of funds, because treatment was given free of charge, and the failure to find a suitable replacement for Hirschberg, who disagreed with the LMS's administration of the hospital and had some personal problems.[16]

It was almost 30 years later that the LMS attempted to provide medical services in Hong Kong again, prompted by the arrival of Dr. William Young from Canada.

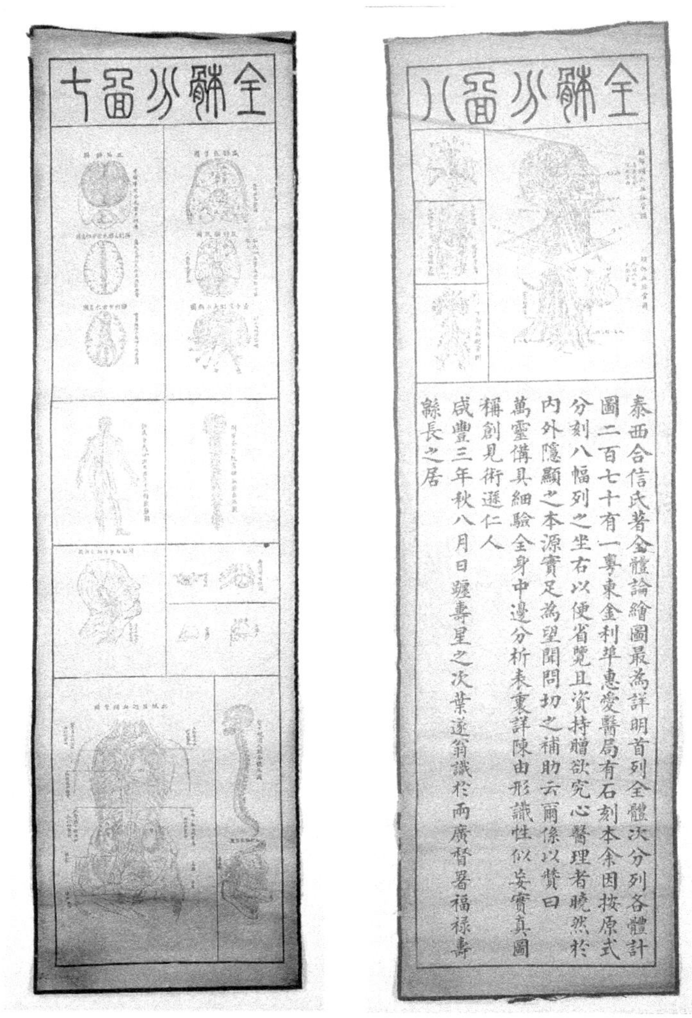

Figure 1.3a and b ***Outline of Anatomy and Physiology*** **by Benjamin Hobson**

Source: Wellcome Collection. Attribution 4.0 International (CC BY 4.0)

2. The Colonial Surgeon and Government Medical Officers

Establishing Sanitary, Medical, and Health Services in Hong Kong

In the early days of the founding of the colony in Hong Kong, having a medical and sanitary service was far from the minds of the administrators. Captain Charles Elliot, who took possession of Hong Kong after the First Opium War in 1842, had hoped that the colony would become "an Emporium of the Far East." After he announced that Hong Kong was to be a free port, many British merchants from Macau moved to Hong Kong to take advantage of British protection and free trade.

Hong Kong was often described as a "barren island" then, with a few fishing villages and a population of about 7,000. The City of Victoria developed very rapidly after the ratification of the Treaty of Nanking on 26 June 1843, when Henry Pottinger became the first governor and commander-in-chief of Hong Kong. A new city required considerable infrastructure, such as roads, houses, and docks. Fortunately, there was no shortage of labor because Chinese workers flocked to Hong Kong from the mainland looking for work. As the city was to be a free port, there was a problem as to who would pay these expenses. The British merchants believed that the British home government should pay, and a grant was offered by the British government for only a few years. As a result, the civil administration was kept to a minimum and very little was left for sanitary services and nothing for medical services. Unfortunately, Hong Kong failed to develop into an Emporium of the Far East as Elliot and Pottinger had hoped, because of the opening of other treaty ports in China and the widespread piracy in the surrounding waters of the island. Most British merchants, in addition to their trade, were involved in smuggling Indian-grown opium into China, to increase their profits. Until World War I, around 30% to 50% of Hong Kong coffers came from the opium trade. Funding for sanitation or medical care remained scarce.

Nevertheless, the City of Victoria grew. By 1852, the population had increased from around 7,000 in 1842 to 23,000, and by 1862, to around 120,000. Since Hong Kong is a hilly island, the only land where houses could be built inexpensively was along a narrow strip of land on the northern side of the island. The government encouraged racial segregation. As the population mushroomed, there was a lack of building lots. The poor Chinese, who previously occupied areas just west of the Central District, were asked to move further westward and up the hill to Taipingshan, vacating their land for the arriving Europeans. The government's resumption of the area was carried out in a way that flagrantly violated the rights of property ownership. It simply took over the lots owned by the Chinese and sold them to the Europeans, telling the Chinese that the lots they purchased in 1842 were only temporary, as the Treaty of Nanking had not been ratified then. The Chinese owners would be relocated to Taipingshan, where the land would be leveled, and streets marked out and they would enjoy a "rent holiday" for five years.[1] The scarcity of land for building resulted in tremendous overcrowding in the small Chinese tenement houses. The lack of water supply and refuse and sewage disposal rendered Hong Kong unsanitary, but especially so in Taipingshan. It was a place where infectious diseases would propagate rapidly to become an epidemic. Indeed, various diseases, such as "Hong Kong Fever" (which later proved to be malaria), dysentery, and other diarrheal illnesses, were rampant in early Hong Kong.[2] The high absenteeism among the police force from these illnesses led the government to employ a Colonial Surgeon to be responsible for the health of the colony.

Dr. Alexander Anderson was the first Colonial Surgeon in 1843, but he resigned after one year and died shortly after. The first few Colonial Surgeons lasted not more than one or two years on the job, because they either died while in service or retired because of ill health. Many difficulties faced the Colonial Surgeon. Not only was the job hazardous because of exposure to infectious diseases, but it also carried considerable hardship, as the doctor had to travel to different places on horseback to attend to many patients in different parts of Hong Kong. There was no public hospital in Hong Kong then. At first, the government paid Seamen's Hospital for admitting sick civil servants and police. In the end, the governor was persuaded to believe that having a public hospital was indeed a money-saving exercise. A bungalow was rented as the temporary Government Civil Hospital in 1849.[3]

In 1859, Dr. John Murray was appointed Colonial Surgeon. He remained on the job for 13 years (1859–1872), breaking the trend of early retirement and early death. The hospital was moved to another house (where Tsan Yuk Hospital is today), with much better ventilation but not so in other amenities. As Colonial Surgeon, Murray was successful in reducing the mortality of Europeans, which had hitherto been high in Hong Kong. The salary of a Colonial Surgeon at £600 per year, about one-eighth that of the governor, was the lowest on the colonial administrator ladder in Hong Kong.[4] In 1872, at the age of 48, Dr. Murray decided to retire to England.[5] He passed away in 1903.

The appointment of a Colonial Surgeon and the establishment of Government Civil Hospital marked the beginning of public medical and health services, which were vital for the health of Hong Kong people. In the beginning, these medical services were only used by the Europeans, as the Chinese did not trust Western medicine. The Chinese did not go to hospitals when they were sick, and traditional Chinese medicine (TCM) practitioners did not attend patients in hospitals. This practice changed in 1869 after a horrendous local scandal appeared in the British media and rocked England. Dying Chinese men, unattended, were found among the dead in several small rooms for holding coffins behind Kwong Fook I Tsz Temple. Governor Sir Richard Graves MacDonnell (governor of Hong Kong, 1866–1872) was forced to respond, and he granted a piece of land for the local Chinese elite to build a hospital for the Chinese.[6] Tung Wa Hospital (now Tung Wah Hospital) was opened in 1872 and practiced only TCM.[7] It became highly popular among the local Chinese.

In the 1840s, Western medicine was still in a primitive stage of development. Western medical therapeutics included bloodletting, purging, and treating with heavy metals such as arsenic and mercury. These measures often made patients sicker by causing anemia, loss of electrolytes, and poisoning. Only surgical procedures offered some help. Unfortunately, it was before the era of antiseptic technique, and surgical mortality was high. However, Western medicine advanced very rapidly in the second half of the nineteenth century. The discovery of germs can cause diseases and the use of antiseptic technique and anesthesia in surgery led to markedly reduced surgical mortality and the use of antisepsis in delivery also lowered maternal mortality. Moreover, in 1842, poor sanitation and overcrowding were discovered by Edwin Chadwick in England as major causes of ill health in England.[8] Subsequent legislation and reforms improved sanitation and housing, especially for the lower social class in England. These and other advances led to the superiority of Western medicine.

The appointment of the following physicians: Philip Burnard Chenery Ayres, John Mitford Atkinson, Francis Clark, William Hunter, and Arthur Robartes Wellington, to the government Medical and Sanitary Services in Hong Kong from 1873 to just before World War II, represented the next stage of development. These individuals were equipped with the up-to-date knowledge of Western medicine and sanitation when they arrived. Their work improved the sanitation and the health of the population and laid the foundation of the modern public health, medical, and sanitary services in Hong Kong.

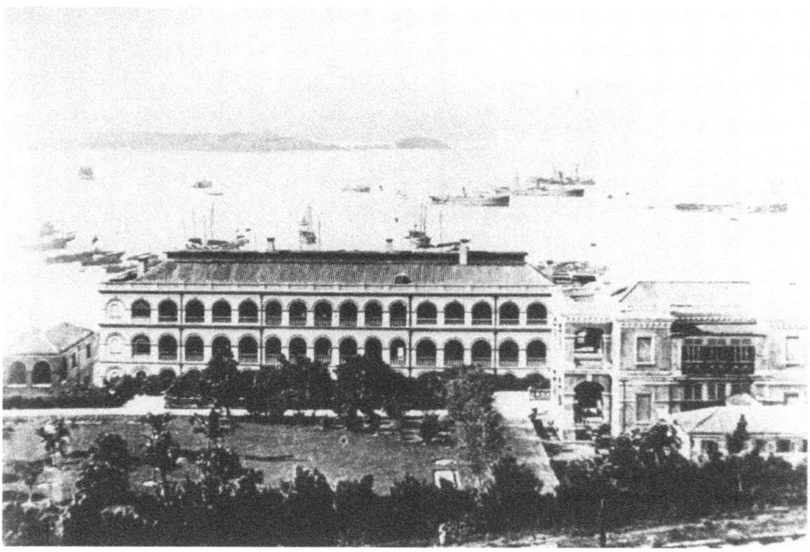

Figure 2.1 Government Civil Hospital c 1910
Image courtesy of Hong Kong Museum of Medical Science (HKMMS)

Philip Burnard Chenery Ayres (1840–1899)

MD (Lond), MRCS (Eng) and LRCP (Edin), CMG

Dr. Philip Burnard Chenery Ayres was the first Colonial Surgeon in Hong Kong who survived 25 years on the job. Born in 1840 in England, the eldest son of the chief medical officer of Civil Hospital in Mauritius, Ayres received his medical education at the University of London and the University of Edinburgh, and held an MD (Lond), MRCS (Eng) and LRCP (Edin). After graduation in 1865, he had a series of appointments as health officer and surgeon in the colonial administration system in different colonies, mostly in Mauritius, and Bengal and Assam in India. In 1873, he was appointed Colonial Surgeon and Inspector of Hospitals in Hong Kong.[9] As Colonial Surgeon, he was responsible for patients in Government Civil Hospital and Lock Hospital (for female patients with venereal diseases), sick civil servants, police force and convicts, and for preparation of annual medical reports. He also attended private patients to supplement his income because of the low salary.

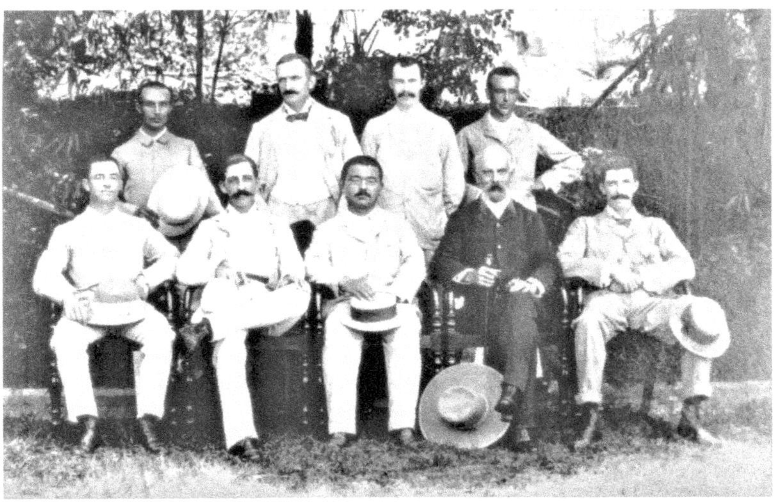

Figure 2.2 Dr. Philip Burnard Chenery Ayres (sitting, R2), Dr. Kitasato (sitting, center) and Dr. Lowson (sitting, R1) with the rest of the team fighting against plague, 1894

Image courtesy of HKMMS, photo donated by Mrs. F. M. Ashburner

A conscientious man, shortly after his arrival, Ayres made his first survey of Taipingshan, an area where few officials had ever ventured, accompanied by the surveyor general, Mr. John MacNeile Price. Both of them became desperately sick after their house-to-house visit and nearly lost their lives. They found that although at first glance the town of Victoria appeared cleaner than most Asian towns, beneath the surface it would be difficult to find a filthier place. Much to his alarm, he discovered pigs being kept by the hundreds in residential houses all over the town, and pigsties under the beds on the second and third floors and even in kitchens. The government had granted many people licenses to keep pigs, even though the upper floors of their dwellings were constructed of thin boards, with wide interstices between the boards that allowed the pig urine to drop to the floor below. The ground floor tenants could not wash their floors because they were mud. The floors above could not be washed without "half drowning" the inhabitants below. Five to ten families often lived in one tenement house of two to three storeys, built on a lot 13 to 16 feet wide and 40 to 60 feet deep, which he "would not consider fit to put pigs in by any decent person."[10]

The meagerness of the water supply meant that personal cleanliness was not possible. Women of the lowest social class rarely washed themselves and men washed only their exposed parts. Washing of clothes was carried out once or twice a month at most, and usually once every several months. Ayres also reported that many houses in Taipingshan had a well either in the main room or in the kitchen on the ground floor. These wells were invariably only one or two feet away from the house drain or downspouts, and raw sewage would filter through the earth and mix with the water in the wells. In some cases, the water smelled or tasted so bad that it could not be used for drinking.

In his annual report for the year 1874, Ayres put in truthfully all the above findings and warned that every necessary condition existed in Taipingshan "for the development of cholera or fevers of a typhoid character; if the seeds are once sown, they will have a fair start," and that "… the houses of the lower classes whose filthy habits are well known, or in future years these plagues will be endemic in the Colony, and probably end in an epidemic of unenviable renown…." Ayres's report of 1874 was censored by the colonial secretary, who deleted the offensive sections on sanitation before sending it to the Colonial Office.

As inspector of hospitals, Ayres visited Tung Wa Hospital. He was very critical of its sanitary condition and the treatments that patients were receiving. In his 1874 report, Ayres also wrote about the hospital: "The treatment of surgical cases shows an amount of ignorance which is much to be deplored. Seeing that the institution was endowed with such a large sum of money by the Colonial Government I think that the directors might be asked to set apart one ward of their hospital for the treatment of patients by foreign doctors."[11]

In 1881, there was a disagreement between Governor John Pope Hennessy and General E. W. Donovan, Commander of British troops in China and Hong Kong. Donovan objected to an ordinance which would extend the area in which Chinese houses could be built, because these houses were usually filthy and unsanitary. He referred to Ayres's original report of 1874, which inexplicably appeared, and it caused considerable alarm in the Colonial Office. Because of this, the Colonial Office sent Oswald Chadwick, a sanitary engineer, and the son of Sir Edwin Chadwick, to assess the sanitation in Hong Kong. Edwin Chadwick was well known for reporting the association between insanitary conditions and ill health and poverty, and high death rates in England. The 1882 report of Chadwick,[12] which vindicated Ayres's 1874 account of the insanitary conditions in Taipingshan, provided the blueprint for sanitary reforms in Hong Kong.

It was most unfortunate that, for over a decade following Chadwick's visit, Hong Kong was governed by a series of short-term governors and colonial administrators.[13] Even though the seriousness of the problems was recognized, the reforms were not implemented. Thus, there had been very little improvement in the sanitary condition despite Chadwick's recommendations. In 1893, after a house inspection, Ayres wrote in his annual report of the hopeless lack of progress: "The floors were reeking with filth, the drainage was very bad, the smell abominable. In some of the houses were dark holes in which there were quantities of decomposing and putrid meat, fat, and bones and one of them filled with maggots. The staunch was unbearable. I found [these houses] in the same condition I had reported twenty years ago."[14]

In 1894, Ayres's long-predicted epidemic of "unenviable renown" descended on Hong Kong with a fury. The horrendous plague killed around 2,550 people and affected an unknown number of residents. As almost half of the population left Hong Kong for the mainland during the epidemic, it was impossible to determine the total number of people affected. Plague returned to haunt Hong Kong almost every year for the next 30 years. The last cases were reported in 1929.[15]

In 1894, Hong Kong had only four full-time doctors and one part-time doctor in the medical service, for a population of around 240,000. During the epidemic, Dr. John Mitford Atkinson, the Superintendent of Government Civil Hospital, was on leave in England. The Superintendent of Gaol (jail) then was a full-time medical officer but not available to look after patients at Government Civil Hospital. The part-time doctor, the Port Health Officer, was unable to look after the plague patients, as the job of ship inspection kept him busy. The plague patients were cared for mainly by Dr. Ayres and Dr. James Lowson, Assistant Superintendent of Government Civil Hospital.[16] One doctor each was seconded from the army and navy to help. The very demanding work and the anxiety wore Ayres and Lowson down by the end of the 1894 epidemic, after which both doctors went on leave. Ayres retired in 1897, one year after he returned to Hong Kong from his leave, because of continuous ill health.

Ayres contributed to the medical and health services in Hong Kong in many ways other than being a doctor to the police and civil service and responsible for the public health of the colony. He conducted periodic medical examinations on the inmates of brothels as required by the Contagious Diseases Ordinance of 1867,[17] an ordinance enacted to reduce the high prevalence of venereal diseases in Hong Kong. The ordinance was only applicable to brothels that serviced foreigners and not those that serviced the Chinese, as Chinese women objected to being examined by a foreign doctor. Those found to have venereal diseases during the periodic examination were admitted to Lock Hospital for treatment until they were "cured." At the time, the most common venereal diseases were syphilis and gonorrhea. Because the causative organisms had not yet been discovered, there was no method of confirming the diagnosis. Nevertheless, because of Ayres's conscientious work, the prevalence of venereal diseases among the police force and the armed forces was reduced considerably. The prevalence of these diseases among the inmates of brothels was lowered to such an extent that many beds were empty in the new 1878 Lock Hospital. When the temporary Government Civil Hospital was partly burned down that year, instead of building a new hospital, Ayres advised the government to turn the new Lock Hospital into the new Government Civil Hospital.[18]

During Ayres's prolonged service, proper lunatic asylums (as psychiatric hospitals were called at the time) were built to accommodate Chinese and European mentally ill patients separately. He also saw the appointment of a colonial veterinary surgeon and the establishment of a vaccine institute to safeguard public health.[19] Government Civil Hospital received the first few trained nurses from hospitals in London in 1889,[20] greatly improving the standard of inpatient care.

Contrary to popular belief, the Sanitary Board, a body that was responsible for the sanitary state of the City of Victoria, was formed as a result of Ayres's proposal and not at the recommendation of Chadwick. Chadwick only requested reorganization of the sanitary staff and rationalizing the chain of command. The Sanitary Board was first established in 1883 by Ordinance 7, and the original members were only officials: the Registrar General, the Colonial Surgeon, the Captain Superintendent of the Police, the Sanitary Inspector, and the Surveyor General as chairman. In 1886, four unofficial members were added. In 1888, the Sanitary Board was reconstituted under the 1887 Public Health Ordinance with two more unofficial members. Ayres was the chairman. He became increasingly disenchanted with the Sanitary Board, because the plague of 1894 revealed that many provisions of the 1887 Public health Ordinance had been played down at the request of one or other local factions. He commented bitterly, "As for the Sanitary Board ... it seems fast relapsing into the 'do nothing' principle until the Unofficial Members get all that they demanded, constituting themselves the public representatives and being in reality only that of a very small portion of the public, and the necessity of its reform in some way is fully demonstrated."[21]

After the 1894 plague, Ayres worked hard to reorganize the Medical Department and to reform the Sanitary Board according to the recommendations of the committees appointed to inquire into the workings of these two institutions.[22] As a result, the first Medical Officer of Health, Dr. Francis Clark, was appointed. Ayres was also the first Colonial Surgeon to suggest that some medical services should be provided to the poor Chinese, but it was only years after his retirement that Chinese Public Dispensaries were established, and the Chinese received free consultation from the licentiates of HKCM.[23]

Ayres created some controversy in his claim of the harmlessness of opium use. He wrote in his annual reports of the results of his experiments on inmates in gaol showing that opium smokers did not experience any withdrawal symptoms from deprivation and that only smoking large amounts of opium could lead to addiction.[24] This, unfortunately, led to the impression that Ayres was in favor of opium smoking. He was not. He found that addiction to opium produced fewer social and medical problems than did addiction to alcohol among Europeans. Not infrequently the alcoholics ended up in gaol or in a "lunatic asylum." His observations made him an enemy of all missionaries who tried to break the opium trade in China.[25]

The Colonial Surgeon and the medical officers had the lowest pay on the colonial administrative ladder and had to work the longest hours, and there was no hour of the day that they would call their own. Ayres wrote, "The Doctor, without reference to the many hours he has been on duty, is expected to present an alert and cheerful appearance, to be sympathetic, courteous, and kindly in his manner, gentle and skillful in the handling of his patients. When he has probably been many hours over the twenty-four without sleep and in much anxiety and mental worry over many cases he has in charge, yet from Government downwards when it comes to pay, the Doctor is the last person to be considered. Though when he is wanted, no one is more anxiously looked for or is received with greater delight and relief."[26] This comment resonated in the minds of many medical officers then and even now.

Hong Kong was indebted to Dr. Ayres especially from the sanitary point of view. His constant zealous appeal of the importance of sanitation contributed to the reforms that finally took place. He wrote, probably correctly, in his last annual report for the year 1896, "what all my reports could not do the epidemic [referring to the 1894 plague] has done."

Dr. Philip Burnard Chenery Ayres was awarded the CMG (Companion of the Order of St. Michael and St. George) in 1893. He was also a prominent Freemason, and a Master of his lodge. After his retirement in 1897, he was presented a Plague Gold Medal by the Hong Kong community for his service during the 1894 plague. The Japanese government awarded him a ring in acknowledgement of the services he rendered to the Japanese Mission, headed by Professor Shibasaburo Kitasato, when they were in Hong Kong during the plague epidemic of 1894, searching for the cause for the scourge.[27] Before he left Hong Kong, Ayres received many valedictory addresses from the Hong Kong community and from several sectors of society, in appreciation of his remarkable skill, devotion, and sacrifice.

Sadly, he did not enjoy a long retirement and passed away in 1899, two years after his departure from Hong Kong.

John Mitford Atkinson (1856–1917)

MB (Lond), DPH (Cantab)

Dr. John Mitford Atkinson, son of the Rev. S. Atkinson of England, was educated at London University and received his medical education from London Hospital. He graduated in 1881 with an MB (Lond) and entered Colonial Service in 1887, when he was appointed Superintendent of Government Civil Hospital in Hong Kong.[28] In 1894, he obtained a DPH (Cantab) while on home leave. When Dr. Ayres retired in 1897, Atkinson succeeded him and assumed the title of Principal Civil Medical Officer (PCMO), a new name for Colonial Surgeon. He served Hong Kong from 1887 to 1912, a total of 25 years. He sat on both the Legislative and Executive Councils during his career in Hong Kong.[29]

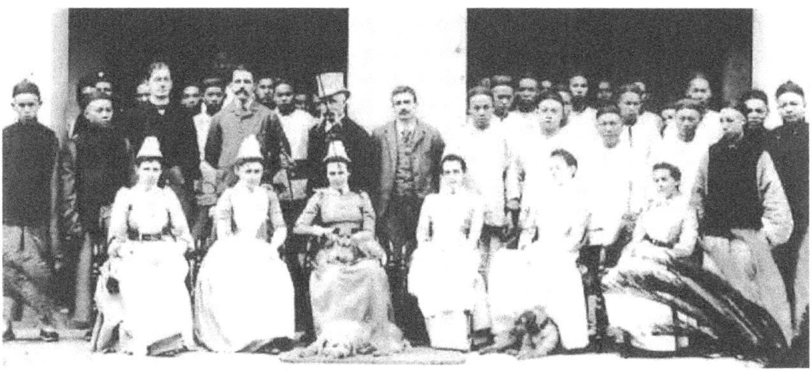

Figure 2.3 Dr. John Mitford Atkinson (second row, L4) and Dr. P. B. C. Ayres (L5, with top hat) and staff of Government Civil Hospital, 1897. The nursing sisters of the hospital are sitting in the front row.

Image courtesy of HKMMS; photo donated by Mrs. F. M. Ashburner, the granddaughter of Dr. James Lowson.

A skilled administrator, Atkinson got on well with Ayres. They were able to recruit trained nurses from London to replace the local untrained nurses, thereby raising the standard of nursing care in the hospital, as discussed. His lasting contribution was the institution of classification of diseases to hospitals in Hong Kong. He established a requirement that all patients discharged and those who died should have a diagnosis in a standardized way. There was no standardization of classification of diseases up to then to assess changes in disease pattern or the effects of intervention. Atkinson introduced a system devised by William Farr, an English public health official, after the inaugural International Statistical Conference at Brussels in 1853. This system was later called the International List of Causes of Death—the precursor of the International Classification of Diseases (ICD) that we use today after its many revisions.[30] Atkinson was the first medical officer who distinguished the three different types of malarial fever and compiled a separate admission and mortality table for different malarial fevers.[31]

Atkinson was awarded a gold cigarette case mounted with the imperial arms in diamonds from the Tsar,[32] as an appreciation of the expert care the Russian sailors received in 1905 after the Russian cruiser *Varyag* sank. *Varyag* was engaged in a battle against five Japanese cruisers during the Battle of Chemulpo Bay at the start of the Russo-Japanese War (1904–1905). The crew of the *Varyag*, who bravely decided not to surrender but to sink the cruiser, was saved by three ships, a British, a French, and an Italian. Many of the Russian crew were taken to Hong Kong, and the sick ones were admitted to Government Civil Hospital.[33]

An excellent clinician, Atkinson often described in his annual reports interesting cases on their presentations and his management. He published several articles on plague and malaria in *The Lancet* or in the *British Medical Journal*,[34] contributing some new knowledge to these diseases. He also investigated a hemorrhagic septicemia outbreak in the cattle in Dairy Farm in Pokfulam and demonstrated the infectious nature of the disease when the same disease was induced in a healthy cow after he injected the blood from an infected cow.[35] Careful disinfection and cleansing of the farm stamped out the disease.[36]

During the plague epidemic of 1894, Atkinson was on home leave, taking a course in public health, which would become important for his position in Hong Kong. When plague recurred almost every summer after the outbreak in 1894, affecting the life and trade of the city greatly, the people in Hong Kong were ready for any measures that would bring about an end to these epidemics. As the Sanitary Board was not functioning even before the plague, there was a great deal of discussion about whether it should be abolished. In the end the Sanitary Board remained, and the first Medical Officer of Health, Dr. Francis Clark, became the Sanitary Board chief executive officer, entirely independent of the control of the Medical Department—a model similar to that in England.[37] In 1902, Oswald Chadwick and Dr. William John Simpson, an expert in tropical medicine, were invited to Hong Kong at the request of Governor Sir Henry Arthur Blake (governor 1898–1903) to advise him on the prevention of plague. In addition to a series of recommendations on sanitary reforms, the two experts drafted the Public Health and Buildings Ordinance of 1903 and advocated that the Sanitary Board be chaired by a sanitary commissioner who should head the Sanitary Department. The sanitary commissioner should have expertise in sanitation and be knowledgeable in the prevention of infectious diseases. Because of the lack of funds to appoint a sanitary commissioner to head the Sanitary Department, Governor Blake decided to place the Sanitary Department and the Medical Department under the administration of the PCMO, who should have expertise in both disciplines. In 1903, Atkinson, the PCMO who had both qualifications, was asked by the governor to take over the responsibility of the Sanitary Department.[38]

Such an administrative arrangement did not last long. In 1906, the Sanitary Department was heavily criticized by the press for its handling of the 1903 Public Health and Buildings Ordinance. There were also complaints about officers entering houses during daytime without warning and irregularities of contractors striking bargains with inspectors and clerks of the Sanitary Department.[39] To investigate these allegations, Governor Sir Matthew Nathan (governor 1904–1907) appointed a commission in 1907.[40] The commissioners found widespread corruption among the subordinate staff in the Sanitary Department and brought formal charges against 14 British inspectors.[41] Poor Atkinson had been overwhelmed by having the administrative responsibilities of two relatively large departments and at the same time single-handedly heading a hospital, Victoria Hospital for Women and Children. It is hardly surprising that he had overlooked irregularities in the Sanitary Department. The report came out when Atkinson was on leave, and it disturbed him greatly. He criticized it as nonjudicial and not based on evidence. He regretted that the whole staff had been stigmatized because some inspectors had demeaned themselves by accepting bribes.[42]

In 1908, the Sanitary Board was reorganized once again. A cadet officer was appointed the head of the Sanitary Department and ex officio president of the Sanitary Board, accountable to the governor for the expenditure of the funds voted by the Legislative Council. For the next three decades, the Sanitary Department and the Sanitary Board had little medical input, as they were divorced from the Medical Department.[43]

Medical officers, despite their efforts to become involved, were unable to enforce sanitation rules.

In 1912, Dr. John Mitford Atkinson retired from the Colonial Service and settled in London. For a while, he practiced as a consultant in tropical diseases. In 1915, he was appointed head of Richmond Military Hospital, converting the old workhouse and infirmary into a modern war hospital. During that winter, in addition to this job, he devoted evenings to ambulance and first-aid work. By then, his health began to fail and he resigned from the project. On 23 May 1917, he suddenly developed chest pain, which he had been suffering for a while, and passed away on the same day.[44] He left his wife, who was the head nurse of Government Civil Hospital of Hong Kong, and two sons, aged 17 and 18.

Francis William Clark (1864–1940)
MB, MD, MRCS and LRCP (Lond) and DPH (Cantab), JP

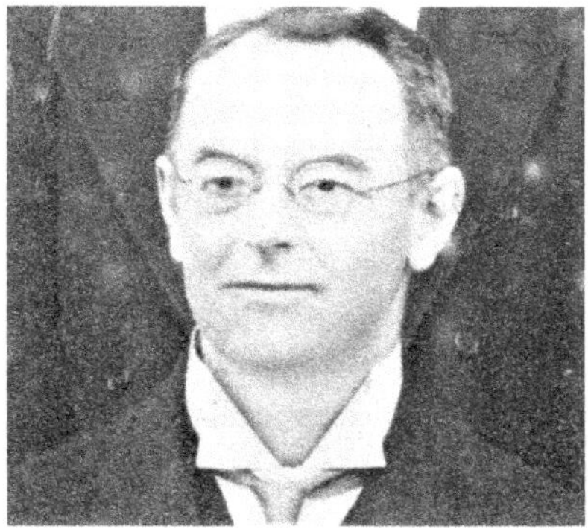

Figure 2.4 Dr. Francis Clark, Dean of the Faculty of Medicine, HKU (1912–1915)
Source: Hong Kong University Archives, HKU

Dr. Francis William Clark was the first Medical Officer of Health in Hong Kong. Born in London, educated at Durham University and later at St. Bartholomew Hospital, Clark had a distinguished student career and was awarded several scholarships during his university days. He obtained his MB degree in 1892, and MD in 1900. He also held diplomas of MRCS and LRCP (Lond) and DPH (Cantab). He spent some time in private practice before becoming Assistant Medical Officer of Health of Port of Tyne. In 1893, he was engaged as Medical Officer of Health and Superintendent of Fever Hospital at Lowestoft. In 1895, he was appointed Medical Officer of Health, the first such appointment in Hong Kong.[45] He served Hong Kong from 1895 to 1915, a period of 20 years.

The job of a medical officer of health is different from that of a medical officer. A medical officer of health was the watchdog of public health, such as prevention and control of infectious diseases, malnutrition, insanitary environment including houses, ensuring clean water and food supply, and keeping good vital statistics of the population. Clark arrived in Hong Kong one year after the 1894 plague epidemic, its epicenter at Taipingshan. He was aware of his many duties and set to work immediately on the problem of insanitary dwellings in Taipingshan, which was thought to be one of the causes of the plague epidemic. During the epidemic, Governor Sir William Robinson (governor, 1891–1898) had cordoned off a large area in Taipingshan where dwellings were considered insanitary. These houses had since been demolished and cleared, streets remarked, and lanes set aside for public use. In 1896, Governor Robinson ordered a commission to further define and classify unsanitary properties and to determine the full extent of the problems in Taipingshan.[46] After deliberating on the commission's findings, the Sanitary Board, of which Clark was a member, drafted a unanimous recommendation: an Insanitary Properties Ordinance to reduce the degree of overcrowding in the city. This ordinance was sanctioned by the Legislative Council in 1899.[47] It was also during Clark's tenure that the recommendations of Chadwick, who visited Hong Kong twice in 1882 and 1902, on reforms of water supply, drainage, sewage, and refuse disposal were gradually being implemented. The death rates from enteric fever[48] and other water-borne infectious diseases progressively declined as a result.

It was largely his sustained efforts that training and registration of midwives in Western methods of delivery took place, leading to reductions in maternal and infant mortality. In 1896, he noted that 20% of total deaths in Hong Kong were infants under one year of age. The infant mortality among the Chinese was high, 745/1,000, compared with 147/1,000 among the non-Chinese.[49] At that time many Chinese did not register births, especially if it was a girl, but registration of death was mandatory for burial. Clark investigated the cause of the disparity in infant mortality between the races, recognizing infant mortality rates among Chinese were likely overestimated. On many dead Chinese infants, he saw burn marks on the heads, arms, and legs, a common remedy used for treating fever and diarrhea by the Chinese.[50] Clark believed that the Chinese midwives or *wan pos* were responsible for the high infant mortality seen in Hong Kong. In 1900, he observed that the Chinese infant mortality rate had soared to 928/1,000, and although this unbelievably high rate was most likely due to unregistered births, Clark blamed the Chinese parents for their neglect and even invoked the horror of infanticide.[51] Clark pressed for registration of Chinese midwives. His drafted bill, however, was considered premature by the unofficial Chinese members of the Legislative Council, because the 14 midwives qualified in Western methods at that time could not possibly meet the demand.[52] Clark also wanted to have the 1896 Births and Deaths Registration Ordinance amended to allow for postmortem examination in cases where the cause of death had not been identified, but the Chinese members of the Legislative Council strongly opposed the bill because postmortem was against Chinese custom.

In 1903, Joseph Chamberlain, the Secretary of State for the Colonies, finally acted on this problem and requested an enquiry on the causes and possible remedies for the high infant mortality.[53] The results show infection and malnutrition were common causes of death. The committee recommended education of Chinese mothers in the basic hygiene of infant rearing and better-trained midwives. Based on these findings, an annual training program for six Chinese midwives was launched in Alice Memorial Maternity Hospital under Dr. Alice Sibree. In 1910, all midwives had to be registered by the Midwives Ordinance, as Clark had hoped.[54] As all midwives required a defined period of training, a larger training institute for nurses and midwives which could accommodate up to 24 students, was established in 1911 at Alice Memorial Maternity Hospital.[55] The infant mortality for Chinese was reduced to 345/1,000 in 1939.[56]

Clark was one of the first doctors in Hong Kong who believed in the malaria-mosquito theory. He assisted Dr. John Christopher Thomson to set up a study of mosquitoes and found the *anopheles* species which was responsible for carrying the malarial parasites in Hong Kong. To control mosquitoes, Clark and the Public Works Department carried out "nullah-training": concreting streams to prevent water from stagnating to form ideal mosquito-breeding pools. The authorities were impressed with the results and publicized its effectiveness.[57] In an article by Sir Ronald Ross in *The Times* on 24 July 1920, Francis Clark of Hong Kong was named one of the three British pioneers in the modern method of prevention of malaria; the other two were Malcolm Watson of Klang and Andrew Balfour of Khartoum.[58]

Clark, who represented Hong Kong, had been active in the Far Eastern Association of Tropical Medicine, and was elected the first general secretary of the association in 1908.[59] Beriberi, a disease due to thiamine deficiency, was common in Hong Kong and in East Asia in the nineteenth century and the first part of the twentieth. The death rates due to beriberi were high, fluctuating between 50/100,000 and 200/100,000 from 1901 to 1938 in Hong Kong.[60] In 1910, Clark recommended fresh fish or beans to supplement the rice diet of beriberi patients, because studies found that in Hong Kong and China, beriberi was associated with the consumption of polished white rice without supplementation of other foods.[61] As the disease carried considerable economic implications, the Far Eastern Association of Tropical Medicine focused on it as a central concern in a series of ten congresses held in Asia between 1910 and 1938. At the inaugural meeting in Manila in 1910, Clark put forth a resolution that since there was sufficient evidence to show that beriberi was associated with the continuous consumption of white rice as a staple diet, governments must act. This resolution, however, made little difference to the beriberi problem in Hong Kong.[62] It was not possible to eradicate the disease when no one, including coolies, was ready to trade a familiar luxury of polished white rice for rough or parboiled rice, and there was serious opposition from the vested interest groups.

Since his arrival Clark had taken a keen interest in the medical students at the Hong Kong College of Medicine (HKCM) (Chapter 3). He lectured on various subjects, including tropical diseases, hygiene, and physiology. He was the third and the longest-serving Dean of the College, a post he held for 16 years (1896 to 1912), and was devoted to his students. When HKCM became the Faculty of Medicine of The University of Hong Kong (HKU) in 1912, he became Professor of Medical Jurisprudence, founding Dean of the Faculty of Medicine, and warden of the university residence, now Lugard Hall, until 1915. He oversaw the transition of students from the College to the University so that they would not be disadvantaged. The students remembered him fondly and recorded in *Caduceus* what a bonus it was to have the Medical Officer of Health as the dean and warden of the University. From 1912 to 1915, the grounds were free of mosquitoes from the constant inspection and supervision of Dr Clark.[63] Clark worked on an honorary basis for the University at the time because of the poor financial situation of the institution.

The graduates of HKCM were not allowed to practice in Hong Kong because it was not recognized by the General Medical Council in Britian. Clark saw the need for the services of these graduates in Hong Kong, which desperately needed young doctors in Western medicine. The graduates were well-trained except for lack of laboratory experience. Since only 10% of deaths in Hong Kong had known causes then, he thought the graduates would be very useful to determine the causes of death especially of the "dumped bodies," bodies left on the street after death. His promotion of the graduates of HKCM was one of the reasons for their employment to staff Chinese Public Dispensaries.[64] Recognizing the importance of public health education, Clark as Medical Officer of Health, gave several lectures on prevention of diseases caused by insect bites,[65] including malaria.[66]

Clark was a member of the Royal Sanitary Institute, a member of the Pathological and Clinical Societies in London. A prolific writer, his contributions to various medical journals such as the *British Medical Journal* and *Medical Magazine* had been numerous.[67] His main recreation was yachting, and he was the commodore of the Corinthian Yacht Club since its formation in 1906.[68] He was also a Freemason.

In 1915, after working for 20 years in Hong Kong, Dr. Francis Clark resigned and returned to England with the good wishes of his students and many friends and colleagues. He returned to China in 1922 to work in the British embassy in Mukden. From 1924 to 1929, he served as Senior Medical Officer in Weihaiwei during the final period before its return to China in 1930. Clark retired in 1929 and died in 1940 in England.[69]

Dr. Francis Clark was the first Medical Officer of Health in Hong Kong and one of the best. He enforced sanitary reforms and pushed for registration of midwives. He enforced measures to eradicate mosquito breeding grounds to prevent malaria. As Dean for HKCM, he was also instrumental in making a breakthrough for the licentiates to practice medicine locally, enabling them to have a future in Hong Kong.

William Hunter (1875–1909)

MB, CM, FRIPH (London)

Dr. William Hunter was born in 1875. He graduated in medicine from The University of Aberdeen in 1896 and received postgraduate training in several prestigious institutions, including King's College, West London Hospital, Leipzig University, and the University of Berlin. As a distinguished scholar, Hunter received medals, scholarships, and fellowships during his student days. He was particularly interested in laboratory medicine, as reflected in his postgraduate training: a laboratory assistant in the Pathology Department in Aberdeen University, and in the Neuropathological Laboratory in King's College in London. In 1900, he became assistant bacteriologist in London Hospital and later Director of the Pathological Institute.[70] When he was appointed by the Hong Kong government as Government Bacteriologist at the recommendation of Sir Patrick Manson in 1902, he was highly qualified for the job.

Hunter was appointed by Governor Blake at a time when plague continued to punish Hong Kong year after year. The governor had metropolitan experts, such as Professor William Simpson and Oswald Chadwick, coming to Hong Kong to advise him on plague, but he wanted to have his own expert to carry out research on this scourge and other infectious diseases. Having some surplus funds for two years, Governor Blake decided to build an institute and have a bacteriologist to direct the research.[71] Hunter astutely requested the most up-to-date equipment for research as one of the conditions for employment. The equipment, salary, and travel expenses came to the relatively large sum of HK$40,000.[72] This far-sighted proposal was most unusual for a colony that had only primitive facilities for medical care. Since plague was so detrimental to trade, the large budget to build the Bacteriological Institute to prevent the disease was approved readily by the Legislative Council without any questions. Whether the appointment was a wise one for a young bacteriologist to work in an environment without infrastructure and support from the rest of the medical staff, who were naturally hoping for more funds to improve the poor facilities in their hospital, did not enter the mind of the busy governor.

When he first arrived in Hong Kong, Hunter established a temporary laboratory at Kennedy Town Infectious Diseases Hospital. While the Bacteriological Institute was being built, he moved into a nearby new building on Hill Road, which was the future public morgue.[73] Due to damage of the equipment during transit to Hong Kong, the laboratory set-up was delayed for several months.

Hunter supervised the construction of the Bacteriological Institute. Completed in 1906, it boasted four laboratories, two on the top floor and two on the ground floor in the main block. There was an animal house for making vaccines, and a dormitory for the staff. His clinical work included postmortem examination of all the bodies in the public mortuary to determine cause of death, bacteriological examination of clinical samples sent to the Institute, and regular examination of quality of water and milk. For many years, the Institute was the place to examine for plague bacilli in rats collected daily by rat catchers, and it produced vaccines against smallpox, cholera, and other infectious diseases when necessary for local use.[74]

After Hunter's arrival, Governor Blake appointed him a member of the commission to inquire into the excessive infant mortality among the Chinese. The commission reported that about 50% of the infants died of *trismus* or lockjaw, which had been known to be due to tetanus bacilli infection. This finding led Pathology Professor C. Y. Wang at HKU to investigate the problem. In 1927, Wang discovered live tetanus bacilli in sealing-cord powders that were customarily applied to the umbilicus of the newborn by Chinese women.[75] Prohibition of the practice led to almost complete disappearance of *trismus* in newborns.

Hunter did not confine his studies to infant deaths, he also studied the causes of adult deaths. The Chinese did not allow postmortems unless required by law. Because of the draconian sanitary regulations, ill people without relatives were often thrown out onto the streets and left to die, or their bodies were simply "dumped" after death during epidemics of plague or smallpox, to avoid being found as contacts, and to prevent their houses from being disinfected. Hunter examined the cause of death of these bodies shortly after his arrival. Between March 1902 and February 1903, Hunter examined 2,816 bodies. He divided the causes into two groups: general and local. Of those with general diseases (N=1,636), the majority died from infection. The common causes that year were plague (473), cholera (379), and tuberculosis (151). Other infectious diseases included smallpox, typhoid, dysentery, beriberi, malaria, tetanus, leprosy, and syphilis, acquired and congenital. Beriberi was classified as an infectious disease even though no micro-organism had been isolated then. Anemia, premature death, still birth, burn, death by hanging, and suffocation were also considered general causes of death. The local diseases (N=1,099) were divided by systems: nervous, circulatory, respiratory, digestive, lymphatic, urological, and reproductive. He based his classification on microscopic and bacteriological findings.[76] This was the first postmortem study ever carried out in Hong Kong.

His second task was to confirm rats as a vector for the transmission of plague. He performed bacteriological examinations of rats collected every day in Hong Kong. Although it was generally accepted by then that *Yersinia pestis* causes plague, it was not yet accepted that rats were the vector of transmission. A special rat postmortem room was established in the public mortuary. The study began in March 1902, shortly after his arrival, and the bacteriological examination was conducted by four Japanese doctors on all dead mice found in the city. When the Japanese doctors left, three graduates from HKCM carried on the work. During that year, he found a high correlation between the number of rats infected with plague bacilli and the number of human cases of plague. The rise in the number of infected rats preceded human disease for about one week.[77] The findings were the same in subsequent years, confirming the relationship between the disease in rats and in humans and that rats were likely vectors for transmission of the disease.

Plague was also found in cats, and Hunter believed that they contracted the disease from devouring infected rats. He went on to study whether other animals were also susceptible to infection and the portal of entry of the plague bacilli in humans. He carried out the study on animals in Dairy Farm in Pokfulam and the slaughterhouse in Kennedy Town and found that pigs, calves, sheep, monkeys, and fowl were also susceptible to plague infection. He cautioned that people should be careful with the possibility of food infection and postulated that the gastrointestinal tract rather than the skin was a more frequent portal of entry of the plague bacilli.[78]

In addition to plague, he investigated the vectors for the liver fluke, *Clonorchis sinensis*, which caused recurrent pyogenic cholangitis, a prevalent disease in Hong Kong at the time. He also studied the etiology of beriberi and concluded that it was not an infectious disease, because he was unable to isolate pathogenic bacteria from beriberi patients.[79]

He trained the staff working in his laboratory. The Certificate of Laboratory Instruction he issued for the staff he trained received recognition as fulfilling the conditions for the Diploma of Public Health from some universities in England[80] and by the Committee of Management in the Colonial Office.[81] In 1905, three years after arriving in Hong Kong, he published four original articles and three case reports. Although this output may seem modest to us today, one must consider that he started from scratch—from supervision of the building of the laboratory—and he carried a very heavy clinical load. To accomplish what he had accomplished, he must have had worked long hours, day after day.

Despite his high productivity, Hunter's temporary appointment had to be renewed every three years and did not seem to be leading to a permanent position that he had been hoping for. Published in prestigious journals such as *The Lancet* and the *British Medical Journal*, his work was beginning to gain recognition at home. It must have been devastating for him to learn that even his re-appointment was in question after five years, in part because Governor Blake had been replaced by Governor Nathan, who had less interest in health issues. Hunter was told that Hong Kong was too small a place to afford a research institute when, in fact, his reappointment was opposed by the Principal Civil Medical Officer.[82]

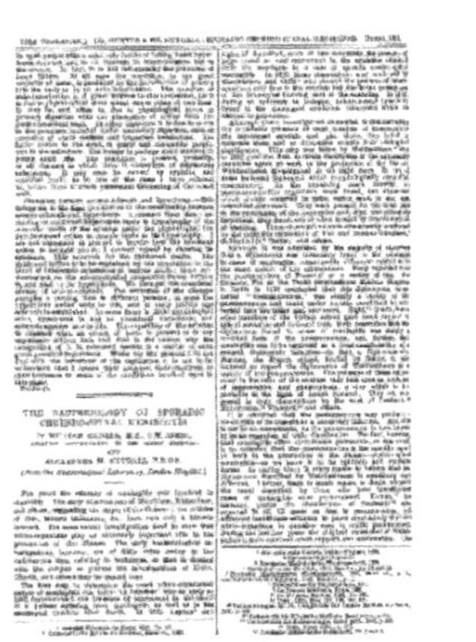

Figure 2.5 Dr. William Hunter's *Lancet* paper on the bacteriology of sporadic cerebrospinal meningitis

Source: *The Lancet*, June 1 (1901): 1504

Although Hunter's appointment was finally renewed in 1908, he died suddenly in 1909, at 34 years of age. The telegram from Governor Lugard to the Colonial Office was terse and cryptic: "Regret to inform you of the death of Hunter Bacteriologist."[83] The cause of death was not revealed.

Despite the short career, Dr. William Hunter accomplished a great deal in Hong Kong. He was instrumental in getting the Bacteriological Institute built, initiated the first series of autopsies in Hong Kong to confirm the cause of death of the "dumped bodies," began a research program applicable to local medical problems, and trained technicians. He achieved more than what was expected of him. The Bacteriology Institute continued to serve the people of Hong Kong by providing public health services in disease prevention, surveillance programs for plague and other diseases, vaccine production, and supervision of water and milk quality for the community. Few in Hong Kong recognized its role in public health and its contribution. After World War II, the name was changed to Pathological Institute. When Pathological Institute was relocated to a new facility at Sai Ying Pun Polyclinic in 1960, vaccine production continued in the old building until the 1970s. In 1990, the building was declared a protected monument, and in 1996, it was turned into a museum under the auspices of The Hong Kong Museum of Medical Sciences Society.

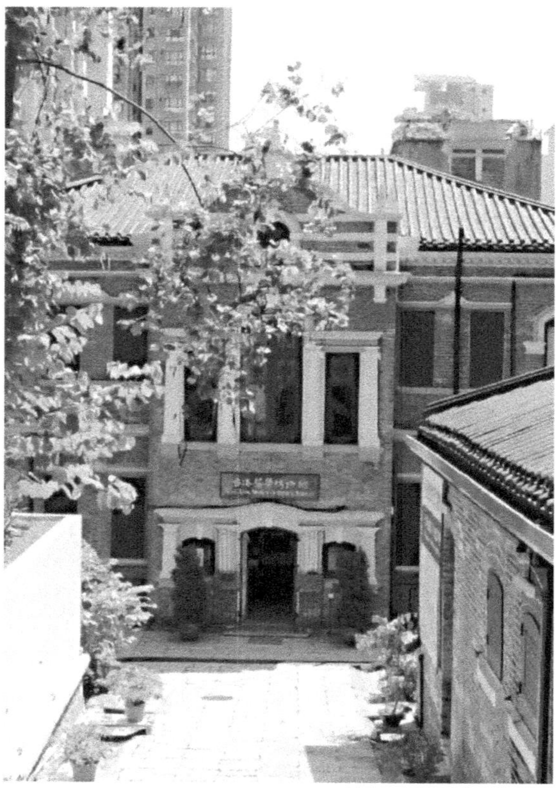

Figure 2.6 Bacteriological Institute, now The Hong Kong Museum of Medical Sciences
Photo taken by Moira Chan-Yeung

Arthur Robartes Wellington (1877–1961)

MD, DTM&H (Cantab), DPH (Cantab), CMG

The next person that made significant changes to the Government Medical Department in Hong Kong was Dr. Arthur Robartes Wellington. He was born in Canada in 1877 but received medical education at Kelly College, Tavistock, and at St. Mary's Hospital, London, qualifying in 1902. He took the course in tropical medicine and public health in Cambridge and received both a DTM&H (Cantab) and a DPH (Cantab) in 1905.[84] The same year he joined the Sarawak Medical Service in British North Borneo.[85] Though he enjoyed the pioneer work, he left for Singapore at the end of the first contract because of his wife's ill health. In Singapore, he was Health Officer and worked in St. John's Island, undeterred by the fact that his two predecessors had died from typhus.

In 1908, when he was in the malaria-ridden states of Selangor and Perak in the Federated Malay States, he contributed greatly to the control of malaria and also venereal disease and typhus. At that time mosquitoes had been found by Dr. Ronald Ross as the vector for transmission of malaria.[86] Wellington worked closely with Dr. Malcolm Watson on controlling mosquitoes, using civil engineering methods. As a result, Watson was knighted in England for his work, but Wellington was not, the latter being modest by nature. In 1919, he was promoted to Chief Health Officer of the British Federated Malay States. His engagement as Director of Medical and Sanitary Services of Hong Kong began in 1929 and ended in 1937.

In Hong Kong, Wellington was appointed to the Legislative Council and became the official advisor to the government on all matters of public health, medicine, and sanitation. He was also tasked with the reorganization of medical and sanitary services. After studying the health system in Hong Kong, Wellington proposed that all government public health activities other than scavenging, conservancy, and public works be placed under the control of the Director of Medical and Sanitary Services.[87] The plan was referred to the Sanitary Board, but it took several years before reorganization finally occurred in 1936. In the reorganization, the Sanitary Board was replaced by the Urban Council, which would have an expanded range of services. The Medical Department and the Sanitary Department were combined. The Director of Medical Services was responsible for health officers, veterinary surgeon, and sanitary

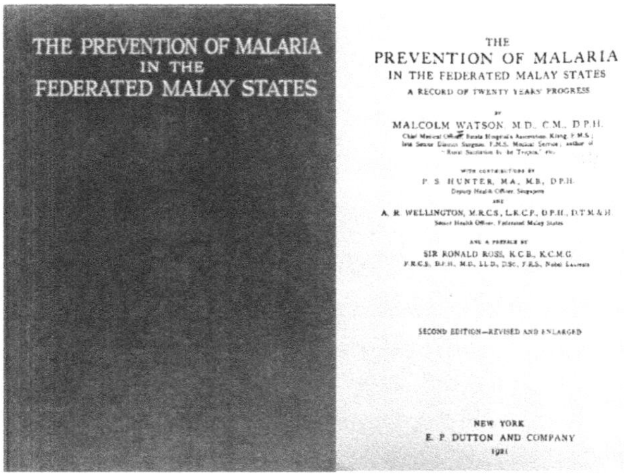

Figures 2.7a and b. Book on prevention of malaria by Malcolm Watson, F. S. Hunter, and A. R. Wellington

Source: Photograph of the book *The Prevention of Malaria in the Federated Malay States* taken by Wong Tai-wai

inspectors, as well as acting as the vice-chairman of the Urban Council. The responsibilities of the Urban Council, Medical, Sanitary, and Public Works departments were clearly defined.[88] The Medical Department assumed tasks of the operation of government hospitals and dispensaries, inspection of Chinese and subsidized hospitals, bacteria research, detection and control, quarantine, and prevention of diseases, registration of births and deaths, vaccination programs, venereal disease clinics, and school health programs.[89] After the reorganization, the Sanitary Department, now under the same director as the Medical Department, benefited greatly from medical input in creating and implementing vital public health policies in Hong Kong.

In 1934, having dealt with the reorganization of medical and sanitary services in Hong Kong and Kowloon, Wellington turned to medical and sanitary services in the New Territories, that were poorly developed. In 1902, the government only had a clinic in Tai Po to care for the police force in the New Territories. After the building of the Kowloon-Canton Railway (KCR) had started, a small dispensary was established at the southern end of the Beacon Hill tunnel, built especially for the railway. This dispensary and Tai Po clinic cared for all the workers of the KCR.[90] For the purpose of medical administration, Wellington divided the New Territories into the western and the eastern medical districts, headquarters at Yuen Long and Tai Po, respectively. The western medical district had a population of 49,848 and included four districts of the mainland (Tsuen Wan, Ping Shan, Au Tau, and Lok Ma Chau) and nearby islands, Lantau, and Cheung Chau. The eastern medical district, with a population of 46,864, included five districts of the mainland (Sha Tau Kok, Sheung Shui, Tai Po, Sha Tin, and Sai Kung), the Po Toi group of islands and Tseung Kwan O Bay.[91] The division of the New Territories into two medical districts enabled Wellington to develop a long-term strategic plan on expanding medical services in there.

In the early 1930s, two voluntary organizations, St. John Ambulance and New Territories Medical Benevolent Society (MBS), established clinics in different parts of the New Territories. In 1933, there were no fewer than 10 medical clinics, each included its own nurses and midwives provided by either one of the two voluntary organizations. During 1934, the government also established four dispensaries in the New Territories: Lady Ho Tung Welfare Center, Sham Tseng Dispensary, Tai O Dispensary, and Sai Kung Dispensary. As a result, there were duplications of services in some areas. Wellington arranged for the two voluntary organizations to combine into one and, together with the government, they ensured that there was only one clinic in one area, and new clinics were set up in areas that did not have such a service. In the second half of the 1930s, Shing Mun Dam was built for the construction of Jubilee Reservoir. A small hospital was erected in Shing Mun even before the beginning of the construction of the dam, in anticipation of medical problems presented by the influx of workers. At the time the most prevalent medical problems in the New Territories and for the workers of the KCR and Shing Mun Dam were malaria, dysentery, beriberi, and injuries.[92]

Wellington also saw the completion of Queen Mary Hospital in 1937.[93] It was built to replace Government Civil Hospital, which had become too congested and in too crowded an environment to serve as a teaching hospital. Today, Queen Mary Hospital is the flagship hospital in Hong Kong and one of two teaching hospitals. Wellington had greatly improved the standard of medical and health services, especially in hospital care. Before he retired, he organized a Technical Committee for the Reorganization and Improvement of Official Hospital and Clinical Facilities. The committee recommended another 2,500 hospital beds, as well as increased outpatient and welfare services. Although this proposal was approved by the Colonial Office and the Hong Kong government, the start of World War II interrupted the implementation.[94]

Another major contribution of Wellington was in malaria control. Malaria was endemic and a regular unwelcome summer visitor in Hong Kong. Between the late 1880s and early 1890s, the incidence of malaria in the civilian population was around 400/100,000, and had a death rate of approximately 200/100,000.[95] As noted before, Dr. John Christopher Thomson discovered that the *Anopheles* mosquito, the species responsible for transmission of malaria, was present in Hong Kong.[96] Although individual physicians, such as Dr. Francis Clark and Dr. Ho Nai-hop, the Chinese Medical Officer working in Tai Po station, knew how to control mosquitoes using methods such as "training nullahs" to prevent stagnation of water and pouring oil on the surface of water that could not be drained, the public had no knowledge of the disease and of the mosquitoes. There was also no colony-wide program to control mosquitoes.

As the Chief Health Officer in the Federated Malay States, Wellington had extensive experience in malaria control and knew the experts in this area. He was able to secure the services of malariologists Dr. Robert Best Jackson and his assistant, Mr. Deb, from British Malaya to head the Malaria Bureau in Hong Kong. These two specialists had a long experience of operating together in anti-malarial work, and they formed the nucleus of antimalarial branch of the Medical Department and trained local recruits.[97] Even before Jackson's arrival, Wellington began to provide public education on malaria and mosquitoes and on other infectious diseases.[98] He likened the antimalarial campaign to a war. He said, "War against mosquitoes like war against man is a scientific problem ... Every effort must be made to bring untoward influences to bear upon the enemy's front line, the adult mosquitoes, and upon his reserve, the larvae...."[99] Wellington and Jackson devised campaigns based on their experience in Malaya. Wellington delegated the responsibility of overseeing the permanent sanitary and drainage works to an engineer in the Public Works Department. A team of coolies was hired and supervised by the assistant malariologist to carry out oiling of breeding pools that could not be drained.[100] The Malaria Bureau carried out regular analysis of larval specimens from different parts of the colony. This program of eliminating the breeding grounds of mosquitoes was comprehensive and highly effective. The mortality from malaria in Hong Kong dropped from 203/100,000 in 1901 to 35/100,000 in 1937 (Figure 2.8), accounting for 8% to just 1% of all deaths in the respective years.

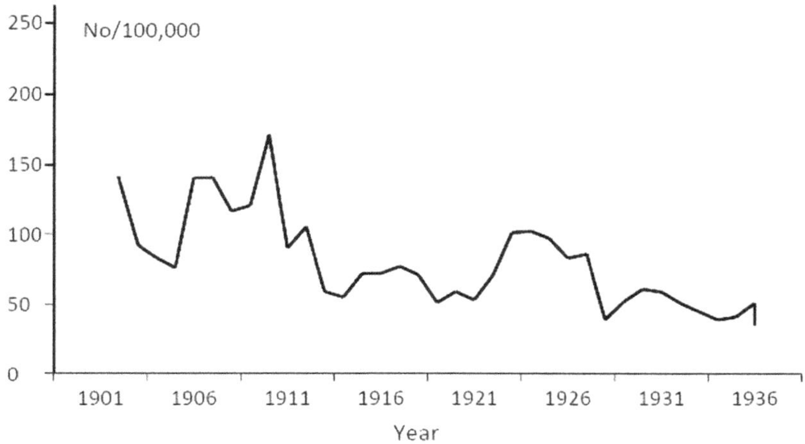

Figure 2.8 Deaths from malaria (no./100,000) in Hong Kong, 1901–1938
Source: Moira Chan-Yeung, *A Medical History of Hong Kong, 1842–1941*, 210

While conducting a general mosquito survey of Hong Kong, the Malaria Bureau also investigated other mosquito-borne diseases: filariasis, yellow fever, and dengue fever. Fortunately, these diseases were not found in Hong Kong. The bureau also identified two more species of *Anopheles* mosquitoes, *Anopheles minimus* and *Anopheles jeyporensis,* that were responsible for malaria transmission locally.[101]

During a short period of 7 years, Wellington reformed medical and sanitary services in Hong Kong, and altered the administrative division for medical services in the New Territories. For the first time, he established the Malaria Bureau and placed malaria under control. His distinguished service as the Director of Medical and Sanitary Services in Hong Kong was recognized by the award of CMG in 1934.[102]

Dr. Arthur Robartes Wellington was a founding member of the Royal Society of Tropical Medicine and Hygiene. A past president of the Malaya-branch of the British Medical Association, he represented Malaya and Hong Kong at health conferences in various parts of the world and was a delegate to several League of Nations conventions. He enjoyed golf and swimming and was a great lover of verses. Wellington retired in 1937 and died in 1961 in Nice, France. He was succeeded by Dr. Percy Selwyn Selwyn-Clarke.[103]

3. Physicians Who Propagated Western Medicine

Founding the Alice Memorial Hospital and Hong Kong College of Medicine

After the closure of Medical Missionary Society Hospital, there was a lapse of 30 years before the LMS began to provide medical services to the impoverished in Hong Kong again. This began with the arrival of a Canadian doctor, Dr. William Young, in Hong Kong in 1881. Dr. Young was struck by the number of sick people and medical neglect among the deprived Chinese.[1] He contacted the local LMS and a small Medical Mission Committee was formed, initially with three local businessmen. The committee was chaired by an accountant, Mr. Henry William Davis, who donated funds for the operation of a dispensary, Nethersole Dispensary, named after his mother.[2] The dispensary, located in one of the rooms of Taipingshan Chapel of the LMS, was opened on 4 October, 1881. Dr. William Young attended the clinic from 7:00 a.m. to 8:30 a.m. two days a week, offering free medical services. During the first three months of its operation, 927 patients visited the clinic, receiving treatment. Encouraged by the clinic's success, the committee requested the LMS to build a hospital and send a full-time doctor.[3]

In early 1882, when Dr. Ho Kai and his English wife, Alice Walkden, returned from England after his training as a doctor and a barrister, the Medical Mission Committee of the LMS approached him about a charity Chinese Hospital. Ho Kai was keenly interested and became a member of the committee. To build the hospital, the committee decided that the LMS would make a contribution up to HK$14,000 from the sale of its Queen's Road Chapel for the acquisition of a site for the hospital, and the senior missionary of the LMS in Hong Kong would be a member of the managing committee. The major challenge was finding enough funds to build the hospital.

In 1884, the funding problem was solved by Ho Kai. He generously offered to pay for building the hospital in memory of his wife who had just passed away.[4] A site was purchased on the northeast corner of Hollywood Road and Aberdeen Street for HK$22,000, of which

HK$14,000 was paid for by the society and the rest by public subscription. Opened on 16 February 1887, Alice Memorial Hospital would provide medical consultation, medicine, and accommodation free of charge, except for food, for the sick of all creeds and nationalities.[5] Local doctors consented to provide medical services free of charge, even though the LMS had intended to send out a missionary doctor to take charge of the hospital.

As the population rapidly grew in Hong Kong, so did the demand for medical services. Alice Memorial Hospital was always full. Mr. Davis donated funds again to build Nethersole Hospital, situated at 1 Bonham Road, again to honor his mother.[6] It was opened on 5 September 1893 for women only,[7] and Alice Memorial Hospital became a hospital for men only. When there was a demand for maternity beds, Ho Kai and a group of prominent Chinese raised funds to build the first maternity hospital in Hong Kong—Alice Memorial Maternity Hospital—at 6A Bonham Road. It was completed in 1904.[8] Shortly after that, there was another proposal to build yet another hospital by Ho Miu-ling, the sister of Ho Kai, to relieve the congestion. Ho Miu Ling Hospital was completed in 1906 at Breezy Path.[9] In 1929, Alice Memorial Hospital was rebuilt near the other three hospitals. As a result, all four small hospitals were situated next to each other. They had a total of 126 beds, and in 1954 they were incorporated under one name—Alice Nethersole Ho Miu Ling Hospital—and under the administration of the LMS.[10] These hospitals continue to serve the people of Hong Kong today but in a new location at Tai Po.

The four doctors who contributed their free medical services to the hospital initially included local prominent physicians in the community: Drs. Patrick Manson, William Young, William Hartigan, and Gregory Jordan. They were remarkable men who were also interested in the founding of a medical college to teach local students. When the hospital was opened in February 1887, there were students interested in entering the medical college, even though the college was not officially opened until October 1887.[11]

To relieve his busy private practice, Manson recruited Dr. James Cantlie from Britain as his partner. Cantlie arrived in Hong Kong on 30 August 1887. He, too, was interested in disseminating Western medicine among the Chinese. A meeting was called when eight people: Drs. Patrick Manson, James Cantlie, Ho Kai, Gregory Jordan, Johann Gerhard Gerlach, William Young, and the Rev. John Chalmers from the LMS, and

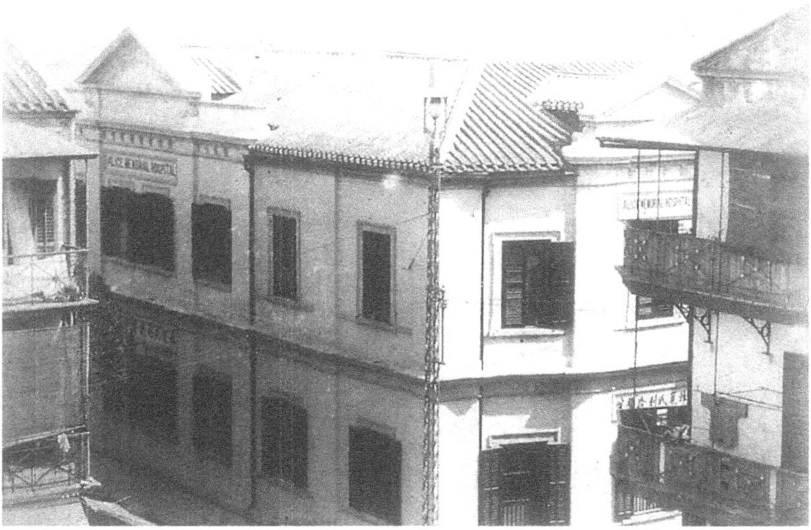

Figure 3.1 Alice Memorial Hospital, 1887
Image courtesy of Alice Ho Miu Ling Nethersole Charity Foundation

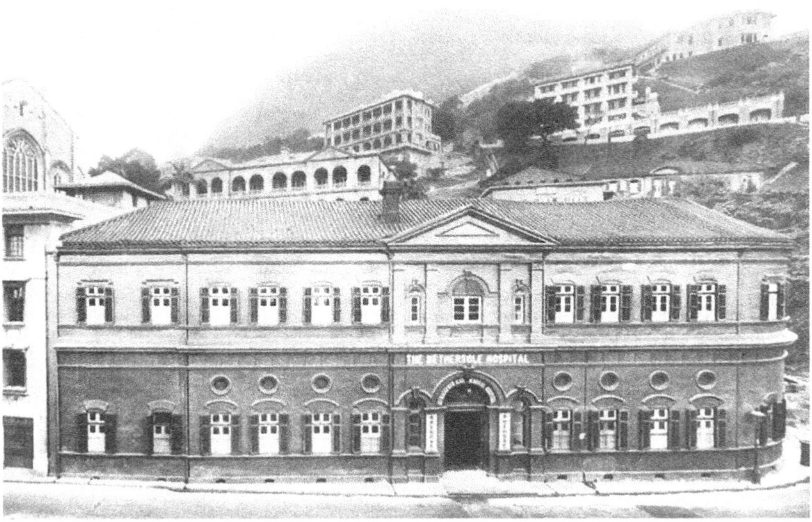

Figure 3.2 Nethersole Hospital, 1893
Image courtesy of Alice Ho Miu Ling Nethersole Charity Foundation

Mr. W. E. Crow, who was Apothecary and Analyst of Government Civil Hospital, were present. During this meeting, Hong Kong College of Medicine (HKCM) for Chinese was formally founded; all those present at the meeting formed the senate and Manson as dean.[12] Since the medical school had no building, Alice Memorial Hospital provided rooms for lectures and demonstrations and wards with patients for bedside teaching.[13] There were, however, no facilities for laboratory studies. As secretary, Cantlie took over the day-to-day running of HKCM.

The College had the support of Governor Des Voeux as its President and Li Hongzhang, Viceroy of Zhili and Huguang as its patron.[14] It had a senate that was responsible for academic matters and a teaching staff, a council for the business part of the College, and a court as a public interest monitor. It had no endowment, and the government did not provide any grant for the operation of the College. The regular income came only from students' fees, and many students were on scholarships.[15] It operated on a shoestring budget. The lecturers included local private practitioners, the Colonial Surgeon, and other officers of the Government Medical Service. More volunteer faculty was added later, including the first Medical Officer of Health, Superintendent of Alice Memorial Hospital, and medical officers of the army and the Royal Navy.[16] One of the first two graduates from the College was Dr. Sun Yat-sen.

After the departure of Manson and Cantlie from Hong Kong in 1889 and 1896 respectively, the enthusiasm for the College waned and so did the morale of the College. HKCM was not recognized by the General Medical Council in England, and graduates were not allowed to practice in Hong Kong, according to the Medical Registration Ordinance of 1884.[17] The reason given was that HKCM's medical curriculum was "not the equivalent to the minimum course required in England." The lack of adequate clinical and laboratory facilities was clearly one of the factors that mitigated against the College securing recognition from the General Medical Council.

When the University of Hong Kong was founded in 1911, HKCM was incorporated into the University to become the Faculty of Medicine.[18] The last meeting of the Court of the College took place in January 1915.

In its 28 years of existence, HKCM had admitted 128 students, and of these, 60 graduated.[19] Unable to practice locally, many licentiates left for Southeast Asia or China, where they could practice.[20] HKCM and the outcome of its licentiates had been documented in detail by Professor

Faith Ho in her book, *Western Medicine for Chinese: How the Hong Kong College of Medicine Achieved a Breakthrough*, published in 2017 by Hong Kong University Press. At least two of the licentiates received further training in Edinburgh and returned to Hong Kong; their contributions to the development of medicine locally will be discussed later in this book. Later, some licentiates were able to serve Hong Kong by working in government positions such as Chinese Public Dispensaries and the Bacteriological Institute.

This chapter is devoted to the key physicians who were associated with Alice Memorial Hospital and HKCM. The first four individuals were related to the founding of these two institutions: Ho Kai, Patrick Manson, James Cantlie, and Gregory Jordan. Manson and Cantlie provided much of the medical expertise necessary for the initiation and development of the HKCM and up-to-date medical knowledge to local practitioners. Jordan took part in teaching various subjects in HKCM since its inception; he became Pro-Vice-Chancellor of HKU when it was founded in 1911. John Christopher Thomson, a medical missionary from the LMS, was not one of the founders, but he cared for the students and was crucial in keeping the College going until he retired from Hong Kong in 1909. Lastly, the story of one of the graduates of HKCM, Dr. Ho Ko-tsun, who dedicated his whole life as a general practitioner to look after the residents in Wanchai, is also recounted. These physicians were devoted to Western medicine and desired to see it being propagated for the benefit of the local residents. Their contributions to medical services and medical education in Hong Kong had been invaluable and led to the general acceptance of Western medicine in the local population.

Ho Kai 何啟 (1859–1914)

MBCM, MRCS and LRCP (Lond), JP, KCMG

Sir Kai Ho Kai was one of the most prominent figures in Hong Kong during his time. Although he was qualified in medicine and in law, he did not practice medicine but law for his living. He donated to the construction of Alice Memorial Hospital and helped raise funds to build the Alice affiliated hospitals. He was one of the founders of the HKCM and raised funds to establish HKU. In addition to his role in initiating medical education and in building hospitals, Ho Kai left a profound and lasting influence on the well-being of the community in Hong Kong as a member of the Sanitary Board and the Legislative Council.

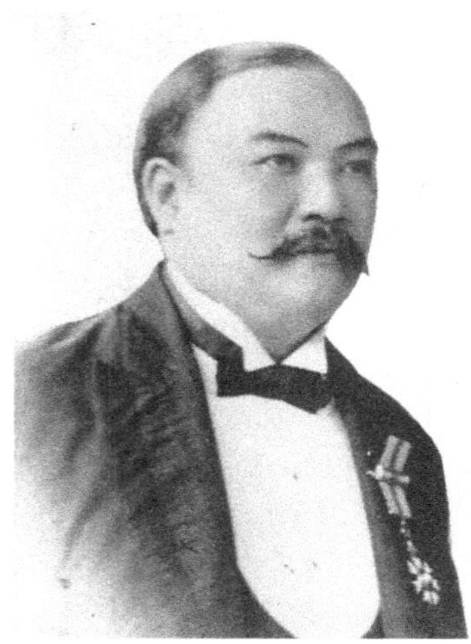

Figure 3.3 Sir Kai, Ho Kai
Image courtesy of HKMMS, donated by Alice Ho Miu Ling Nethersole Charity Foundation

Ho Kai was born in 1859, the fifth son of the Rev. Ho Fuk-tong, and grew up in a large family with 11 children. One of his sisters, Ho Miu-ling, a devout Christian and very intelligent and well-educated young woman, married Ng Choy (also known as Wu Ting-fang), the first Chinese to be appointed to the Hong Kong Legislative Council and a well-known calligrapher, politician, and diplomat of the Republic of China.[21]

A brilliant scholar, Ho Kai entered Class 4 in Central School (Queen's College today) at the age of 11. He reached Class I (top form) in two years. In 1872, at the age of 13, he studied at Palmer House School, Margate, Kent. In September 1875, he registered at the University of Aberdeen. In 1879, at the age of 20, he received his medical degree, MBCM, and went to St Thomas' Hospital to take up clinical training. He became the first Chinese qualified physician from The University of Aberdeen. At the persuasion of his future wife, Alice Walkden, he entered Lincoln's Inn to study law and was called to the bar in 1881. In the same year he passed the examination for membership in the Royal College of Surgeons of London (MRCS, Lond) and was also awarded the licentiate of the Royal College of Physicians (LRCP, Lond). The couple were married in 1881 and returned to Hong Kong in early 1882.[22] Sadly, she died three years later from typhoid, leaving a daughter. Ho Kai remarried and had 17 children from the second marriage.

On his return to Hong Kong in 1882, Ho Kai set up a medical practice. Much to his annoyance, he could not make a living as a doctor. No Chinese would pay to see a Western doctor, and no European would consult a Chinese doctor in Western medicine. He turned to his other skill and set up a law practice. He was admitted as a barrister in the Supreme Court on 29 March 1882, the second Chinese to join the roll. Shortly after he settled in Hong Kong, he became deeply involved with community affairs and in public service. He was appointed a Justice of the Peace in 1882, and a member of the Sanitary Board in 1886, a position he held for about 10 years. In 1890, he became the third Chinese to sit on the Legislative Council. He served the Legislative Council until 1914, a record of 24 years.[23] In addition, he was on a large number of boards and committees, such as the Public Works Committee, Standing Law Committee, Examination Board, Medical Board, Po Leung Kuk Committee, District Watch Committee, Tung Wah Hospital Advisory Committee, and the boards of schools. He never begrudged the time he had to serve on these committees and boards. For these numerous services to the community, he was awarded a CMG in 1902 and knighthood in 1912.[24] This presentation will focus mainly on his contributions to medicine.

As he was a doctor and a Christian, it was not surprising that he was approached by the Medical Mission Committee of the LMS about establishing a charity hospital to provide Western medical care to the poor Chinese. When his wife passed away, he donated funds to build Alice Memorial Hospital, in memory of her, as noted.[25] Ho Kai remained on the Medical Mission Committee for many years. He and his friends were responsible for raising funds to build two out of three affiliated hospitals and operating funds for all of them.

Ho Kai was highly supportive of training Chinese young men in Western medicine and to introduce it to the Chinese community. He was one of the founding members of HKCM for Chinese.[26] He taught forensic medicine in the College for a number of years. Well known for his reputation in the Chinese community and his ability to raise funds, Governor Sir Frederick Lugard (governor of Hong Kong, 1907–1912)

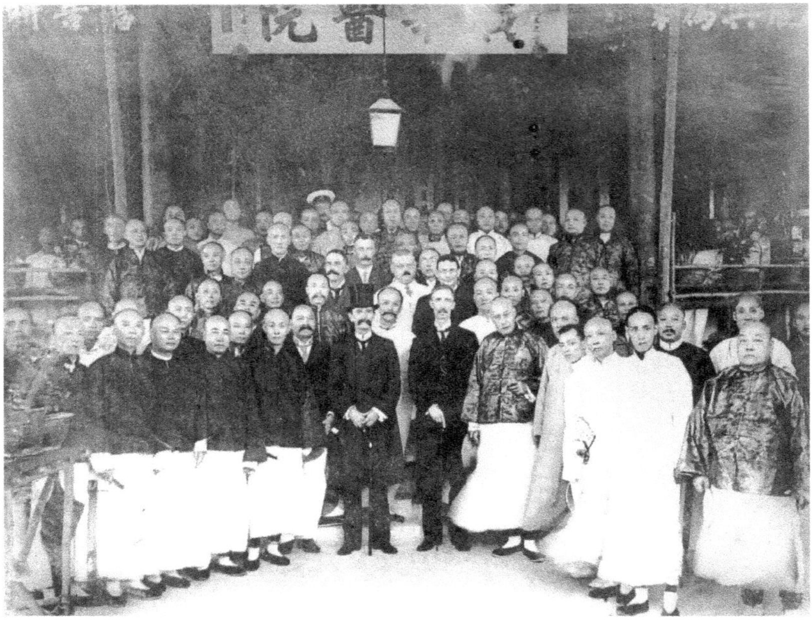

Figure 3.4 Ho Kai (wearing a tie) standing next to Governor Lugard (with top hat) on his right at the opening of Kwong Wah Hospital, 1911
Image courtesy of Tung Wah Hospital Archives

assigned to him the task of raising funds from the Chinese community for constructing the university buildings.[27] Thus his contribution to medical education extended to the founding of HKU and the Faculty of Medicine.

Ho Kai was concerned with the high maternal and infant mortality in Hong Kong.[28] He agreed with the recommendations of Dr. Francis Clark, the first medical officer of health of Hong Kong, to train midwives in Western methods of delivery. Also, at that time there were virtually no facilities to care for Chinese women for confinement. Nethersole Hospital was small; similarly, the maternal bungalow in Government Civil Hospital had very few beds. Victoria Hospital for Women and Children, theoretically built for all races, was located at the Peak and used by Europeans only because Chinese were not allowed at the Peak.[29] Ho Kai and his friends raised funds for building Alice Memorial Maternity Hospital, which was completed in 1904. They requested a female doctor to be in charge of the hospital.[30] The LMS sent a female medical missionary, Dr. Alice Sibree, to head Alice Memorial Maternity Hospital.[31] Sibree organized midwives training in Alice Memorial Maternity Hospital and successfully introduced Western methods of delivery to the Chinese community and won their support (Chapter 6).

Ho Kai's term of 10 years on the Sanitary Board and 24 years on the Legislative Council were highly appreciated by the Chinese community, as he represented their interests.[32] His strong opposition to the Public Health Ordinance of 1887 for sanitary reforms recommended by Chadwick in his Memorandum of Objections[33] was controversial. He believed that "the Ordinance made the mistake of treating Chinese as if they were Europeans because it was based on the one implemented in England. The Chinese should be governed as much as possible in accordance with their manners and customs ..." As a result, the enacted Public Health Ordinance of 1887 was very much watered down.[34] In helping to protect the interest of the Chinese landlords, Ho Kai perpetuated the continual overcrowding and unsanitary living conditions in Hong Kong.

During the 1894 plague epidemic, Ho Kai and the chairman of the board of directors of Tung Wa Hospital (later Tung Wah Hospital) were the two members on the Sanitary Board who did not concur with enacting into law the severe measures to control the epidemic, including house-to-house search for cases and cleansing of "infected" houses. However, their opposition was ignored. The enactment of draconian measures into law resulted in the Chinese community hiding cases of plague from officials and "dumping" dead bodies on the streets. As a member of the special committee to enquire into the workings of Tung Wa Hospital in 1896, Ho Kai was highly supportive of sanitary reforms and the introduction of Western medicine to the hospital, but Chinese medicine should continue to be used.[35] He became the chairman of the founding directors of Kwong Wah Hospital (one of the hospitals in the Tung Wah Group of Hospitals) in 1907, which was opened in 1911.

Thoroughly westernized after years abroad, Ho Kai had his queue cut off and adopted a Western style of clothing (Figure 3.4). He even became a Freemason along with his brother-in-law, Ng Choy, one of the first few Chinese to be admitted into Lodge St. John No. 618 SC—the first Scottish Lodge of Freemasonry established in Hong Kong.[36] Despite this, Ho Kai was very much a Chinese at heart, a monarchist loyal to the throne, and supportive of the Reform Movement in China initially.[37] His advice was often sought by some high-level Qing officials. In fact, he had written several essays on political reforms in China, such as "Critical Essay on China, the Sleep and the Awakening," which was published in

1887, in both English and Chinese. He contributed much to the literature on reformation in China.[38] He was disappointed when he received no response from the Chinese government. The failure of the Hundred Days' Reform and the Boxer Rebellion might have led Ho Kai into believing that removal of the Manchu government through revolution was necessary, as proposed by Dr. Sun Yat-sen, a student of HKCM and his protégé. In 1894, Ho Kai helped Sun draft the aims of the Xing Zhong Hui, (Revive China Society), and it was thought that he might have taken part in planning the ill-fated uprising that aimed at obtaining Guangzhou as a base for future revolution but ended in disaster. He was named an adviser to the government of the Republic of China when it was proclaimed in 1911.[39]

Ho Kai was, at times, in financial trouble, as he spent most of his time in public service rather than earning his living. He had to support a large family of 17 children, 10 sons and 7 daughters, and he was very generous with donations. To supplement his income, he went into business ventures, which did not always work out. For example, he and his son's father-in-law, Au Tak, were the joint owners of the Kai Tak Bund, which later became Kai Tak Airport. The land failed to be developed for a long time and, in 1924, the company they formed went into liquidation and the land was taken back by the government.[40]

Sir Kai Ho Kai retired in April 1914. He was honored by Chinese merchants and influential members of the Chinese community, who paid tribute to him for his long and devoted service. They were grateful that he had never hesitated to speak out on what he thought was the best for them.[41] Ho Kai died in July 1914, intestate and in debt.[42] The governor helped with the education of his sons for a while, but it was his brother-in-law, Ng Choy, who looked after his children, and his colleagues and friends who took care of the immediate expenses. Ho Kai's enormous influence and contributions to Hong Kong had not been fully appreciated, according to Professor Gerald Choa, who, after extensive research, wrote a biography of him entitled *The Life and Times of Sir Kai Ho Kai*. It was published in 1981 by The Chinese University of Hong Kong Press.

Patrick Manson (1844–1922)

MB, MD, MRCP, FRCP, FRS, DSc, KCMG, GCMG

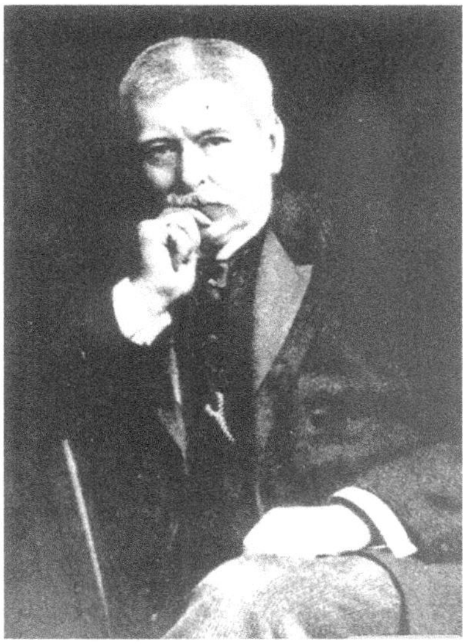

Figure 3.5 Sir Patrick Manson, Dean of HKCM 1887–1889
Image courtesy of HKMMS, photo donated by Alice Ho Miu Ling Nethersole Charity Foundation

Sir Patrick Manson was the "Father of Tropical Medicine" and was well known in the medical circle in Hong Kong as the founder of HKCM for Chinese, the precursor of the Faculty of Medicine, HKU. He was a role model for researchers of the modern era, especially for those in infectious diseases.

Manson was born in 1844 at Oldmeldrum, in Aberdeenshire, Scotland, where his father, a banker, owned a huge estate. As a young man, Manson was keenly interested in natural history. He received his medical education at Aberdeen University and graduated with an MB degree in 1865 and an MD a year later. In 1866, at the age of 22, he took up a post as Medical Officer to the Chinese Imperial Maritime Customs in Takao, Formosa (present-day Kaohsiung, Taiwan). His official duty was to inspect ships calling at the port and to treat the crew with medical problems. He attended a local missionary hospital where he saw a variety of diseases, including elephantiasis and leprosy, which he had never encountered at home. He also treated European patients who usually suffered from liver disease due to excess alcohol. In 1871, he was advised by the British Consul to leave for Amoy (Xiamen) because of unrest in the region.[43] It was in Amoy that Manson carried out the most fruitful fieldwork that rendered his name immortal.

In Amoy, he was Medical Officer of the local Imperial Maritime Customs. He also served the local Chinese at Baptist Missionary Society Hospital and Dispensary. There, he was joined by his younger brother, Dr. David Manson, for two years. At the time, malaria, typhoid, dengue fever, leprosy, and beriberi were endemic in Amoy. Years of careful observation and meticulous record keeping turned Manson into an excellent clinician and diagnostician despite having no mentor or supervision. He operated, under chloroform anesthesia, on patients with elephantiasis, especially those disfigured from enlarged limbs and scrotum. By operating behind a large glass window on street level so that passers-by could convince themselves that he was working for the good of the sick, he gained the trust of the local people.[44] He relieved patients suffering from colic due to bladder stones by surgical lithotomy and tackled liver abscesses by putting in drainage.[45] He even invented a special trocar for draining liver abscesses.[46] In Amoy, Manson trained many young local Chinese as surgeons and dressers, who established their practice elsewhere. He also popularized vaccination.

In 1875, after spending nine years in China, Manson went home on leave. In London, he married Henrietta Isabella Thurburn, and at the same time, he learned eye surgery, which was important for practice in China because of the high prevalence of eye diseases, especially cataract. He was disappointed in the lack of new knowledge of tropical diseases in England. However, when he was studying in the British Museum Library, he encountered a report of a patient in India who was suffering from chyluria, similar to his patients with elephantiasis. This patient was found to have a nematode worm, *Filaria sanguinis hominis* in the chylous urine and in blood microscopically.[47] When he returned to China, he had with him a new and more powerful microscope.

Back in China he was delighted at finding microfilaria in the blood of patients with elephantiasis and that they were present invariably at night, peaking at around midnight, coinciding with the feeding time of mosquitoes when humans were sleeping.[48] He had his gardener, who was infected with filariasis, sleep inside a mosquito house that he built specifically for this purpose. At around midnight, the door was opened for 30 minutes to allow mosquitoes to go in. In the morning the mosquitoes were found with their abdomen engorged with his gardener's blood. Manson dissected and examined the mosquitoes under the microscope and found microfilariae.[49] Manson did not know much about mosquitoes but thought that the infected mosquitoes would die, and microfilariae would then go into water and humans got the disease by drinking the infected water.[50] Despite this, the discovery that disease could be transmitted through insect bites was staggering, given that it opened up a completely new spectrum of diseases with the meager resources available to him. He wrote the classic paper on his research, "Role of the Mosquito as a Nurse," and published the results in the *China Imperial Maritime Customs Medical Reports*. He relayed them to the Linnean Society, the world's oldest active society devoted to natural history, in London.[51]

This was by no means Manson's sole scientific discovery in Amoy. He was also the first one to describe paragonimiasis, a trematode (fluke) infection of human lungs due to the consumption of raw or undercooked crab or crayfish. He later identified this to be *Paragonimus westermani* and proposed that this lung fluke required an intermediate host for the completion of the life cycle.[52]

In 1883, Manson moved to Hong Kong, thus bringing to a close the most productive period of his research on filariasis and other tropical diseases. In Hong Kong, Manson established a profitable private practice in partnership with Dr. William Hartigan. Within a short time after his arrival, he carefully documented the disease, which was labeled "sprue," presenting with diarrhea and malabsorption, in Europeans in the tropics. He called the disease "a climatic disease."[53] While in Hong Kong, Manson was very much the leader of the medical community. He established the Hong Kong Medical Society which later became the British Medical Association (Hong Kong branch).

At that time, the death rate among the Europeans was high in Hong Kong mostly due to infection. To reduce infection and to improve nutrition, Manson and his friends founded Dairy Farm in Pokfulam to breed imported cattle to provide fresh milk which was then pasteurized for the community.[54] He believed a clean milk supply was only second in importance to a supply of clean water. He recruited farmers and animals from his Aberdeenshire compatriots. Hens, ducks, and geese came the same way.[55] Manson was appointed in 1886 to the Sanitary Board.[56]

In early 1887, Manson was called to Tientsin (Tianjin) to attend to Li Hongzhang, Viceroy of Zhili and Huguang. Li thought that he was dying from cancer of the tongue, but Manson found that it was only a sublingual abscess, which he drained. Li was cured and Manson was well rewarded by Li's gratitude. The trip to Tientsin took six weeks, and was tedious by pony and junk.

Manson had always been interested in educating Chinese young men in Western medicine. He and a few other doctors proposed the establishment of HKCM for Chinese after the laying of the foundation stone for Alice Memorial Hospital, on 3 June 1886. The establishment of the College, as noted, not only had the support of the Governor of Hong Kong but also Li Hongzhang, Viceroy of Zhili and Huguang, who became the Patron of the College.[57] Manson became the first Dean of the College in 1887.

As his practice flourished, Manson recruited Dr. James Cantlie, another Scot, to share his practice in 1887. When Manson retired to England two years later, Cantlie succeeded him as the second Dean of the HKCM. Manson had hoped to retire after he returned to England, as he thought he could afford to do so. He speculated on land in Hong Kong, as many people did during that period, and purchased IL47 C and D, the site where Phase Three Pacific Place is today, but the land value did not escalate as he had hoped. He sold the land in 1899, 10 years after he had left Hong Kong, without making much profit.[58] As well, the Chinese currency fell in value and his large income was reduced. He had to give up the idea of retirement.

Manson began his practice in London and became a member of the Royal College of Physicians (MRCP). In 1889, he was appointed physician to Seamen's Hospital at Dreadnought. Two years later, he was given a teaching post at Albert Dock Seamen Hospital, where he identified many tropical diseases, such as sleeping sickness, bilharzia (schistosomiasis), and malaria. He postulated mosquitoes as the vector for transmission of these diseases. In 1894, he began to work with Dr. Ronald Ross on the vector of transmission of malaria. He guided Ross, who was working in India, on every step of the research that ultimately led to the discovery of mosquitoes as the vector for transmission of the malaria parasite.[59] In 1900, Manson conducted a crucial experiment to confirm the hypothesis. He allowed infected mosquitoes to bite his own son, who was a student at Guy's Hospital. Within 15 days, his son developed malaria and the parasites were found in his blood, thus confirming his theory.[60] Manson was elected a fellow of the Royal College (FRCP) in 1895 and of the Royal Society (FRS) in 1900.

Manson was convinced of the need to have a special school to teach tropical diseases. In 1899, he founded The London School of Hygiene and Tropical Medicine and lectured there.[61] He was also the first president of The Society of Tropical Medicine and Hygiene, founded in 1907 by James Cantlie, who had also returned to London from Hong Kong.

Kristin Hussey, who studied Manson's life and work and his home at 21 Queen Anne Street, gave us a glimpse of how Manson functioned and his interaction with his family and home environment.[62] A tour of his five-storey house showed that the top floor housed the "muck room," his laboratory, where he kept all kinds of animals which harbored parasites, such as rats and guinea pigs. He also experimented on live animals including dogs, monkeys, and birds, as incubators for parasites. The patient consultation room was situated on the ground floor of his house, where he created an exotic oriental atmosphere and at times might even dress up as a Chinese mandarin. He was well known for his unique diagnostic method: the use of a blood film to detect parasites. His parlor and dining room, just a few steps from his consulting room, was a busy social place visited by his patients and dignitaries. After the founding of The London School of Tropical Medicine and Hygiene in 1899, his Queen Anne Street home became the hub of activity for the school. Even the school committee met there more frequently than in the school itself. The whole family worked for Manson, involved in all his activities. They helped to ensure his professional and social success, and there was no division between domestic and business or scientific space in the house.[63]

Manson received numerous honors for his original scientific achievements in his lifetime and was awarded a CMG in 1900 and knighted in 1903.[64] He retired from the Colonial Office Medical Advisership in 1912, and passed away in 1922.[65] HKU named a building after him, the Patrick Manson Building, which was opened on 8 March 1973, and housed the Medical Library, the Student Center, and the administrative offices of the Faculty of Medicine.[66]

Sir Patrick Manson was not only a great clinician, a competent surgeon, and a passionate teacher, but he was also a very creative and imaginative thinker. He was the first to prove that an insect can be the host for a parasite that causes human disease. His discoveries laid the foundation for tropical diseases prevention—by controlling the vectors in eradicating diseases such as malaria, schistosomiasis, and filariasis. The world owes Mansion a great deal.

James Cantlie (1851–1926)

MBChM, FRCS, KBE, KStJ

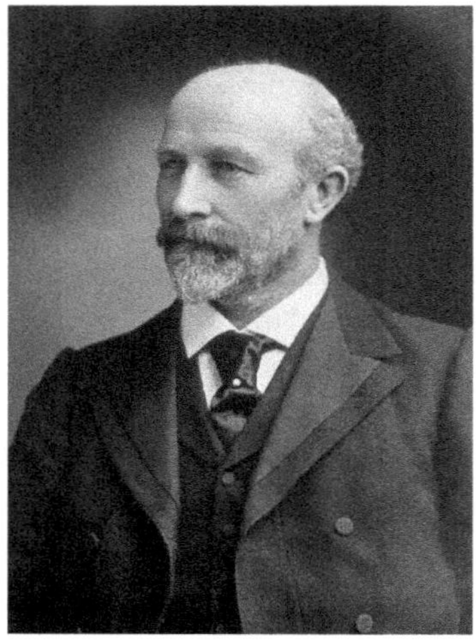

Figure 3.6 Sir James Cantlie, Dean of HKCM 1889–1896

Source: Wellcome Collection (4.0 International CC BY 4.0)

Sir James Cantlie was well known among the Chinese as the British doctor who secured the release of Dr. Sun Yat-sen who was kidnapped by Qing officials of the Chinese embassy in London. Sun was snatched from the streets of London and imprisoned in the Chinese embassy, where he would be smuggled home and executed. Cantlie's achievements in medicine, however, are no less remarkable and important.

He was born in Banffshire, Scotland, in 1851, the eldest son of a wealthy farmer, who took a great interest in those less fortunate than he was, and Cantlie resembled his father in this respect. Cantlie received his education at the University of Aberdeen and studied both arts and science. Then he went into medicine and graduated MBChM in 1873 with honorable distinction. He became a Demonstrator in Anatomy at Charing Cross Hospital and continued his surgical training in the same hospital. He became interested in first aid and joined the St. John Ambulance Association, where he became an instructor. In 1883, Cantlie volunteered for service in Egypt where he encountered a cholera epidemic, which aroused his interest in tropical diseases. Back in London, Cantlie was concerned with the poor physical condition of the urban poor and their unsanitary surroundings. His controversial paper in 1885, "Degeneracy among Londoners," in which he argued that the poor health of the Londoners was due to air pollution. While history proved that he was way ahead of his time in postulating air pollution as a cause of ill health, the wide criticism he received then made him quite unhappy, and when he received Manson's invitation to join the latter's practice in Hong Kong, he accepted.[67]

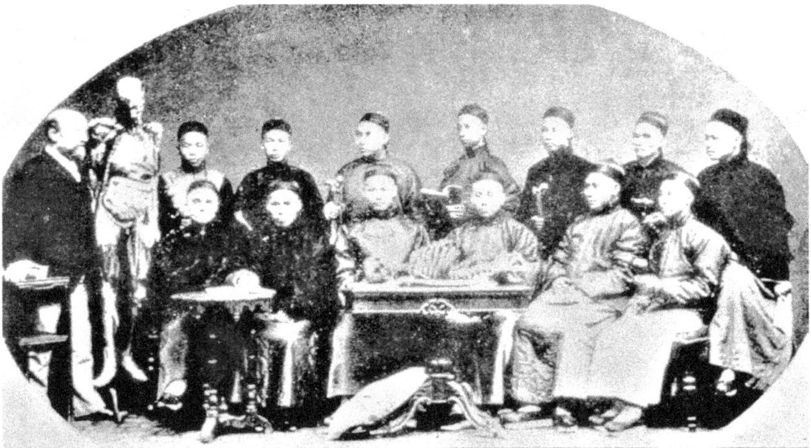

Figure 3.7 Dr. James Cantlie teaching anatomy to students of HKCM, 1893
Source: Wellcome Collection: Cantlie's work and activities in Hong Kong

Cantlie's contributions to Hong Kong from 1887 to 1896 were incredibly numerous. He and his wife both put themselves to work tirelessly to serve the people of Hong Kong until their departure. Although it is generally believed that Manson was the founder of HKCM for Chinese, in the biography of Cantlie, *The Quality of Mercy: The Lives of Sir James and Lady Cantlie*, the author, Jean Cantlie Stewart, his daughter, wrote that it was Cantlie who called the first meeting that led to the formation of the College 34 days after his arrival in Hong Kong.[68] However, she did not mention that there were already several meetings on the establishment of HKCM. It was after Cantlie's arrival that HKCM was formally founded. Cantlie contributed greatly by designing the curriculum for the HKCM according to his experience of Charing Cross Hospital and became dean after Manson's departure. Dr. Sun Yat-sen, one of the first two students who graduated from the College, was a protégé of Cantlie. In October 1896, shortly after his return to London, Cantlie received a message from Sun of the latter's kidnapping by the Qing authority. Cantlie contacted Manson, who had returned to London earlier. Together the two doctors worked hard to secure Sun's release.[69] The families of Cantlie and Sun are still in contact with each other.[70]

Cantlie established an excellent reputation as a surgeon in Hong Kong. The treatment of liver abscess, which was a common condition due to ameba or bacteria, by draining the pus was first carried out by Manson but the technique was perfected by Cantlie. Cantlie also tackled partial hepatectomy and was the first to postulate that hepatic lobulation was based on vascular supply and not on surface markings and recommended partial hepatectomy should be carried out accordingly.[71]

Cantlie contributed in numerous other ways to Hong Kong. He and his family lived on the Peak. He was in high demand, traveling to different locations to see patients and found that invariably the care patients received in their own homes was inadequate. To solve the problem, Cantlie rented a house on the Peak to accommodate his sick patients, which was not legal. In the end, Peak Hospital was built with the approval of the government.[72] Initially he asked his wife, Mabel Cantlie, to act as his nurse; this proved to be inadequate and overburdened her. In 1888, he asked Maude Ingall, a trained nurse and a relative, to come to Hong Kong. She became the first trained private nurse in the colony. Soon Governor Des Voeux caught up with the idea after he had Maude Ingall working in Government House for a while. As a result, trained nurses were brought in from England not only for private nursing for wealthy Europeans, but also for the Government Civil Hospital, greatly improving the standard of patient care in the hospital.

Cantlie was keenly interested in improving the sanitation in Hong Kong and was appointed by Governor Des Voeux to the Sanitary Board. At the time, it was difficult to pass any important ordinance in relation to public health because of vested interests of the unofficial members on the Sanitary Board and opposition from the community. Cantlie did have two proposals finally approved. The first one was to place filter beds into water supply to remove bacteria and parasites to reduce the diseases they cause; the second was to build a vaccine institute to produce vaccine for Hong Kong.[73] Vaccination, using the crust from a smallpox lesion, had been well accepted by the Chinese because it was a longstanding practice in China. The use of cowpox vaccination reduced the severity of reactions. The cowpox vaccine, however, was imported from England, and it was not uncommon for Hong Kong to run out of supply. The proposal to build a vaccine institute was approved and opened by Governor Des Voeux in 1891. In addition to producing smallpox vaccine, the vaccine institute later also manufactured antiserum for cholera, typhoid, paratyphoid, and meningococcal infection. In 1906, it was incorporated into the Bacteriological Institute.[74]

During the bubonic plague of 1894, Cantlie assisted Dr. Alexander Yersin in search of the plague bacillus.[75] In 1895, after the 1894 plague epidemic, he was one of the five commissioners appointed to inquire into the workings of the Medical Department. As a result of the commissioners' recommendations, Hong Kong appointed its first Medical Officer of Health, and the internal organization of the Medical Department improved.

A less well-publicized aspect of Cantlie's work relates to leprosy. In his report "Conditions under Which Leprosy Occurs in China, Indo-China, Malaya, the Archipelago, and Oceania" (1897), he depicted Chinese coolies as the sole agent responsible for the spread of leprosy in the Pacific region. Thus, he was responsible for much of the imperial fear of Chinese migrants. He believed that leprosy was a sexually transmitted disease and highly infectious, but he did not advocate deporting these patients. He suggested to the government to secure permission from the Chinese authority to establish a leper colony in one of the islands near the border. When he visited a European-style leprosarium in Macau, he and his wife were taken aback by the profound misery in there. They were so moved by the finding that they returned every year, bringing with them provisions and treating those that required therapy.[76]

Cantlie had never neglected first aid work which was one of his interests. In Hong Kong he joined the medical volunteers as surgeon-captain. He trained Chinese medical students of HKCM to form four bearer units (ambulance service) for St. John Ambulance.[77] He was also very much involved with the establishment of the Hong Kong Public Library.[78]

After nine years in Hong Kong, the Cantlies returned to London, where he set up his private practice. By then he had gained a reputation as an expert in tropical diseases, having published many articles on these diseases, especially for treating liver abscesses. His experience of plague in Hong Kong led to his appointment in 1896 as an adviser to the Indian government when plague broke out in Bombay (now Mumbai).[79] In London, he supported Manson in establishing The London School of Hygiene and Tropical Medicine in 1899, and became the first surgeon and lecturer in tropical surgery at the school. Cantlie founded The Society of Tropical Medicine and Hygiene with Dr. George Carmichael Low in 1907 and established the *Journal of Tropical Medicine and Hygiene* with Dr. William Simpson, who was an expert in tropical diseases and had been invited by Governor Blake to advise on management of plague in Hong Kong in 1902. Cantlie remained one of the journal's editors for 23 years.[80] In addition, he wrote many books on medicine and surgery, among them a textbook on naked eye anatomy. He also wrote about ulcer, veins, ligation of arteries, gunshot wounds for a medical dictionary, and articles on beriberi, plague, tropical surgery and diseases.[81]

His association with the St. John Ambulance Association and emergency medical aid remained, and he acted as an adviser to the War Office. During World War I, he and his wife became commandants of the British Red Cross Society to coordinate volunteer medical aid. He organized a humanitarian corps to aid those in distress because of disease or poverty. For these services, Cantlie was made a Knight of the British Empire (KBE) and Knight of Venerable Order of St. John (K.St.J) in 1918. His wife was appointed OBE for her wartime work with Voluntary Aid Detachments under the Red Cross.[82]

Sir James Cantlie died in 1926, after a severe cerebral hemorrhage.[83] A statue of Sir James, which had been cast with funds mainly from the government of the Republic of China, was exhibited at the Royal Academy of Art in London before being shipped to China to be displayed in one of the museums.[84]

Gregory Paul Jordan (1858–1921)

MB CM (Edin), MRCS (Edin.) Hon. LLD

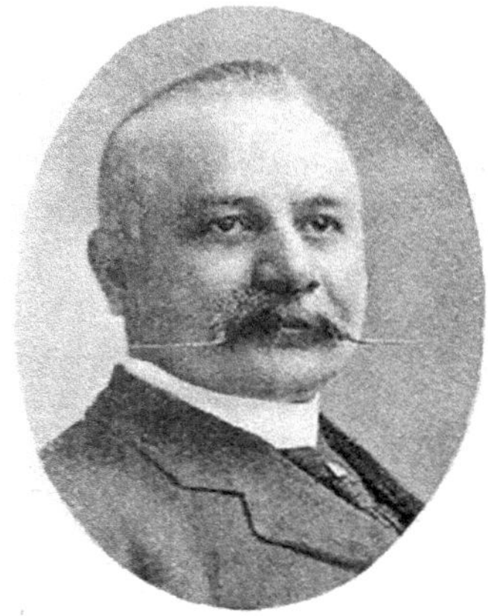

Figure 3.8 Dr. Gregory Paul Jordan
Source: Wikipedia common

Dr. Gregory Paul Jordan served as a half-time Port Health Officer in Hong Kong for 31 years and was a highly successful and much-demanded private practitioner. Nevertheless, he always involved himself in public affairs: he provided free professional service to patients in Alice Memorial Hospital and founded, with others, the HKCM, taught its students and later students of the Faculty of Medicine, HKU. He was Acting Vice-Chancellor of HKU for two years. Some people in the community referred to him as "a man overlooked," as his contribution was not widely recognized.[85] Jordan Road in Kowloon was not named after him but after Sir John Newell Jordan, envoy extraordinary and minister plenipotentiary from the United Kingdom to the Qing Empire (1906–1910).

Gregory Jordan was an Armenian born in 1858 in Calcutta (now Kolkata). The Jordan clan had moved to India from New Julfa, Armenia, a number of years prior. Gregory's father was a stocks and shares broker whose business was based in Hong Kong and Shanghai. His father traveled regularly to Calcutta, where all eight of his children were born. Gregory Jordon received his early education in Calcutta and was sent to Edinburgh University for his medical education. After obtaining his MBCM (Edin) in 1880, and MRCS in 1884, he went for further training at St. Thomas's Hospital, London, and in hospitals in Vienna and Paris. After completing his studies in 1885, he arrived in Hong Kong, where his uncle, Paul Chater (later Sir Paul Chater), a highly successful businessman, lived.[86]

Once in Hong Kong, Jordan worked very hard to secure his future. At that time, Dr. William Stanley Adams, who was the first salaried half-time Port Health Officer and Medical Inspector of Emigrants, and had a private practice partnered with Dr. James Orr Henderson, as Adams and Henderson, wanted to go on leave. He asked Gregory to stand in for him as the Port Health Officer. When Adams returned, Dr. P. B. C. Ayres, Colonial Surgeon, asked Jordan to act temporarily on his behalf, as he was going also on leave. Thus, Jordan became Acting Colonial Surgeon within one year of his arrival in Hong Kong. Jordan discharged his duties very well. In 1888, when Adams went on leave again, he again asked Jordan to deputize for him. On return this time, Adams did not resume his duty, and Jordon became the half-time Port Health Officer until 1919, close to his retirement.[87]

At that time, there were more than 4,000 ships a year arriving in Hong Kong (up to 15 a day), each containing several hundred travelers. As Port Health Officer, Jordan had to board every vessel arriving in the harbor and assess the health of the passengers as they disembarked. It was also his duty as "Medical Inspector of Emigrants to inspect intending emigrants and to supervise all matters related to the comfort and well-being of emigrants both before their departure and on their voyage." It was really a miracle that after 31 years in such service that he was spared any of the serious epidemic diseases, such as cholera and plague. This post brought lucrative business to his practice—examination of crews, treatment of passengers, issuing certificates and bills of health—all outside the duties of Port Health Officer. Jordan described the post as the foundation of his whole career, and he doggedly remained loyal to his port health job.[88]

Jordon entered into partnership with Adams in 1887 in the practice located in Pedder Street. By the beginning of 1888, Jordan was very much in charge even though the practice was listed as Adams and Jordan. His practice thrived. Many local celebrities and their families, such as Chater, his uncle, and Sir Robert Ho Tung, another successful entrepreneur and philanthropist in Hong Kong, were his patients. Jordan spoke fluent Cantonese and Mandarin and was a trusted and highly respected doctor among the local Chinese community. According to Dr. George H. Thomas, one of his students from the HKCM,

> He [Jordan] was particularly popular with the Chinese community, who almost worshiped him. His name was mentioned with awe, respect and affection. No one who was really ill could afford not to consult him, at least once. His personality was no less remarkable than his reputation. He

> was stout and of short stature, but he possessed a magnificent head and a confidence-inspiring countenance, enhanced by his striking mustache and his deep, resonant but soothing voice.[89]

When Jordan was having difficulty keeping up with his appointments, the Chinese community pulled together and purchased a car for him, so that he was able to continue attending to his patients and his port health duties.[90] By 1900, Jordan's practice had two more doctors, Drs. James Herbert Swan and Robert Gibson. They both stayed for a short period, but on their departure, two other doctors: Dr. Charles Forsyth and Dr. Friedrich Piers Grone, joined the practice. The latter two stayed longer and Forsyth remained for 25 years. By 1914, the practice had grown considerably and attended by five doctors: Jordan, Forsyth, Grone, C. E. Aubrey, and L. Woods.[91]

Jordan was one of the doctors who offered his free professional service to Alice Memorial Hospital when it first opened, before the arrival of a medical missionary. He was also one of the founders of HKCM and taught tropical medicine. When Governor Sir Frederick Lugard planned to establish HKU, Jordan was one of the few who were involved in the negotiation of incorporating HKCM into the University as the Faculty of Medicine. In 1913, Jordan was nominated Pro-Vice-Chancellor of the University, a position he held until 1921.

From the beginning, the University had been short of funds; it was underfunded and under-endowed. At the end of the 1910s, it faced a major financial crisis. Charles Eliot, the first Vice-Chancellor, had been seconded by the Foreign Office to become a diplomat in 1918, and the University came under the administration of Jordan as Acting Vice-Chancellor for two years. Jordan had no experience with the financial management of the University. The University's finances were so grossly mishandled that the University Court was unable to accept the university accounts of 1919–1920. The Governor appointed a Commission of Inquiry under the chair of E. H. Sharp, a barrister. As a result, the government injected HK$1 million to cover the University's bank overdrafts. In addition, a finance committee under the University Ordinance was established to ensure that future university expenditures could not be undertaken without the sanction of the committee.[92]

In January 1921, Jordan retired from HKU as Pro Vice-Chancellor. His successor, Sir William Brunyate, presented Jordan with an honorary doctorate of laws in recognition of his service. After the ceremony, students carried him from the Great Hall to his car and towed the car from Pokfulam into town. The students were enormously fond and respectful of him because he collected HK$20,000 from his friends to furnish the Student Union Building.[93]

In addition to his participation in public affairs, Jordan was a Freemason, which also helped him to establish himself very quickly in Hong Kong. He was initiated into the Freemason movement early when he was in Edinburgh. In Hong Kong, he became a member of Perseverance Lodge, where his brother was the master and his uncle and Colonial Surgeon Dr. Ayres were its past masters. By 1904, Jordan became District Lodge Grand Master.[94]

Dr. Gregory Paul Jordan left for England shortly after his retirement in 1921. Unfortunately, he did not have much time to enjoy his retirement, as he passed away from a heart attack on 4 December 1921.[95] The library that he had hoped to create at HKU for the Student Union was completed with the help of his uncle. Jordan Memorial Library was opened by his wife, Mrs. Marion Jordan, on 16 September 1922.

John Christopher Thomson (1863–?)

MBCM (Edin) and MD (Edin)

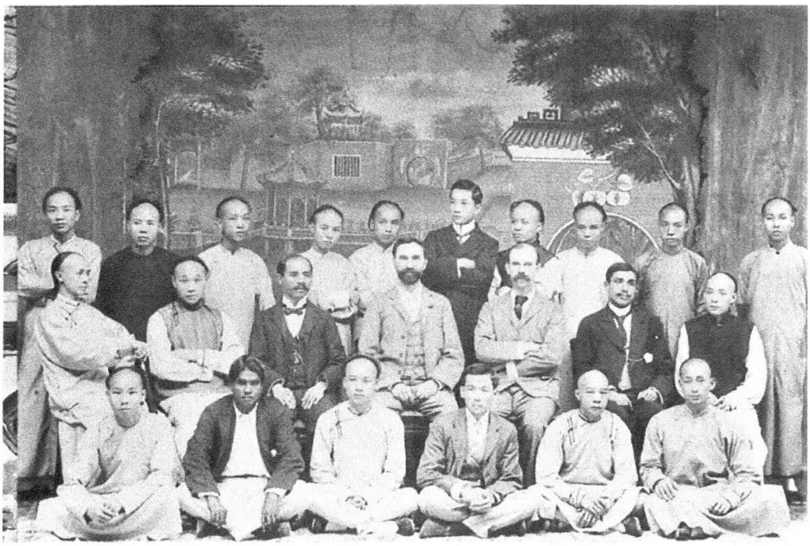

Figure 3.9 Dr. John Christopher Thomson (middle row, center), with Dr. R. M. Gibson (R3) on his left with students of HKCM, c. 1903
Image courtesy of HKMMS, photo donated by Alice Ho Miu Ling Nethersole Charity Foundation

Dr. John Christopher Thomson was a missionary doctor sent by the LMS to Alice Memorial Hospital to be its first Medical Superintendent. Later he left missionary service and joined the Government Medical Department as a medical officer. Few people in Hong Kong have heard of his name, but his contributions to HKCM and Tung Wa Hospital had been invaluable. Although he was not a founder of HKCM, it was through his effort that the College was able to keep going until it was incorporated into HKU in 1911.

Thomson was born in 1863 in Lockerbie, Scotland. He graduated from the University of Edinburgh MBCM (Edin) in 1888 and was awarded an MD (Edin) in 1892. He was the medical missionary sent by the LMS as the first Medical Superintendent of Alice Memorial Hospital, which was founded in 1887 as a charity hospital. According to the constitution of Alice Memorial Hospital, the LMS would send out a missionary doctor to manage the hospital, but all local doctors were welcome to practice in it.[96] It was only in 1888 that the LMS appointed Thomson. Before Thomson's arrival in 1889, the local doctors had formed a medical committee with Dr. Gregory Jordan as secretary. The hospital was managed as any hospital in England. The medical staff was unhappy with the appointment of a medical missionary, newly graduated from a medical school, as superintendent of the hospital. However, Thomson was not someone who could be intimidated by a group of powerful local medical practitioners. He had a mission to accomplish for the LMS. With great tact and tenacity, he gradually took over control of the hospital, and when Dr. Patrick Manson left Hong Kong, Thomson took over Manson's duties.[97] He learned the local language, organized Nethersole Dispensary, and began evangelical work in the hospital.[98] By taking over control of the hospital, Thomson ensured its long-term survival, which would require the support of a well-funded society for its continuity rather than being dependent on a group of loosely organized local doctors.

As Superintendent of Alice Memorial Hospital, Thomson was on the teaching staff of HKCM.[99] He immediately threw himself to work. First, he taught pathology, then he lectured on *materia medica* and therapeutics over a period of more than eight years. He was a missionary at heart and was keenly interested in students. He introduced a series of evangelistic activities in the hospital to include the medical students. In 1891, he succeeded Ho Kai as Secretary of the College and held that position until his retirement in 1909. Later he also took over the role of Director of Studies, holding both positions. The inability of the graduates to practice in Hong Kong and the difficulty to secure endowment and funds for building its own campus left many disheartened. The government had over the years failed to give an operating grant to HKCM. According to Francis Clark, the College's continuing operation was due to Thomson's energy, indomitable perseverance, and willingness to serve.[100] Both Thomson and Clark were highly supportive of their students and believed that they were well trained and should be qualified for work in Hong Kong.[101] Later, in his capacity as Inspecting Medical Officer of Tung Wa Hospital, Thomson brought in students or graduates of the College to help Dr. Chung King-ue alias Chung Boon-chor, a Chinese doctor trained in Western medicine, appointed by the government as the resident surgeon to introduce Western medicine into Tung Wa.[102] To his students, Thomson had been a father, always guiding and encouraging. To the graduates, he had been their friend and someone they would seek help from. Thomson continued

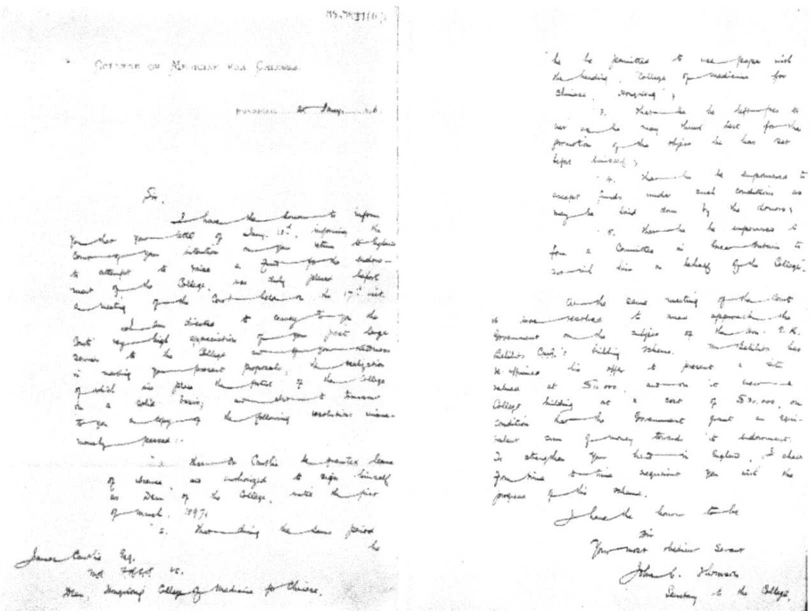

Figure 3.10a and b Letter from Dr. Thomson to Dr. Cantlie on 20 January 1896 of his appreciation of the latter's intention to raise funds for the HKCM for Chinese

Source: Wellcome Collection

to serve the College until his departure in 1909.[103]

In 1897, Thomson resigned from his position as Superintendent of Alice Memorial Hospital, as he was unsure of its future. He briefly attempted private practice,[104] but the bubonic plague epidemic in Hong Kong resulted in anti-foreigner sentiments and his practice did not flourish. When a new position came up in the Government Medical Department offering an annual salary of HK$3,600 with HK$700 in lieu of quarters and HK$216 for conveyance,[105] he applied for the job.[106] His duties at the Medical Department varied over the years but his main role was as Inspecting Medical Officer of Tung Wa Hospital, and Medical Officer of Kennedy Town Infectious Disease Hospital, Gaol, and the KCR. During the 1902 bubonic plague outbreak, when he was in Kennedy Town Infectious Disease Hospital, he made two relevant observations. The ingestion of carbolic acid for treatment of plague was not useful, and plague bacilli in the blood were found in 11% of plague patients, and these were severe cases.[107]

After the 1894 bubonic plague, a commission was appointed in 1896 to inquire into the workings of the Tung Wa Hospital, where only TCM was practiced. Many weaknesses were discovered, especially in the sanitation of the hospital and in treatments received by patients, which were considered unscientific, useless, or even dangerous by doctors of Western medicine.[108] There had been no improvement in the high mortality of its inpatients, which had remained at around 50% since its founding in 1872. The Hospital Board of Tung Wa Hospital had no medical doctor, only wealthy Chinese elite. The Board had engaged in many charitable works and also in many political activities in Hong Kong and in China. It acted as the mouthpiece for the Chinese community locally and was in contact with Chinese officials of the Qing government.[109] The commissioners recommended that the hospital should discontinue its political activities and focus on its medical work, which included improving sanitation and introducing Western medicine. To ensure these changes took place, the government appointed Thomson to supervise sanitary reforms and Dr. Chung King-ue, the resident surgeon, to introduce Western medicine. Patients admitted to the hospital were to be given the choice of either TCM or Western medicine.[110]

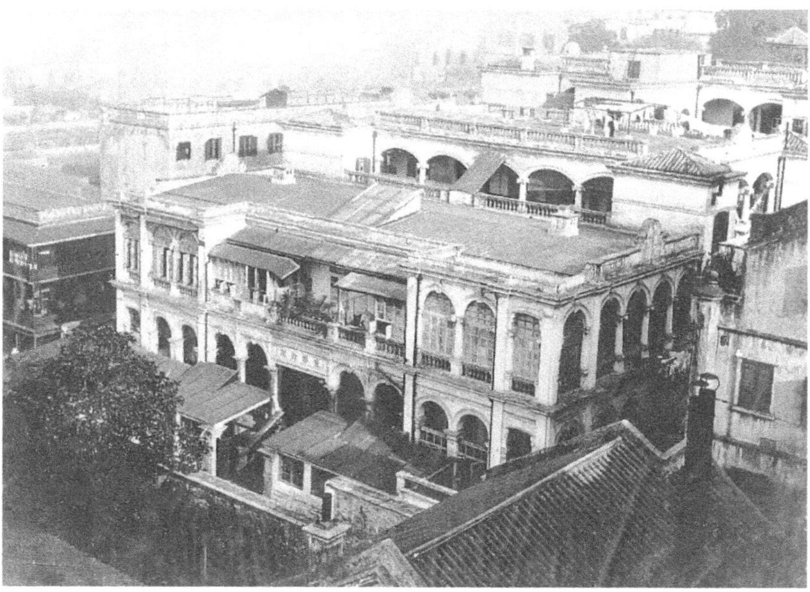

Figure 3.11 Tung Wah Hospital in 1902
Image courtesy of Tung Wah Hospital Archives

The introduction of Western medicine to Tung Wa Hospital was an important milestone in the development of the hospital. As a result of the inquiry, Tung Wa Hospital had no option but to discontinue its political pursuits and expand in its medical activities. Kwong Wah Hospital, Tung Wah Eastern Hospital, and a number of clinics were established in the ensuing period. This Tung Wah Group of Hospitals continues to play a major role in providing patient care to the Hong Kong medical system. It is of interest to see how Thomson effectively implemented the changes without arousing the antagonism of the local Chinese elite.

A major issue was the failure of recognition and isolation of infectious cases, leading to the spread of the disease in the hospital and the community, as in the plague epidemic. Thomson established a receiving ward, where all new cases were admitted, and an isolation ward, where all infectious cases were sent. In the receiving ward, patients were examined by Chung and reviewed by Thomson to ensure that the correct diagnoses had been made and appropriate treatment had been given to the patients. Cases of bubonic plague and smallpox were sent to Kennedy Town Infectious Diseases Hospital as soon as possible.

Thomson separated patients with various special diseases, such as malarial fevers, diarrhea and dysentery, beriberi, and general medical cases, to be accommodated in different wards. This lessened the degree of cross-infection and rendered management of patients easier. The wards with small rooms that could only accommodate two people were used for women and children or for isolation purposes. Two new wards were built on the compound for surgical patients.

He also discussed with Chung the causes of deaths of those who died on the wards and those brought in already dead in the mortuary. Friends or relatives who brought the body in were interviewed by Chung, who tried to determine the cause of death from the deceased's symptoms. When foul play was suspected or an obscure case of public health importance was found, coroner orders for a postmortem examination would be sought.[111] This was the first time that Tung Wa Hospital had the cause of death of each patient determined and recorded.

The ventilation in the hospital was improved. Thomson had holes cut in partitions whenever possible, to improve circulation of air. To prevent overcrowding, the maximum number of patients allowed in each ward was determined by the size of the ward. Other sanitary measures included removal of commodes from the wards as soon as possible. All clothing of patients was changed twice a week and all bedding once a week. All soiled clothing had to be removed immediately, and all soiled old quilts were burned and replaced. Jeyes Fluid, a disinfectant, was used to clean the wards and the bathrooms frequently. He carried out inspections of the hospital twice a week to make sure that it was clean and sanitary. Clean quarters were provided for Dr. Chung and the hospital staff.[112]

The hospital was to keep good records of the number of admissions, discharges, and deaths daily, as well as the number of bodies brought in dead with diagnoses.[113] The mortality of inpatients of Tung Wa Hospital, which had been around 50%, decreased to about 35% to 40% for those who received treatment with TCM. For those who received treatment with Western medicine, the mortality was 15% to 20%.[114] After a while, the Chinese patients knew what treatment to ask for when they were admitted to Tung Wa Hospital. Over the years, Thomson brought in students from HKCM, such as Tang King-fai, Leung Chik-fan,[115] and Ho Ko-tsun[116] to help Dr. Chung, as the inpatients of Tung Wa Hospital increasingly opted for treatment with Western medicine.

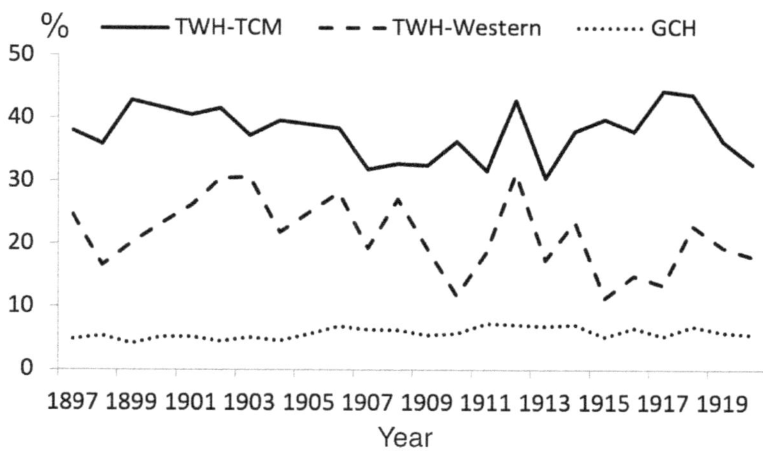

Figure 3.12 Inpatient mortality of Tung Wa Hospital by TCM and by Western treatment

Source: Moira Chan-Yeung, *A Medical History of Hong Kong*, 1842–1941, 77.

Thomson was a conscientious and firm individual, and at the same time, courteous and sympathetic. As a result, he received full cooperation from the Hospital Board, which always came up with funds for changes needed in the hospital. The introduction of Western medicine proceeded smoothly and, in 1908, the director of Tung Wa Hospital even permitted teaching Western clinical medicine in the hospital—this was a major shift in the attitude of the Hospital Board and a success that could largely be attributed to Thomson's efforts.

Thomson had another major contribution. Malaria was an endemic disease in Hong Kong. In the late 1880s and early 1890s, the incidence of malaria in the civilian population was around 400 / 100,000, with a 50% death rate.[117] During a period of leave in England, Thomson learned about malaria and mosquitoes. On his return to Hong Kong in 1900, he carried out a systematic study on mosquitoes. With cooperation of the police force to collect 12 mosquitoes each week for one year from each of the 36 police stations in Hong Kong, Kowloon, and the New Territories, Thomson received 31,350 mosquitoes during the year. He found that on average, 96.3% of the mosquitoes belonged to the *Culex* species and 3.7% to the *Anopheles* species. He was the first to identify in Hong Kong three species of *anopheles* mosquitoes which carry the malarial parasite: *Anopheles sinensis*, *Anopheles maculates,* and *Anopheles fatigans*.[118] His work gave support to the new malaria-mosquito theory and received acclaim in London. The Secretary of the State of Colonies also expressed appreciation for his work.[119]

For some reason, Thomson did not continue with malarial research. In 1909, he retired from government service because of debilitating sprue and left Hong Kong.[120] His service, which was carried out with courtesy and consideration, was quite different from some British colonists of the time, and was highly appreciated by the Chinese community. In the farewell ceremony, the Hospital Board of Tung Wa Hospital presented him a silver tea set to express their appreciation.[121]

Dr. John Christopher Thomson was another physician whose enormous contributions to the development of medicine in Hong Kong had not been recognized or appreciated appropriately. This is a belated celebration of his life in gratitude of his highly effective administration, his dedication to his students and to his work, and his humanity shown to the people of Hong Kong.

Ho Ko-tsun 何高俊 (1878–1953)

OBE, LMSH

Dr. Ho Ko-tsun was born in 1878 into a Christian family. His grandfather, Ho Fuk-tong, was the first Chinese to be ordained by the LMS in Hong Kong. His uncle, Dr. Ho Kai, a doctor and lawyer, donated funds for building Alice Memorial Hospital and was one of the founders of HKCM for Chinese. Ho Ko-tsun studied at Queen's College before entering HKCM in 1896. He received the Belilios Scholarship for his study and graduated in 1902.[122] Even as a senior student, he was a public vaccinator (1901) and an assistant to the resident surgeon of Tung Wa Hospital (1902).[123]

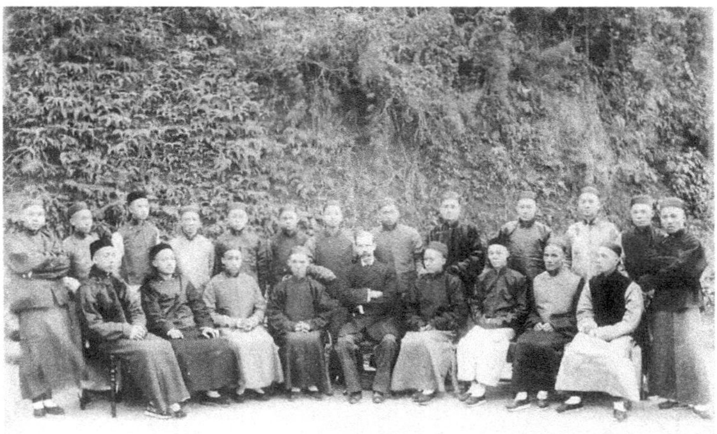

Figure 3.13 Dr. Ho Ko-tsun (standing, L2) and other students of HKCM, 1897

Image courtesy of HKMMS, donated by the Alice Ho Miu Ling Nethersole Charity Foundation

When he graduated from the College, job opportunities were limited, as the College license was not recognized by the Medical Registration Ordinance in Hong Kong. Early in 1902, the new government bacteriologist, Dr. William Hunter, arrived in the colony and was in need of assistants to help with dissection of dead rats to ascertain if they were infected by plague. Ho and two other graduates of the College were employed as assistants to the bacteriologist. Their competency on the job was commended by Hunter in his report.[124] After leaving the public mortuary in 1903, Ho joined Nethersole Hospital as a house surgeon. At that time, Dr. Robert M. Gibson was the Medical Superintendent; a year later, Dr. Alice Sibree joined the staff to take charge of the new Alice Memorial Maternity Hospital. Sibree was the first women doctor who introduced Western midwifery to Hong Kong. Ho would collaborate with her later in developing maternity service for local residents in Wanchai. The year 1904 marked the beginning of Ho's decade-long association with HKCM as a tutor in anatomy and surgery.[125] In 1907, he left Nethersole Hospital to be in charge of the Eastern District Chinese Public Dispensary at Wanchai. In the following year, he started a private practice in Central[126] but he continued to tutor HKCM students.

Between 1907 and 1911, Ho was busy with several extracurricular projects. His interest in sports led him to start Tai Yuk Primary School in Hollywood Road in 1908. The premises served as a primary school during the day and offered classes for sports training in the evening. He was the honorary principal of the primary school and the elected president of the sports training organization. At the school, he also taught hygiene and first aid. His lecture handouts for students were published later as a book entitled *Basic Red Cross First Aid*. Dr. Wan Man-kai and the inspector of schools, Mr. Edward Alexander Irving, indicated in the preface of the book how lay people would benefit from such work.[127] The school was closed during Japanese Occupation.[128] In 1910, Ho became a founding member of the Hong Kong Chinese Swimming Association.

Being patriotic, Ho joined a group of Guangdong doctors to support the revolutionary efforts of Dr. Sun Yat-sen.[129] After the revolution, not surprisingly Ho was invited by the Guangzhou government to join the Ministry of Health as Vice-Minister to Dr. Li Shu-fan, who was at the helm (Chapter 5). As public health was something new to China, they had to set up the whole system from scratch. For example, Ho had to promulgate rules and regulations for licensing of hospitals and healthcare workers.[130] Prevention of infectious diseases, plague in particular, was also an important responsibility.[131] Ho advocated teaching medicine in Chinese and submitted a proposal to the government to send young scholars overseas to learn medicine and to return to the country as physicians and translators, bringing with them Western science.[132] In 1913, General Long Jiguang, an army leader of Yuan Shikai's faction took over the Canton (Guangzhou) government. Many officials, including Ho, were arrested and put in jail.[133] This effectively ended Ho's political career in new China.

When Ho returned to Hong Kong in 1916, he headed the Eastern District CPD again until his retirement in 1949. The CPD had its origin from the plague epidemic in 1894 when "dumping" dead bodies to avoid compulsory disinfection of the affected household had become prevalent. Two Chinese members of the Sanitary Board, Mr. Fung Wa-chun and Mr. Lau Chu-pak, came up with the idea of setting up district offices to deal with the problem. Thus, in 1905 the first two CPDs were established in the Western District and Eastern District (Wanchai), staffed by the licentiates of HKCM. Their duties were to dissuade people from dumping dead bodies, to determine the cause of death of these bodies, and to provide care for plague patients. CPDs were controlled by a central CPD committee. Eventually the roles of the CPDs expanded to include general medical care based on Western medicine, and vaccination.[134] As CPDs were welcomed by the community, more CPDs were established in other parts of Hong Kong Island and Kowloon. By the 1930s, there were nine CPDs serving the urban population. After World War II, all CPDs were taken over by the government to become government outpatient clinics.[135]

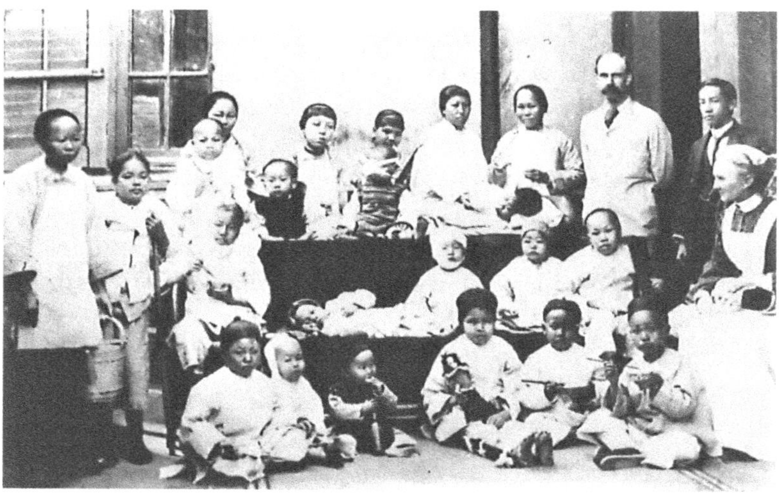

Figure 3.14 Dr. Ho Ko-tsun (back row first on the right) when working as Resident at Nethersole Hospital; Dr. R. M. Gibson, Medical Superintendent, standing next to him.

Image courtesy of HKMMS, donated by the Alice Ho Miu Ling Nethersole Charity Foundation

When Ho first joined the Wanchai CPD in 1907, it was located in a small ground floor shop on Queens Road East. Ho encouraged the local residents to raise funds for a larger CPD. In 1911, a building was constructed at Stone Nullah Lane to accommodate the CPD and a plague hospital. By 1919, when there were hardly any plague cases, the plague hospital was converted into a maternity unit,[136] and Dr. Alice Sibree was invited to supervise the midwifery work. It was such a great success that the CPD committee, which controlled all CPDs in Hong Kong, decided to build a bigger maternity unit in Western District, which became Tsan Yuk Hospital (Chapter 6). As the number of deliveries at the Wanchai maternity unit increased with time, a new maternity floor was added in 1931 from subscriptions of the Chinese community.[137] Ho was also associated with the development of the CPD in Kowloon City.[138] In 1949 he was awarded an OBE for his long service for the poor in Wanchai, especially during Japanese Occupation when, owing to shortage of funds, he undertook the work of the maternity hospital in addition to his other duties. He continued his service throughout the occupation, shouldering much of the financial burden himself.[139]

Ho also played a leading role in the local medical community. In 1920, Dr. Kwan King-leung organized a dinner gathering to discuss the formation of a local Chinese medical association. It was unanimously agreed that the Hong Kong Chinese Medical Association be formed. The first president and vice-president were Dr. Wan Man-kai and Dr. Kwan King-leung respectively; Ho became the vice-president in 1923. One of the agenda of the newly formed association was the establishment of a Chinese private hospital to counteract racial discrimination in some existing local hospitals.[140] A limited company was formed and a property acquired in Happy Valley. In 1922, Yeung Wo Nursing Home came into being with Ho as the elected chairman of the board of directors.[141] The nursing home later became Hong Kong Sanatorium and Hospital under the management of Dr. Li Shu-fan.

Dr. Ho Ko-tsun retired in September 1949, after more than three decades of service at the Wanchai CPD. When the dispensary was taken over by the government, Ho was still living at the staff quarters on the second floor. The Secretary for Chinese Affairs did not want to evict him, for he had done so much for the local residents, who also petitioned for him to stay.[142] After retirement, Ho worked for one year at Red Swastika Society Free Clinic at Dragon Terrace, until failing health prevented him to continue. He died in June 1953, aged 75.

His funeral was attended by prominent doctors such as the Hon. Dr. Yeo Kok-cheang, Director of Medical and Health Services, and many local residents. True to his benevolent spirit, in lieu of floral tributes, money was collected for the building of Hay Ling Chau Leprosarium. He was cremated, and his ashes were scattered into the sea—unusual for a Chinese person in that era. Dr. Ho Chung-chung, his eldest daughter and Principal of True Light School, said during the ceremony: "… father placed great emphasis on spiritual and moral values and did not care for material things. All his life was a devoted service to others. He gave more than he took and was absolutely frank and straightforward with a great courage to stand the truth … he was outwardly stern and serious but was warm inwardly, compassionate and full of deep sentiment."[143]

Dr. Ho Ko-tsun is an exemplar of a dedicated *kaifong* (neighborhood) doctor, an altruistic individual who served the local population with great devotion and love.

4. The Early University Medical Educators
Laying the Foundation of the Faculty of Medicine, The University of Hong Kong

When HKU was founded in 1911, it incorporated HKCM into its Faculty of Medicine. One of the first tasks of the Faculty was to ensure that the degree granted would be of sufficiently high standard to meet the General Medical Council's requirement for registration in Britain. The curriculum for the medical degree of HKU was designed accordingly and, as a result, the General Medical Council accorded it full recognition. The Hong Kong government then enacted Medical Registration Amendment Ordinance (No. 31 of 1914), which entitled registration to medical graduates of the University.[1]

Dr. Francis Clark, who was Dean of the College of Medicine, became the first Dean of the Faculty of Medicine, HKU. Thirteen practitioners who taught at the College of Medicine continued to teach in the new faculty.[2] The University intended to gradually replace them with full-time staff. When funds became available, the first full-time medical faculty appointments were Dr. G. E. Malcomson as Professor of Physiology and Biology in 1913, and Dr. Kenelm H. Digby as Professor of Anatomy in 1914. Digby would go on to become Professor of Surgery. When Malcomson left for war duties, he was replaced by Dr. Herbert Gastineau Earle. The next full-time appointment was Dr. Wang Chung-yik, a graduate of the College of Medicine with further training in Edinburgh and London, as Professor of Pathology in 1920, the first Chinese to be appointed professor at HKU.

The Faculty of Medicine had a home in the University even though clinical teaching continued to be carried out at Alice Memorial and Affiliated Hospitals (Nethersole Hospital, Alice Memorial Maternity Hospital, and Ho Miu Ling Hospital). In 1914, Clark proposed that clinical teaching should move from Alice Memorial and Affiliated Hospitals to Government Civil Hospital, which offered more up-to-date facilities.[3] There were no clinical departments yet; medicine, surgery, and obstetrics and gynecology were taught by a few private practitioners.[4]

The University was poorly endowed and was dependent on a less than generous grant from the government and from donations from the public. During the first few years, it was committed to constructing several buildings, including the School of Anatomy and the School of Pathology and Tropical Medicine. In 1918, Charles Eliot, the first Vice-Chancellor, was appointed by the Foreign Office as a diplomat, and the university came under the administration of Dr. Gregory Jordan, Pro-Vice-Chancellor, who became Acting Vice-Chancellor, and Claude Severn, who was Officer Administering for the Government, Pro-Chancellor. Neither of them had experience with finance management. As noted in Chapter 3, the university's finances had been so grossly mishandled that the University Court was unable to accept the university accounts of the year 1919–1920.[5] The Sharp Commission, which was appointed to inquire into the matter, recommended the establishment of a finance committee responsible for approving university expenditure. It also recommended the early establishment of three full-time clinical professorships, one each in medicine, surgery, and obstetrics and gynecology; and that each professor should head his department and control wards, clinical laboratories, and outpatient work. These measures would secure the General Medical Council's continued recognition of the university's medical degree for registration.[6] But the university had no means of doing so until The Rockefeller Foundation came to its aid in 1923.

After establishing Peking Union Medical College in the late 1910s, the China Medical Board of The Rockefeller Foundation found that the project was so expensive that it was not able to establish another medical school in China as it had hoped. When Dr. Richard Pearce, director of the Foundation's Division of Medical Education, visited Hong Kong in 1921, he was impressed with what he saw and felt that it could support an existing institution. In 1922, the Foundation announced a conditional endowment of HK$750,000 for three proposed chairs: in medicine, surgery, and obstetrics and gynecology, which required the university to: 1) build a hostel for medical students and improve the hospital's laboratories; 2) develop a medical library; 3) ensure better coordination between the Faculty of Medicine and the government; 4) obtain the same annual subvention of HK$50,000 from the government; and 5) ensure to have an assistant and a junior officer, paid for out of university funds for each of the new clinical professors.[7] In 1922, the Rockefeller Foundation endowed HK$500,000 for the chairs of medicine and surgery, and in

1923 another HK$250,000 for the chair of obstetrics and gynecology. The Foundation included research funding and established a number of traveling fellowships to allow young doctors to further their education outside Hong Kong.[8] Without funding from the Rockefeller Foundation, the clinical departments in the Medical Faculty, HKU, would have failed to develop, and it might have been difficult for the General Medical Council to continue to recognize the degree offered at the university.

During these early years of the university, there were several individuals who had played crucial roles in developing the Faculty of Medicine at HKU. These included Herbert Gastineau Earle, Wang Chung-yik, and the Rockefeller professors, John Anderson, Kenelm Hutchinson Digby, and Richard Edward Tottenham. They were pioneers, devoted to medical education and to disseminating their medical knowledge to Hong Kong and China. In addition to launching the clinical departments, they attended conferences in China and other parts of the world to share their knowledge and research findings with colleagues elsewhere. They initiated the tradition of research and laid the foundation of the Faculty of Medicine of today.

Kenelm Hutchinson Digby (1884–1954)

OBE, MBBS, FRCS

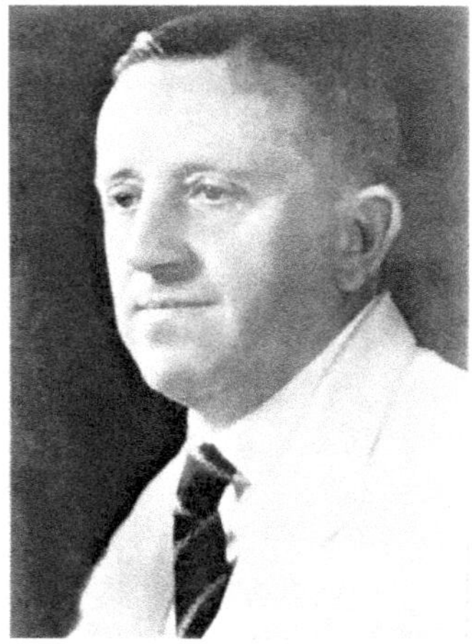

Figure 4.1 Professor Kenelm Hutchinson Digby

Source: "Kenelm Hutchinson Digby," *Elixir*, May 1954: 67.

Professor Kenelm Hutchinson Digby was the longest-serving teacher of the Faculty of Medicine of HKU before World War II. He laid the foundation of the discipline of surgery in the university and, through his students, exerted a great influence on surgical practice in Hong Kong. Digby was born in London in 1884 and obtained his medical degree from University of London in 1907. He was a brilliant student, having won several prizes, including one for anatomy. After graduation, he joined the famous Guy's Hospital as surgical registrar and anesthetist. In 1910, he became an FRCS of England. Before his HKU appointment, he was Principal Officer of Great Central Railway.[9]

Digby became Professor of Anatomy in the infant Faculty of Medicine, HKU, in 1913. His relevant experience included working as Assistant Demonstrator of Anatomy and Instructor of Surgical Anatomy at Guy's Hospital and conducting research in comparative anatomy of the tonsils, Peyer's patch, and appendix.[10] At the time, a chair in clinical surgery had been created in HKU in 1915 with donations from Sir Robert Ho Tung. When the initial holder of the chair, Dr. M. Lobb, resigned, Digby was appointed to the post and headed the two departments, anatomy and surgery, for almost a decade.

In 1915, when the founding Dean, Dr. Francis Clark, left Hong Kong, Digby, then only 31, became the youngest dean in history of the faculty. For the next decade, the deanship alternated between him and Professor Herbert G. Earle of the Physiology Department.[11] During his deanship, the university was in financial difficulty, and more funding was needed for further development. In 1920, Digby wrote to the Rockefeller Foundation in New York for support, with the University Council's approval, at an opportune time when the Foundation had set up the China Medical

Board. As discussed, after some negotiations, the Foundation agreed to fund two full-time professors, one in medicine and one in surgery, in 1922, to be followed by the third one, a chair in obstetrics and gynecology the following year.[12] In 1923, Digby relinquished his post in the Anatomy Department and became full-time Professor of Surgery. He led the department for another two decades until he retired after World War II.

When Digby came to Hong Kong in 1913, he brought with him the tradition of British academic institutions such as Guy's Hospital, which was founded in 1721. He supported with enthusiasm the formation of the HKU Medical Society in January 1914 and its official publication, *Caduceus*, in 1922.[13] All students and staff of the Faculty of Medicine were members of the Society and medical practitioners at invitation. Academic meetings were held by the Society, and students were encouraged to present and discuss scientific papers. In his Presidential Address at the annual meeting of the Society, Digby expressed his philosophy about medical education: students should not be just like gramophones reciting what they had learned from their books and their teachers; the Society should promote original thought and serious debate among its members.[14] He solicited a local donor, Mr. Ho Kwong, to create a prize (Ho Kwong Prize) to be awarded to the best student paper presentation.[15] He pleaded in 1924 with the Faculty of Medicine to take advantage of the Rockefeller professorship to engage in more original scientific research.[16] He believed that research was essential to raise the standard of the university and to increase China's contributions to scientific knowledge. He advised students that the best way to learn about research was to hold a house appointment for one year. Internship was not necessary for registration to practice then, but a year for young doctors to learn about research and to gain some clinical experience. Digby also believed that the university should also offer postgraduate research scholarships for young researchers.

Digby, indeed, walked his talk. His research career began before he came to Hong Kong. He published in 1919 the results of his research studies of the immune function of tonsils and subepithelial lymphatic tissues in the gut, which he carried out in 1913, in a book entitled *Immunity in Health: The Function of the Tonsils and Other Subepithelial Lymphatic Glands in the Bodily Economy*. The book was reviewed by the *British Medical Journal*, and its new insights in the immune function of the tonsil and the lymphatic tissues in the gut were noted.[17] At the time, there was a tendency to take out the enlarged tonsils in children, but Digby did not think such an approach was necessary.[18] He was ahead of his time, as subsequent studies proved that intact tonsils and subepithelial lymphatics were important for children's immunity.

Digby contributed many publications in British academic journals as well as in *Caduceus*. He discovered that some conditions were peculiar to Hong Kong and reported them in the journal. For example, he noted that bile duct stones originating in the liver were common among Chinese in Hong Kong, a condition later referred to as recurrent pyogenic cholangitis and these patients could present as acute abdomen.[19] He observed the unusually high prevalence of nasopharyngeal carcinoma locally[20] and reported a large case series in the *British Journal of Surgery* in 1941.[21] Although his initial attempt to treat the cancer by radium was not successful, he paved the way for radiotherapy after the war. He also suggested, based on cadaver experiment, to treat early pulmonary tuberculosis by intercostal nerve block to collapse the upper lung.[22] As orthopedic surgery was not a separate discipline then, Digby contributed in many aspects to this branch of surgery. For example, he examined the use of ivory as an intramedullary rod in rabbit tibia. It was remarkable that he collaborated with colleagues in physics, mathematics, and engineering to determine the physical and mechanical properties of ivory tubes and compared them to human bones.[23] A new "department" of orthopedics was created under his chief assistant, Dr. Phoon Sek-wah to teach this new branch of surgery.[24] Digby, no doubt, was a pioneer in orthopedic surgery in Hong Kong.[25] After more than two decades of dedicated service, Digby was honored with the King's Coronation Medal in 1937[26] and an OBE in 1939.[27]

When Digby started teaching at HKU in 1913, he had the use of the new School of Anatomy for research and lectures at the west gate of the main campus. In 1915, when he was Ho Tung Chair in Surgery and Professor of Anatomy, he continued to use the School of Anatomy while clinical teaching took place at Government Civil Hospital. In 1923, when he was appointed to the new Rockefeller Chair of Surgery, he had to share the School of Anatomy with the new Professor of Anatomy. He actively raised funds and lobbied the university to have a new building for his department. His efforts bore fruit, and in 1935 a separate School of Surgery was inaugurated next to the School of Anatomy in the main campus. In this new two-storey building were a lecture theatre, laboratories, and a surgical specimen museum. It was hoped that Digby would use the facility to start postgraduate teaching to produce more specialists.[28] When the Department of Surgery was moved to Queen Mary Hospital, the School of Surgery continued to be used. The old building in the main campus was renamed Digby School of Surgery in 1956 to honor him. It was eventually demolished in 1977 to make way for a new university building.[29]

When the Japanese launched the attack at Hong Kong on 8 December 1941, Queen Mary Hospital was turned into a casualty clearing hospital where Digby operated on many wounded soldiers and civilians. When Hong Kong surrendered on Christmas Day, the Japanese Army took over the hospital because it was new and well equipped. The patients in the hospital were hurriedly cleared out by the Japanese despite strong protests by Dr. Selwyn-Clarke, Director of Medical Services of the Hong Kong government. When Digby was asked if he were willing, like many other doctors, to stay outside of camp and work for the health of the community, he was indignant and made an impassioned speech of protest. He would not "co-operate with such vandals as the Japs, such barbarians, such—people, in short, who were capable of evacuating a hospital in such a heartless manner."[30]

In early January 1942, he was sent to the internment camp for civilians in Stanley. Digby and a team of interned doctors established Tweed Bay Hospital inside the camp and provided medical care to the internees with what little resources they had. His tireless work and ingenuity were highly praised by the internees. One internee had a fall and sustained fracture to the femur and vertebra. Digby fashioned a splint using a broom handle and a traction device using an iron. For spine injury, he removed the ceiling fan to create a brace with wood support. The injuries eventually healed satisfactorily.[31] Apart from hospital work, Digby as acting Dean conducted meetings with other Faculty of Medicine internees, to plan for the reorganization of the Faculty of Medicine after the war.[32] For example, a new department of pharmacy and a new dental school were proposed.

In October 1945, after the war, Digby left for England to recuperate, as the internment had taken a toll on his health. He returned to Hong Kong later but had to retire around 1946–1947 from the Chair of Surgery due to ill health. He was made Emeritus Professor in Surgery by the university. After a short spell in private practice, he left for England in 1949. As a true believer in research, he continued his investigation of the function of subepithelial lymphatic glands at the Buckston Browne Research Farm of the Royal College of Surgeons and published his last paper in 1954.[33] He died in February 1954 from cancer of the rectum.

His friends and former students set up the K. H. Digby Memorial Fund to "perpetuate the memory of a great teacher and a perfect gentleman."[34] Dr. S. W. Phoon, a former student, and his chief assistant, noted that Digby took a great interest in the affairs of the students. He acted as a good model for students in bedside manner and in regarding duty before oneself. A man of great humility, he was not afraid to admit ignorance and would take suggestions from students and assistants.[35] Dr. G. H. Thomas, a long-time friend, characterized him as "an original thinker and a born teacher. No student ever feared him ..." and he was extremely polite to his assistants in the operating room.[36] Out of the memorial fund, a Digby Memorial Scholarship was established to help needy students and provide traveling grants. In 1969, Professor G. B. Ong raised an endowment fund to create the Digby Memorial Lecture to be delivered by eminent speakers.[37]

Dr. Duncan Sloss, Vice-Chancellor of HKU, commented: "Professor Digby has had a one-track career, never deviating from the duties of a good surgeon." But Professor Kenelm Hutchinson Digby was more than just a good and innovative surgeon; he was also a passionate educator and will long be remembered as such.[38] Dr. M. B. Osman, acting Professor of Pathology,[39] his former student and assistant, had this to say about him: "The function of a teacher is not just to impart knowledge ... He is merely to suggest an attitude: not to fill notebooks but to thrill a soul ... Prof. Digby somehow or other, with rare surgical skill dissected and displayed my soul."[40]

Herbert Gastineau Earle (1882–1946)

MA, MB, FRCP, FRSM, FRSTMH, Hon. LLD

Professor Herbert Gastineau Earle brought the first major change in curriculum to the Faculty of Medicine, to render it more relevant to the practice of medicine and in line with those offered in the United Kingdom.

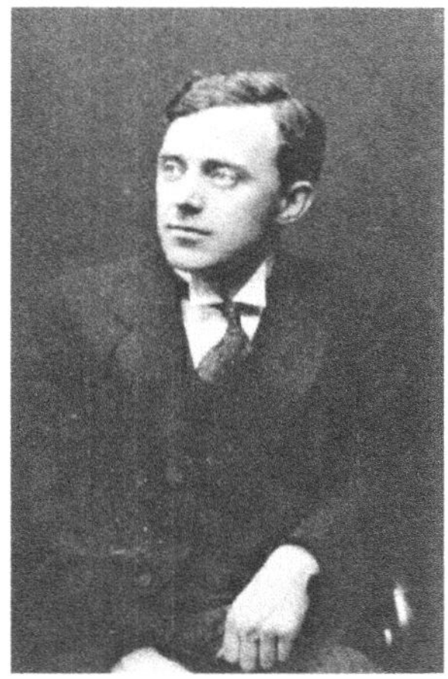

Figure 4.2 Professor Herbert Gastineau Earle
Source: Hong Kong University Archives, HKU

Earle was born in 1882 in London and educated at City of London School and Downing College, Cambridge, where he was a foundation scholar. He gained a first class in the Natural Science Tripos and Bachelor of Arts in 1903, and Master of Arts, Bachelor of Medicine degree in 1913. He was a Demonstrator in Physiology from 1904 to 1915 and Joint Lecturer in Biology at Middlesex Hospital from 1909 to 1915.

He moved to Hong Kong in 1915 as Professor of Physiology and Biology and, in 1918, as Professor of Physiology at HKU, when he became the founding chairman of the Physiology Department.[41] He was Dean of the Faculty of Medicine from 1916 to 1920, and in 1923 and 1925. In 1916, he acted as Honorary Visiting Physician to Government Civil Hospital.

Earle brought with him the experience of working at Cambridge University and a teaching hospital in London and was keenly aware of the reforms in medical education that were taking place in England according to the recommendations of the Royal Commission on University Education in 1913: 1) clinical professors should not be different from professors in other disciplines and should devote the greater part of their time to teaching and research; 2) the departments should be organized as to enable professors to carry on research and give scientific instruction to their students; 3) a "university hospital unit" should consist of a professor with wards under his control, assistants to complement his own knowledge and to assist him in his scientific enquiries, and a laboratory close to his wards; 4) teaching should be carried out through the medium of clinical demonstrations; and 5) students should have access to patients in wards to enable them to learn by practice and experience.

Even before he proposed these plans in 1918, Earle as Dean, introduced some changes to tighten the medical curriculum, to make more specific requirements that a student had to satisfy for a course, and to increase students' contact with patients. Students had to spend specified periods in different areas of medicine, for example, three months each as a junior medical clerk and a surgical clerk and another three months each in senior medical and surgical clerkships. The clinical work took place over the last three years of the curriculum. He also revised the curriculum and reduced the number of examinations from four to three.[42]

Earle identified several defects in the medical curriculum at HKU in 1918: 1) the lack of coordination between the various departments and between courses in the departments, 2) too much didactic work outside the hospital, 3) insufficient beds for inpatient experience, 4) lack of outpatient teaching, 5) inadequate clinical laboratories, 6) no postmortem work, and 7) no research and special postgraduate work. Earle recommended the appointment of three full-time professorships, one each in medicine, surgery, and obstetrics and gynecology. Each professor, as head of his department, would control wards, clinical laboratories, and outpatient work. He would be responsible for organizing teaching and research in his area. In addition to his own teaching, he should seek the help of private practitioners or government medical officers to teach the courses in their area of interest. These ideas also coincided with those recommended by the Sharp Commission. Although Earle wished to implement all these changes to the HKU Faculty of Medicine as soon as possible, it was impossible to do so for lack of funds.[43] When Professor Digby approached Dr. Richard Pearce of the Rockefeller Foundation for possible financial assistance, Earle was initially unhappy with the idea of receiving donations from the US. Being practical, he changed his mind, as it would be better to run a first-rate school with the aid of American philanthropy than a second-rate without it.[44]

The Rockefeller endowment brought new life to the Faculty of Medicine and enabled it to develop the three clinical departments and secure the continual recognition of its degree by the General Medical Council. When the university needed a Department of Biology in 1926, Earle suggested applying to the Rockefeller Foundation. This time it was regrettably declined, as the university failed to live up to its earlier pledges, particularly on the one to build a student hostel next to hospital, because of lack of funds.

In 1928, Earle left HKU to take up an appointment as a general advisor to the Lester Trust and director of the Henry Lester Institute of Medical Research and Preventive Medicine in Shanghai.[45] In China, he was involved in the development of physiological sciences. He became the first director of the Chinese Association for Physiological Sciences and co-founded the *Chinese Journal of Physiology*. He researched into the basal metabolism of Chinese and Westerners and published the results in scientific journals[46] as well as a paper on metabolism in *Caduceus*, which was the magazine of the HKU Medical Society.[47] He was a Fellow of the Royal Society of Medicine (FRSM) and a Fellow of the Royal Society of Tropical Medicine and Hygiene (FRSTMH). In 1936, he was conferred an honorary Doctor of Laws from HKU.[48]

In 1941, Professor Herbert Gastineau Earle retired from the directorate of the Lester Institute on account of age. He remained in Shanghai and was placed in an internment camp at Lunghwa during Japanese Occupation, where he helped the sick internees and their children. Although his health deteriorated by the end of two years in the camp, the first thing he did after the Japanese surrender was to secure the return of the buildings of the Lester Institute from the Japanese. He then decided to visit England and embarked on a hospital ship on 7 May 1946, to be joined by his son, Lieutenant-Colonel E. Earle of the Royal Army Medical Corps, in Singapore. But on 5 June, Professor Earle had a stroke from which he did not recover. He left his wife, a son, and three daughters.[49] China lost a devoted friend who spent the greater part of his life educating its young people in science and medicine and promoting the well-being of its people.

Wang Chung-yik 王寵益 (1888–1930)

MBChM, MD, BSc, DTM&H

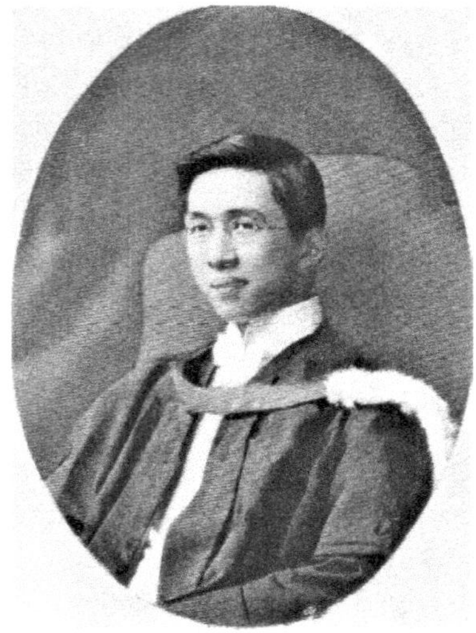

Figure 4.3 Professor Wang Chung-yik
Image Courtesy of HKMMS

Professor Wang Chung-yik was the first Professor of Pathology and the first Chinese professor of the Faculty of Medicine at HKU.

Wang came from an exceptional family in which several of his siblings were educated in Britain or the US. Some became prominent members of society during the late Qing dynasty, when all people in China were still wearing queues. Like Dr. Ho Kai, his father was a Christian and a minister. The Reverend Wang Yuk-cho was a pastor of To Chai Church in Hong Kong associated with the LMS. His grandfather was the first in the family to be converted to Christianity.[50] At the time, many children of Christian families, because of their association with the Church, received education and were able to speak English and became the elite of the community. In China, some of them contributed greatly to the modernization of the Republic.

Wang Chung-yik went to Queen's College and entered HKCM, from which he graduated in 1908. As he was unable to practice in Hong Kong because the license of HKCM was not recognized by the General Medical Council, he left for the University of Edinburgh, where he obtained an MBChM degree two years later.[51] While in HKCM, Wang and Li Shu-fan, also an HKCM student who became a famous surgeon later, shared a room in Nethersole Hospital. They walked together every day to Alice Memorial Hospital for lectures and clinical work. Li described Wang as "a Christian, a most congenial companion, and a young man of brilliance." They became close friends.[52] At the University of Edinburgh, where both advanced their studies, they lived in the same boarding house. Li told a story that the landlady of the boarding house was mystified by the disappearance of her washing board every night and its reappearance in the morning. Apparently, Wang used the board every night to extend his bed out of the window so that he would breathe fresh air all night long, because he might have a "touch" of tuberculosis. Wang was correct, because decades later, he died from the disease.[53]

After graduation, Wang went on to take a diploma course in Tropical Medicine and Hygiene in 1911 and a Public Health course at Manchester University in 1912. The following year he also obtained a BSc in Bacteriology and Comparative Pathology from Manchester University. Having discovered his interest in laboratory medicine and scientific research, he began to work in the Laboratory of the Royal College of Physicians of Edinburgh (RCPE) on a full-time basis supported by scholarships.[54]

While working in the Laboratory of RCPE, he studied tuberculosis in the Scottish population. His thesis, "A Study in Some Phases of Tuberculosis with Special References to the Incidence of Bovine Infection and the Question of Latency and Prevalence of the Disease," won him an MD degree from the University of Edinburgh. Tuberculosis became one of his lifelong research passions. During World War I, he was appointed interim Assistant Superintendent of the Laboratory and was responsible for all the clinical samples sent to the laboratory, in addition to his own research. This clinical exposure prepared him well for his future in Hong Kong. Despite the amount of work, he prepared and submitted the "Reports from the Laboratory for 1915–1920."[55]

At the end of World War I, Wang was becoming known among the pathologists in England. When the position of Professor of Pathology at HKU came up, Wang applied for the job with glowing recommendations from his referees. The appointments of HKU were made in London by a Consulting Committee after approval from the HKU Council. In 1920, Gregory Jordan, Acting Vice-Chancellor of HKU, had authorized the London Consulting Committee to make the appointment without consulting HKU Council. It came as a surprise that the position went to a less qualified British person. The HKU Council refused to accept the recommendation of the London Consulting Committee, which had been endorsed by HKU Senate, although the Senate had no authority in appointing university staff. The London Consulting Committee was under the impression that a Chinese should not be appointed to the professorial rank at HKU. Fortunately, the first appointee resigned, and Wang was offered the position in 1920. It seems that questions were raised about the appointment by the brother of Wang, Dr. Wang Chung-hui, a high-level diplomat in the Chinese Nationalist Party, to bring about the appropriate final outcome.[56] However, over the next 10 years of his employment at HKU, Wang frequently encountered the problem of racial discrimination.

While other professors at the university were paid at HK$8,000 per annum, Wang was paid only HK$6,000 because he was Chinese. In this instance, he had an advocate, Dr. Pearce of the Rockefeller Foundation, who was responsible for the endowment of the three Rockefeller professors for the clinical departments. Dr. Pearce was pleased to see that a Chinese had been appointed to the chair professorial rank in the faculty and told the Vice-Chancellor, Sir William Brunyate, that Chinese professors should enjoy the same salary, housing, and other benefits as other professors. It was only in 1924 that Wang received the same salary and benefits as his colleagues of the same rank.[57]

At the university, Wang started to build the Pathology Department. However, the job came with numerous other duties than teaching. He was Honorary Consultant in Pathology to the Hong Kong government and was responsible for reporting all clinical specimens sent in from different hospitals and clinics and conducting postmortem examination on those who had died on the wards. When the Government Bacteriologist was on sick leave, he was responsible for all the work carried out at the Bacteriological Institute. This meant that he was obliged to perform postmortem examinations on the bodies in the public mortuary and to report on the clinical samples sent to the Bacteriological Institute. He only had one assistant to help him. It is hard to imagine how he managed to find time for his research. Nevertheless, he continued to publish at least one paper each year in *Caduceus* as well as in other journals. Among his publications, the study on infantile tetanus (*Tetanus Neonatorum*) in Hong Kong proved to be most relevant, as *trismus* or lockjaw, due to *Tetanus Neonatorium,* accounted for 50% of infant deaths locally in the early twentieth century. He discovered tetanus bacilli in a number of sealing cord powders, which were used commonly by the Chinese on the umbilicus of neonates and sold in Chinese drug stores.[58] The sealing cord powders were made with burnt ash of red cotton cloth, finely ground cow's dung or human hair, rouge, and dragon bones (mammal fossils), but more common ingredients were earth or manure—a good culture medium for bacteria, including the tetanus bacteria. Prohibition of the sale of these powders resulted in a reduction of infant mortality from tetanus.

Wang wrote a textbook for students, entitled *Handbook of Pathology*, and it was finally published in 1925, after some difficulties in getting funds for printing. The university refused to defray the cost because it was not a research paper. In the end, Robert Kotewall, a businessman and a legislator at the time, and two Chinese gentlemen financed the publication as a result of the efforts of Professor Digby.[59] The book, unlike other pathology books, was not arranged by systems but according to etiology. It was used extensively in Hong Kong and in other parts of the world.[60]

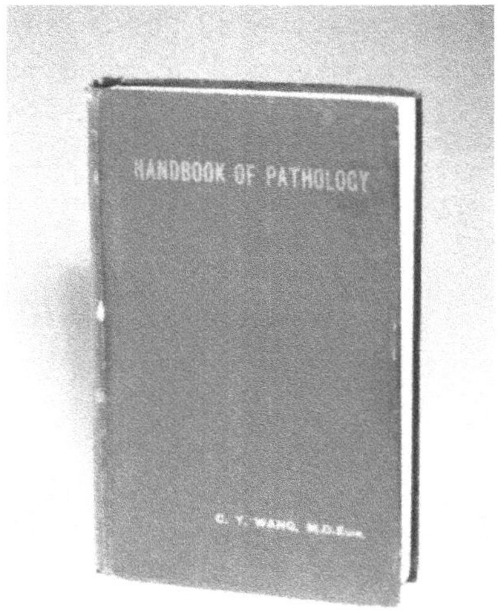

Figure 4.4 ***Handbook of Pathology***
Image courtesy of HKMMS

In the Department of Pathology, Wang built up a teaching collection of specimens for a museum, including microscopic sections. Unfortunately, all these were destroyed during Japanese Occupation.[61] He was elected President of the HKU Medical Society 1922–1923[62] and acting Dean of the Faculty of Medicine.[63]

In 1930, Professor Wang Chung-yik developed tuberculosis laryngitis and was unable to speak. He gave his lectures by writing to be read by his assistant. By September, he was so sick that four of his doctors, including Dr. Li Shuf-fan, wrote to Vice-Chancellor Sir William Hornell that Wang was unfit for work. In the meantime, Wang requested 12 months of sick leave. The university granted him six months leave with half-pay and would reassess his situation at the end of this period. Wang had married Florence Folkard in 1920 before he left Edinburgh. They had two sons. The cut in income and the high medical expenses created hardship for him and his family, but Wang refused to ask the university to reconsider his case. Several professors wrote to the university to request higher pay for Wang. However, the university was divided on this. Vice-Chancellor Hornell met with Mrs. Wang, who denied that she or her husband had ever questioned the university's fairness of the half-pay decision but admitted that she had difficulty making ends meet and an increase in allowance would be of great help. In the end, the head of Finance Committee agreed to increase the sick pay, but 10 days later, Professor Wang died.[64]

Vice-Chancellor Hornell delivered a moving farewell address on 15 December 1930 at the graveside at the Pokfulam Cemetery:

> "... You gave up your life to the sciences and art of Medicine in one of its most vital aspects. You saved others, yourself you could not save. In the plentitude of your life and vigor, a deadly disease got hold of you and in spite of the serenity of your courage and patience and of your grim struggle to live for the sake of those you loved ... You have left behind you the abiding memory of a blameless life of unostentatious devotion. This is your gift to your family, your University and your country. It is no mean one—Fare you well."[65]

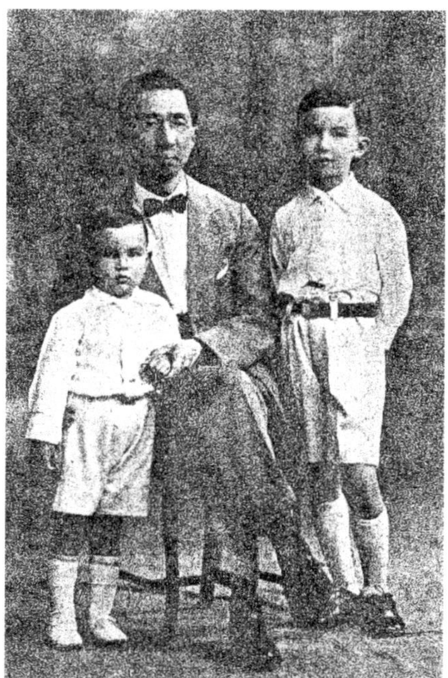

Figure 4.5 Professor C. Y. Wang and his two sons, c. 1930
Source: HKMMS, reproduced with permission, donated by Mrs. Catherine Cheng

John Anderson (1879–1931)

MA, MD, BSc, MRCP, DTM&H

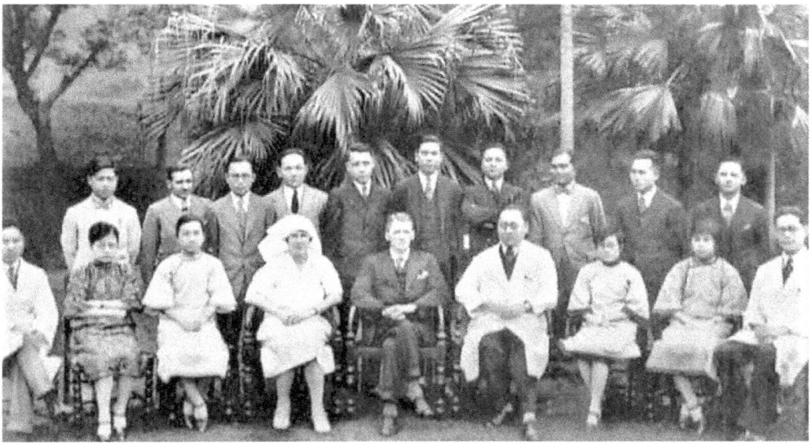

Figure 4.6 Professor John Anderson (sitting center). Dr. T. Y. Li sitting next to him (R4) and Dr. T. J. Hua (R1) and the rest of staff and students in 1928.

Source: HKMMS, reproduced with permission, photograph donated by Dr. Andrew Hua

Professor John Anderson was one of the three Rockefeller professors and the founding professor of the Department of Medicine, HKU. He possessed all the qualities required by a professor of medicine: an astute and compassionate clinician, a dedicated teacher, and an ardent researcher.

He was born in Glasgow in 1879 and received his medical education in the same city, where he graduated as a medalist or prizeman in many subjects. He proved himself to be not only of academic distinction but also of great practical ability. After graduating in 1907, he held resident posts in Glasgow Western Infirmary, Hospital for Skin Diseases, Gardlock Lunatic Asylum, and Ruchill Fever Hospital. He then built a successful private practice in Wallasey, near Liverpool, where he frequently acted as a consultant. At the outbreak of World War I, he was drafted as a medical officer to Gallipoli, where he was regarded as a surgical specialist. He once famously completed an abdominal operation while enemy bombs dropping around his operating tent set the neighboring structures on fire. Towards the end of the war, he became keenly interested in practical bacteriology and pathology. Having already acted as a surgical and a medical specialist, he went on to become an expert in pathology, commanding various field laboratories until the end of the war. He remained in Egypt and Sudan as a general consultant in medical matters to the Director of Medical Services, before returning to England in 1920, where he became a student at the London School of Hygiene & Tropical Medicine. The following year he accompanied Professor R. T. Leiper to British Guiana for a research project on filariasis organized by Sir Patrick Manson and the Seamen's Hospital Society. At the termination of the project, he was appointed Professor of Medicine, HKU.[66]

Recruitment for a professor of medicine began as soon as the Rockefeller Foundation endowment funds were made available. The salary offered was £800 per annum, living quarters provided, and first-class passage going to and returning from Hong Kong.[67] All appointments of expatriate teachers for government schools including HKU had to go through the Board of Education in London at the request of the Colonial Office.[68] The Selection Committee of the Board of Education received a total of nine applicants for this position, but none was found to be suitable. Further advertisement brought one more applicant, Dr. John Anderson, who was highly recommended by people whom he worked with, particularly Professor Leiper, who was very impressed by Anderson's sympathetic handling of people of color and by his courtesy and tact as well as his research ability. So much so that Professor Leiper left the project completely in the hands of Anderson for six months.[69] The Board of Education wisely suggested to the university to appoint Anderson and to start paying him from March of 1923, allowing him to visit English and US institutions to investigate the organization of medical schools before arriving in Hong Kong for the September term.[70]

In the 1920s, HKU was small, and so was the Faculty of Medicine. Clinical teaching took place mainly at Government Civil Hospital. The Department of Medicine, known as the University Medical Unit, was allocated 42 beds and 4 cots in three wards from the total complement of 212 beds in the hospital. After arrival in September 1923, Anderson found that he did not have total control over the use of these beds. Nevertheless, he began to organize his department. In addition to inpatients, he ran the hospital's medical outpatient clinics both mornings and afternoons, and changed some of them into teaching clinics to increase the students' exposure to patients. The clinics attended more than 5,000 patients annually, with the numbers increasing over time.[71]

Anderson had three full-time medical staff assistants. Dr. Li Tsoo-yiu, who had just returned from postgraduate studies under a Rockefeller traveling fellowship in Europe and the US, and joined the staff in February 1927, as an assistant to the Professor. Dr. Li lectured on pediatrics and syphilology and undertook part of the clinical teaching in the wards and the outpatient clinics. Dr. Tseung Fat-im, appointed by Anderson in 1927 as his clinical assistant (resident), turned out to be one of Hong Kong's most notable medical doctors in the mid-twentieth century[72] (Chapter 5). The third medical staff assistant position belonged to the house physician (intern). In 1927, the two house physicians were Dr. Bau Tsu-zung and Dr. J. S. Guzdar, each served for a period of six months and assisted in the supervision of student ward-clerks.[73] Two individuals listed as part-time lecturers were: Dr. G. H. Thomas and Dr. J. Valentine. Dr. Thomas, another well-known doctor in Hong Kong during the first half of the twentieth century, remained in government service throughout his career, serving the poor rather than going into full-time private practice.[74] Dr. Valentine, the Medical Officer in charge of Government Civil Hospital, was a lecturer in therapeutics.

Infectious diseases were widespread in the early twentieth century. Government Civil Hospital, which was a general hospital, had medical wards filled with patients suffering from various infectious diseases and infections. These included bacillary dysentery, amebic dysentery, and other types of parasitic infestations such as hookworm presenting with anemia, malaria presenting with fever, tuberculosis, and venereal diseases, particularly syphilis presenting with a myriad of neurological manifestations.[75] Highly infectious diseases such as smallpox and plague were treated in specialized infectious diseases hospitals.[76]

The 1920s was an era when the "germ theory" of Pasteur and Koch had been confirmed, and different bacteria had been identified as agents causing diseases such as cholera, plague, and venereal diseases. Anderson introduced simple laboratory investigations as diagnostic methods to his students, for example, microscopic examination of body fluids to demonstrate the presence of the responsible organisms, such as parasites in the blood in malaria, and serological test in syphilis. Although antibiotics had yet to be discovered, some drugs were available, such as those for syphilis and parasitic diseases, but side effects were frequent. Chronic noncommunicable diseases such as cancer, stroke, coronary disease, and diabetes were less commonly encountered by students. *Caduceus* recorded that in outpatient clinics, Professor Anderson introduced insulin for treatment of diabetes and thyroid extracts for patients suffering from hypothyroidism.[77]

The university had always permitted their professors to have private clinics to supplement their relatively low salary. Because of his medical skill and his sympathy for patients, Anderson's private clinics with both Chinese and Europeans, increased rapidly in size. Anderson was popular also among his students because of his genial predisposition and eagerness to teach.[78] Although the number of medical students each year was small, varying from 20 to 30 each year, he had to rely on part-time staff for part of the teaching.

Anderson was known for his research on dysentery and filariasis. During his time at HKU, he continued to work on these projects but also took on new ones. In 1924, he conducted a clinical trial using old tuberculin to treat tuberculosis, at a time when there were no effective drugs for treatment of the disease, as well as a study of hookworm larvae.[79] The large clinical load, heavy teaching commitment, and lack of research facilities, did not give him adequate time and space for meaningful research. Nevertheless, Anderson did publish two to three articles in *Caduceus*.[80]

During the short span of six years, Anderson established the Department of Medicine from scratch, giving it a semblance to those in medical schools in England. It offered both inpatient and outpatient services, teaching of medical students with a small team of medical staff and a small research program. In 1929, Professor John Anderson was appointed director of the Henry Lester Institute of Medical Research in Shanghai, to which over £1 million had been bequeathed. Sadly, he passed away two years later, at the age of 52, shortly after completing negotiations for the educational status of the Henry Lester Institute in China, including the formulation of schemes for future research. He willed £250 to HKU to establish the John Anderson Gold Medal, to be awarded to the student who attained the highest aggregate marks in the professional examinations.[81]

On 2 April 1931, in a packed hall, the university held a memorial service to pay tribute to Professor John Anderson, presided by the Vice-Chancellor, Sir William Hornell. The university also sent condolences to the Lester Institute and Professor Anderson's family on the irreplaceable loss.[82]

Richard Edward Tottenham (1889–1971)

MB, FRCP (Ireland), FRCOG (Ireland)

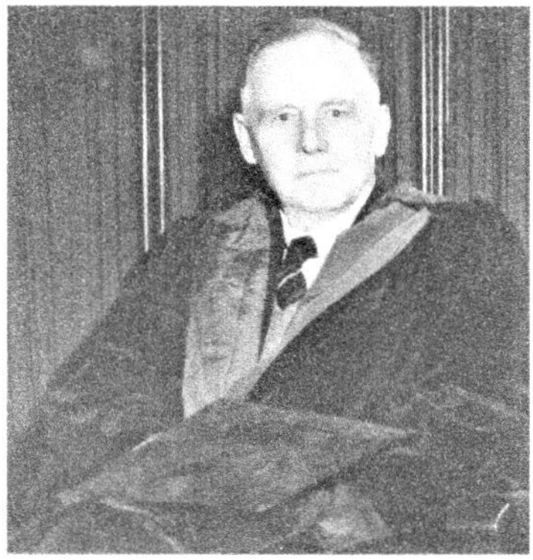

Figure 4.7 Professor Richard Edward Tottenham

Courtesy of the Department of Obstetrics and Gynecology, HKU

Professor Richard Edward Tottenham was born in 1889 in Cork County, Ireland, and attended Trinity College, Dublin, for his education. After graduation, he received further training at the two most prominent maternity hospitals in Dublin. He became a Fellow of the Royal College of Physicians in Ireland in 1919 and a Fellow of the Royal College of Obstetricians and Gynecologists in 1929. He further gained administrative exp-erience as an ex officio governor of Sir Patrick Dunn Hospital in Dublin. In his letter of application to HKU as one of the Rockefeller professors, he stated that he was determined to make the department famous throughout Asia.[83]

The Rockefeller Foundation had agreed to endow three chairs to establish the clinical departments at HKU in 1923:[84] one each in medicine, surgery, and obstetrics and gynecology. The chair for obstetrics and gynecology was endowed about one year after the other two. There were two reasons for the delay. First, while medicine and surgery had been established as separate disciplines in the nineteenth century, obstetrics and gynecology were established only in the following century. The discipline of obstetrics and gynecology rose to prominence when the importance of preventive midwifery, prenatal care, labor intervention, attention to asepsis, and postnatal surgical intervention formed the core of modern medicine in the early twentieth century. The requirement by the General Medical Council of training in obstetrics and gynecology included attendance of 20 labors and clerkship in the ward and outpatient department for at least three months, and a final examination on these two subjects.[85] Second, the government failed to provide an adequate maternity service for training. At that time, the government had maternity beds in Victoria Hospital for Women and Children and Government Civil Hospital, and the facilities for teaching were poor. The total number of beds was under 25, the minimum requirement set by the Rockefeller Foundation for teaching and training. It was only in 1924 that the government agreed to increase the number of beds for obstetrics and gynecology to 25 and the chair was endowed.[86]

On arrival in Hong Kong in 1925, Tottenham found that both the maternal and infant mortality rates were high. This, he believed, was due to the poor education and the lack of acceptance of Western medicine by the impoverished Chinese women. He also found that maternal mortality in Hong Kong was directly related to social status: the lower the social status, the higher the risk of complications and dying from pregnancy.[87] The poor health of women in the lower social class and the large number of children they reproduced drained their energy. The poor sanitation of their living environment bred diseases.[88] The fear of Western medicine and especially hospitals resulted in these women not going to hospitals until they were at death's door. Dr. Alice Hickling (née Sibree) had done a tremendous amount of work to introduce and popularize Western medicine among Chinese women, but there was still a great deal of work to be done.

In his article "Maternity Work in the Colony of Hong Kong" published in *Caduceus* in 1926, Tottenham pointed out that the development of obstetrics and gynecology in Hong Kong was very much in its infancy compared with those in Western countries, where the discipline had already matured. Although he did not wish to "run down Chinese medicine," his distaste for the indigenous treatment was clear.[89] Tottenham was given 25 beds in the maternity bungalow in Government Civil Hospital for teaching and research. Soon he found that the operating room in the bungalow was often used by the Surgical Department and there was little room in the bungalow for teaching.[90]

In the meantime, Dr. Alice Hickling, the supervisor of Tsan Yuk Hospital, had reorganized the hospital according to the principles of the Rotunda Hospital in Dublin. The nursing staff was well trained and quite capable of handling obstetrical complications. The patient population was from the lower social class while those in Government Civil Hospital were from a higher social class, being mostly wives of civil servants. Students would gain more experience from interacting with the poorer patients who were more likely to have complications. Tsan Yuk Hospital was more spacious compared with the Government Civil Hospital. Hickling had her postgraduate training at the Rotunda Hospital and Tottenham had been a staff member at the same hospital. The Rotunda Hospital was established in 1745 by an Irish surgeon and male midwife, Bartholomew Mosse, for poor Irish women who survived the Irish famine in 1740–1741. It eventually became the most renowned maternity hospital in the British Isles in the nineteenth century and set the standard of maternity care.[91] At that time Tsan Yuk did not have a specialist, and the hospital sent sick patients to Government Civil Hospital.[92] At the invitation of Dr. Hickling and Dr. Tso Seen-wan, a barrister who was responsible for raising funds for Tsan Yuk Hospital, Tottenham moved the teaching unit of his department to Tsan Yuk Hospital, satisfying the needs of both parties.

The cooperation between the University Department of Obstetrics and Gynecology and Tsan Yuk continued after Dr. Hickling's death in 1928 and remains today. In 1934, Tsan Yuk Hospital, which was under the administration of the CPD, was given to the Hong Kong government, because the hospital had become too large and too expensive for an nongovernmental organization (NGO) to administer.[93] By then Tsan Yuk Hospital had become such an important and valuable teaching and service center for women's medicine that, for the first time, the government took over the management and assigned an annual budget of HK$20,000 for an institution that was only for the Chinese.

The move to Tsan Yuk Hospital in 1926 allowed Tottenham to start his research program. He studied treatment of eclampsia in pregnancy and compared the outcome of different methods of treatment.[94] He concluded that treatment should be conservative, as practiced by Dr. Earnest Hasting Tweedy in the Rotunda Hospital, and not the hasty delivery of the baby using invasive procedures that often led to complications and death. Whereas Tweedy used morphia to arrest convulsions in eclampsia, Tottenham found that Chinese patients were more susceptible to morphia, and he used olive oil ether per rectum instead. Maternal mortality from eclampsia declined as a result.

Another topic of interest to Tottenham was strictures of the vagina, which were common due to injury from difficult and prolonged labor, infection, or application of caustic material into the vagina. They often led to difficulties in subsequent labor. Sometimes the stricture was so tight and the scar tissue so dense that it was impossible to extract the fetus by forceps. Tottenham performed and described various surgical procedures to relieve the condition.[95] He advocated using cesarean section as the intervention of choice for severe strictures. He introduced cesarean section to Tsan Yuk Hospital in 1925 and popularized the operation in Hong Kong. The prevalence of cesarean section gradually increased in Hong Kong as in the Rotunda Hospital.[96]

He submitted annual reports to the Government Medical Department and to *Caduceus* almost every year from 1926 to 1935, following the example of Rotunda Hospital. He gave a very detailed account of what went on at Tsan Yuk Hospital and the maternity bungalow at Government Civil Hospital during the year: the annual admissions and discharges, the diagnoses, the intervention, the outcome and, if surgical, the complications if any.[97] This is an excellent practice to identify any change in the pattern of disease and the practice in the department and where improvement might be required.[98]

In 1935, Tottenham resigned from HKU, leaving for City and County Hospital in Londonderry, Northern Ireland. Tottenham's resignation came as a surprise to many HKU staff. He and his wife felt that ten years in Hong Kong was enough, especially when the salary offered by the university was so low.[99] On 9 May 1935, members of the HKU Medical Society gathered in the Union Assembly Hall to pay tribute to Professor Tottenham for his contribution to the establishment of the Department of Obstetrics and Gynecology and his teaching to many students. They presented him with an ivory Buddha and phoenix and tiger on blackwood as a sign of their appreciation.[100] He was succeeded by Dr. William Nixon, a very talented young man.

Richard Edward Tottenham, the founding Professor of the Department of Obstetrics and Gynecology, had the wisdom of moving the department to Tsan Yuk Hospital, which had since been the training center of obstetrics and gynecology. By developing the department, he brought modernity to women's medicine in Hong Kong.

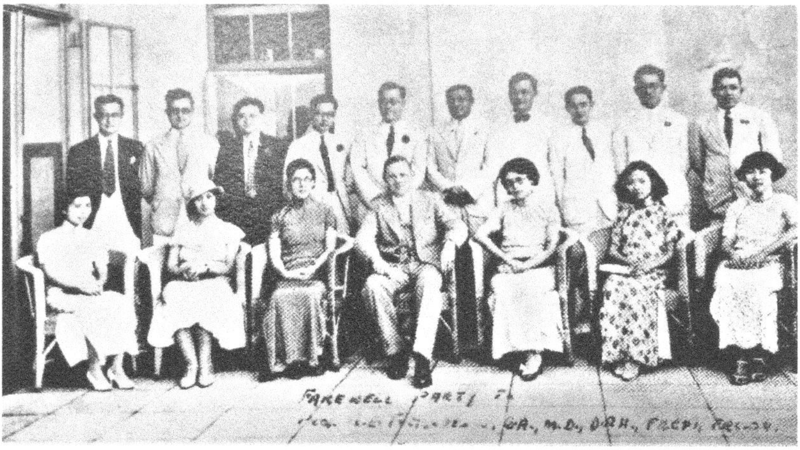

Figure 4.8 Professor R. E. Tottenham (sitting, centre) during the farewell party to him in 1935. Dr. Eva Ho Tung is sitting on his right (L3).
Source: 45th Anniversary book of the Hong Kong Obstetrics and Gynecology Society

5. Private Practitioners with Public Interests
Improving Medical Care and Education

The Chinese in Hong Kong mistrusted Western medicine during its early years as a British colony. They preferred their own ancient Chinese medicine and regarded surgery as barbaric. It took almost a century before Western medicine became the mainstream in Hong Kong. The private practitioners in Hong Kong during the first few decades of its existence were Europeans from Britain to care for the European civilians. The opening of Alice Memorial Hospital (1887) and its affiliated hospitals was a major breakthrough for the local people to appreciate Western medicine. The establishment of HKCM to educate Chinese young men in Western medicine was another major step forward, overcoming the mistrust and the language barrier. During the 1900s and 1910s, the CPDs were established in different parts of Hong Kong, staffed by Chinese licentiates of HKCM. The local Chinese found that Western medicine could cure some diseases that Chinese medicine could not. When Tung Wa Hospital was forced to introduce Western medicine and patients were allowed to choose the form of treatment, those treated with Western medicine had a lower death rate than those treated with traditional Chinese medicine (TCM). As well, after midwives trained in the Western method became available for domiciliary delivery were assigned to the CPDs, maternal and infant mortality rates were reduced. All these factors led to the general acceptance of Western medicine among the Chinese, and Western medicine became the mainstream medicine in Hong Kong before the World War II.

As discussed, the licentiates of HKCM were not permitted to practice medicine in Hong Kong because the College diploma was not recognized by the General Medical Council in Britain. However, there was a great need for the impoverished Chinese to receive medical care. Recognizing that the licentiates were reasonably well trained, the government paid the licentiates to staff the CPDs when the CPDs were established. The licentiates were assigned initially to determine the cause of death of the dumped bodies on the streets, they were later asked to treat and dispense medications to patients in the CPDs.[1] After the war, the government took over these dispensaries as government outpatient clinics. Gradually, several licentiates such as Drs. Ho Ko-tsun, Ma Luk, and Kwan King-leung started their own private practice in Hong Kong. The government did not interfere with their practice, as they saw the need for Chinese private practitioners to attend to Chinese patients who could afford to pay. These licentiates and three other doctors graduating from outside Hong Kong—Drs. Jeu Hawk from the US, Wan Man-kai from Tientsin, and Wu Tin-po from Edinburgh University, founded Yeung Wo Nursing Home in 1922.[2] Most of the Chinese doctors were in solo private practice, only European private practitioners formed group practices.

When HKCM became the Faculty of Medicine of HKU in 1911, the medical degree was recognized by the General Medical Council, as the curriculum of the Faculty of Medicine followed the requirements of the council. The colonial government amended the Medical Registration Ordinance of 1884 to ensure that the medical graduates of HKU were recognized for licensure to practice medicine in Hong Kong.[3]

Table 5.1 shows the number of doctors qualified to practice in Hong Kong by year before World War II and where they obtained their medical degree. The first list of qualified medical practitioners appeared in Hong Kong Gazette in 1904 and yearly thereafter.[4] In 1904, there were 18 qualified medical practitioners in Western medicine, 12 from the United Kingdom, and the rest from Japan, Canada, and Germany.[5] As expected, in 1941, the total number of qualified medical practitioners had grown to 310. Of these, 198 were HKU graduates, 66 were from the United Kingdom, and 46 were from other countries. The latter category mainly consisted of Chinese graduates from Canada, Japan, and a few from Europe.[6] In the decades leading to World War II, medical graduates from outside Hong Kong played a much more important role in providing Western medical care.

Most of the private doctors before World War II in Hong Kong were in general practice. Postgraduate training to become specialists was not available then. There were a few specialists who received their training overseas, such as Dr. Li Shu-fan, a surgeon, trained at Edinburgh University; Dr. Li Shu-pui, brother of Dr. Li Shu-fan, an ear, nose, and throat specialist, trained at University of Vienna;[7] Dr. Arthur Woo, a gynecologist trained at Middlesex Hospital in the UK and the Johns

Hopkins in the United States; and Dr. Eva Ho Tung, an obstetrician and gynecologist, trained at the Rotunda Hospital, Dublin.

Table 5.1 Total number of doctors qualified for practice in Hong Kong by year

Year	Total Registered	HKU Graduates	United Kingdom Graduates	Other Countries Graduates
1904	18	0	12	6
1905	21	0	14	7
1915	38	3	25	10
1925	117	40	62	15
1935	233	159	61	13
1941	310	198	66	46

Source: Moira Chan-Yeung, *A Medical History of Hong Kong, 1842–1941* (The Chinese University of Hong Kong Press, 2018), 242, derived from Hong Kong Government Gazette, 1904, 1905, 1915, 1925, 1935, 1941.

The local medical graduates of HKU usually settled into lucrative private practice, as there was a great demand for Chinese doctors trained in Western medicine. There were of course exceptions. A few practitioners distinguished themselves in the Government Medical and Health Service and used their skills to serve the poor, such as Dr. Lai Po-chuen (Chapter 6) and Dr. G. H. Thomas.[8] There were also a few, who in addition to being successful private practitioners, were active in public service, and devoted themselves to promote medical, social, and educational services in the community. Excellent examples could be found in Drs Li Shu-fan, Arthur Woo, and Tseung Fat-im.

Li Shu-fan 李樹芬 (1887–1966)

MBChB (Edin.), DTM and H (Edin), FRCS (Edin), LLD

Dr. Li Shu-fan lived a remarkable and colorful life, as narrated in his autobiography, *Hong Kong Surgeon*. He was a famous surgeon, a leader of the medical profession, a revolutionary, an academic at heart, an outstanding legislator, a skillful big-game hunter, and a philanthropist. Few people could combine all these roles in their lifetime.

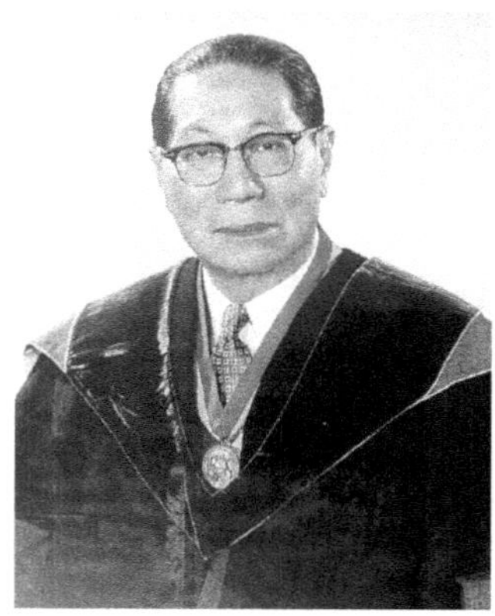

Figure 5.1 Dr. Li Shu-fan
Image courtesy of Hong Kong Sanatorium and Hospital Foundation

He was born in 1887 in Guangdong province. At the age of 12, he joined his father in Boston and lived there for three years before returning to his village. As a child, he knew what he wanted to be—a doctor of Western medicine. After matriculating from Diocesan Boys' School, he was admitted to HKCM in 1903.[9] During the years in the college, he shared a room with Wang Chung-yik, who later became Professor of Pathology at HKU, and they became friends for life.[10] While in the College, Li joined the underground society founded by Dr. Sun Yat-sen to bring about the downfall of the Manchu Empire. When Tong Meng Hui (同盟會, Revolutionary Alliance), a secret society whose membership was punishable by decapitation in China, was founded by Sun, Li did not hesitate to become a member. Li did well in his studies and was awarded an Imperial Government Scholarship to study in Edinburgh, which also guaranteed him an official position after graduation. The Chinese government obviously had no clue of his clandestine activities.[11] In Edinburgh, Li shared a boarding house with his old roommate, Wang Chung-yik. They both graduated with an MBChB in 1910, and in the following year, they were awarded a Diploma of Tropical Medicine and Hygiene. Li then returned to China and was appointed Chief Medical Officer of the Plague Prevention Service of South Manchuria by the Qing imperial government.[12]

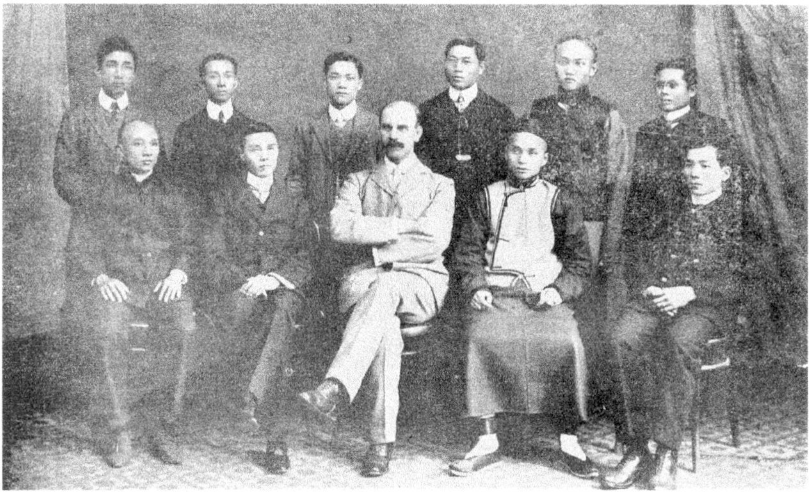

Figure 5.2 Li Shu-fan (standing R3), C. Y. Wang (standing L1) , Dr. R. M. Gibson (sitting, center), and other students of HKCM, 1904
Image courtesy of HKMMS, photograph donated by Alice Ho Miu Ling Nethersole Charity Foundation

In 1911, the uprising in Wuhan led to momentous changes in China. The Qing Dynasty collapsed and the Republic of China was founded. Li was appointed Minister of Health in the new government. However, he did not remain in the position for long. In 1912, when Guangzhou was taken over by General Long Jiguang, Li retired to Hong Kong and entered private practice, but he remained a medical advisor to Dr. Sun Yat-sen.[13]

In 1921 he returned to Edinburgh to take up postgraduate studies and obtained a Fellowship of the Royal College of Surgeons of Edinburgh (FRCS, Edin), specializing in gynecology and general surgery. He visited well-known clinics in Berlin, Paris, Vienna, and Oslo before returning to Hong Kong. On his return in 1923, he was offered the position of President of the Kung Yee Medical College in Guangzhou. There, he successfully organized the medical school after raising funds from a number of cities in North America. At that time civil war was raging in China, resulting in many people being injured. Li operated on many patients with injuries using different types of anesthetics including ether, chloroform, and spinal anesthesia.[14] As medical advisor, he counseled Dr.

Sun Yat-sen to have an exploratory laparotomy when Sun was unwell with a mass in the abdomen. The laparotomy that was carried out at Peking Union Medical College in 1925 revealed that Sun had advanced liver cancer. Li was also asked to treat Mikhail Markovich Borodin, chief Comintern agent in China in the 1920s, who developed pneumonia and refused to be treated except by Li.[15]

At the end of his two years' term as President of the Kung Yee Medical College, Li returned to Hong Kong and began his private practice in earnest.[16] He was approached by three senior Chinese medical practitioners to reorganize Yeung Wo Nursing Home, which was founded in 1922 by doctors of the Chinese community to serve the Chinese. At that time, Tung Wa Hospital, hospitals of the LMS, and Government Civil Hospital were the hospitals that Chinese patients could be admitted to, and these hospitals were always overcrowded. When Li was elected chairman of the board of directors and superintendent of the hospital, he reluctantly agreed to reorganize the hospital because it was running at a heavy annual deficit.[17] He erected a new hospital block, increased the number of beds from 24 to 94, modernized the facilities, installed X-ray equipment, and started a nurses' training program at the hospital. The new building was opened in 1932 by Mrs. Robert Kotewall.[18] In 1935, the hospital was renamed Hong Kong Sanatorium and Hospital.

At the time, almost 40% of patients admitted to Hong Kong Sanatorium and Hospital were suffering from tuberculosis. Anti-tuberculosis drugs had not yet been discovered, and several surgical procedures were used to reduce the size of the lungs to collapse the cavities so that they could heal better. Li's favorite operation was to crush the phrenic nerve to paralyze the diaphragm to collapse the lung. He even devised a special "phrenic avulsion forceps" which was produced by Downs Brothers in London. In Hong Kong, he was the first one to perform thoracoplasty to bring about a more complete and lasting collapse of the lung.[19] During this period, he contributed frequently to *Caduceus* of his experience in clinical practice,[20] such as the use of spinal anesthesia.[21]

Li took a vigorous role in the public life of Hong Kong before World War II. He had been a member of the Sanitary Board, member of the Urban Council and the Legislative Council, President of the Hong Kong Chinese Medical Association, District Chief Surgeon of St. John Ambulance Brigade, a member of the Medical Board, a Justice of the Peace, and a member of the University Court at different times.[22] In each of these organizations, he played an active role. While serving on the Sanitary Board, he brought up many important questions relevant to the well-being of the community. For example, the nuisance of flies in Kennedy Town, inspection of all registered schools in Hong Kong by the school health team, and the issue of "dumping bodies" in Hong Kong.[23] After serving for five years on the Sanitary Board, he resigned when he was appointed to the Legislative Council,[24] from which he also resigned in 1941, just before the Japanese Occupation of Hong Kong.[25]

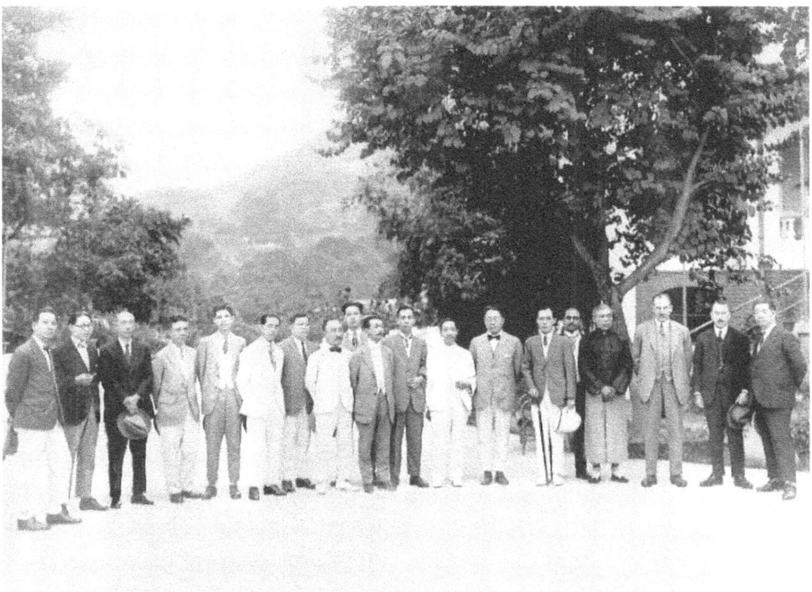

Figure 5.3 Dr. Li Shu-fan (L2), Dr. Ho Ko-tsun (R8), and other directors and guests at the inauguration of Yeung Wo Nursing Home in 1922
Source: HKMMS reproduced with permission

During the invasion of Hong Kong by the Japanese in 1941, Hong Kong Sanatorium and Hospital became a casualty clearing hospital because of Li's experience of war injuries in China. During the first part of Japanese Occupation, Li kept the hospital opened, and the facilities were sometimes used by the Japanese to operate on their own people.[26] As a result, he was able to obtain food and medical supplies for the hospital. However, when he was asked to become President of the Sino-Japanese Medical Association, he escaped to Free China.[27]

After World War II, Li returned to rehabilitate the hospital. In 1948, he went to the US to attend a conference. After consulting experts in the US, he came home with new ideas for further expansion of the hospital. Yeung Wo had only 170 beds then, increasing demand from a growing population necessitated the expansion.[28] The government granted him an adjacent lot on which he built a new wing. When completed, it had air-conditioning and other up-to-date facilities. Soon, Li resumed his public service to become a member of the board of directors of the Hong Kong Anti-TB Association, a council member of the Mission to Lepers Hong Kong Auxiliary, and a member of the Board of Regents of the American College of Chest Physicians in 1956.[29] He remained a member of the Rotary Club and shared his safari experiences with his fellow Rotarians and raised funds for them.

During his long years of medical practice in China and in Hong Kong, Li had contracted many serious infectious illnesses including diphtheria, tuberculosis, typhoid, and almost plague when he accidentally cut his finger while injecting anti-serum to a dying patient with bubonic plague.[30] Luckily, he survived.

Life was not just work for Li. It is well known that he loved hunting and had traveled to the jungles for the biggest and the most fearsome game.[31] During the 1950s, he traveled to different continents and hunted for tigers, lions, leopards, and elephants.[32] After spending four and a half months in different continents, Li "bagged the big five," meaning that he shot a lion, an elephant, a Cape buffalo, a rhinoceros, and a panther, and 20 other animals.[33]

Li's interest in medical education remained throughout his life. In 1961, he donated 80,000 square feet of land in Sassoon Road to HKU,[34] on which the university built the preclinical building and named it after him, in appreciation of his generosity. The following year, he established the Li Shu Fan Medical Foundation, which provided scholarships, bursaries, research grants, research fellowships, and a three-year lectureship in the Department of Pediatrics at HKU.[35] The foundation continues its good work today.

In 1961, Dr. Li Shu-fan was conferred an honorary degree of Doctor of Laws by HKU.[36] In 1964, he published his autobiography, *Hong Kong Surgeon*, giving us an account of his exciting and vibrant life.[37] He passed away in 1966 at the age of 79.[38] His persistent dedication to healing and to the community and his generosity to the Faculty of Medicine at HKU were appreciated by all. His life was one of great achievements and adventures that only those with courage and foresight could accomplish.

Woo Wai-tak, Arthur 胡惠德 (1888–1964)

OBE, MBBS, FRCS

Dr. Woo Wai-tak, Arthur was a prominent gynecologist in Hong Kong. Community service complemented his entire professional life.

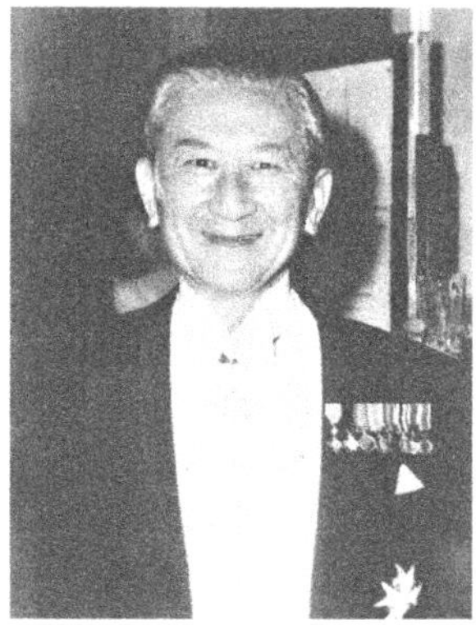

Figure 5.4 Dr. Woo Wai-tak, Arthur in St. John Ambulance uniform

Source: HKMMS, reproduced with permission, photograph donated by Ms. Vivian Li and Professor Faith Ho

Woo was born into a family of Chinese Christians. His grandfather and two uncles were prominent ministers of the Anglican Church of Hong Kong. His father, U I-kai, was a graduate of HKCM in 1895. In 1897, U was appointed house surgeon to Alice Memorial Hospital, but he died of plague less than a year later, on 24 March 1898. It was generally assumed that he was infected during his duties at the hospital. However, it was not so. According to his nephew, Woo Yan-tak, U saw a rat running across the room and he stepped on it instinctively. The rat must have been infected, as U developed plague and died from it. U left his wife, one son (Arthur), and four daughters. Fortunately, Mrs. U was a nurse trained at Alice Memorial Maternity Hospital. She struggled to bring up five children working as a nurse at Government Civil Hospital. Woo's younger sister, Katie, became a well-known educator and the founding principal of St. Paul's Girls' College, which became St. Paul's Co-educational College, one of the elite schools in Hong Kong today.[39]

Arthur Woo followed his father's footsteps. After graduating from the Diocesan Boys' School, he left for the London University, initially to study French and Latin. He then went into medicine and qualified at Middlesex Hospital in 1913. He obtained a Licentiate of the Royal College of Physicians (LRCP) and membership of the Royal College of Surgeons (MRCS) in the same year.[40] He received further training at Chelsea Hospital for Women. While in Middlesex Hospital as a trainee, he designed the Reverdin-Woo needle,[41] a handled needle for surgical use with eye aperture controlled by a thumb stud.

During World War I, Woo served in a military hospital in the UK. After the war, he was awarded a Rockefeller scholarship to study at the Johns Hopkins Hospital in Baltimore in the US. During his training, he worked with some of the most eminent British and American surgeons at the time, including Dr. Preston Maxwell, the future head of the Department of Gynecology at Peking Union Medical College (PUMC) in the UK, and Dr. Charles H. Mayo, a co-founder of Mayo Clinic in Minnesota in the US.

In the early 1920s, PUMC had been rebuilt by China Medical Board of the Rockefeller Foundation. It was a very stimulating place, as it was staffed by men trained at the Johns Hopkins, and they were well known for the research work that they were carrying out at PUMC.[42] Woo was the First Assistant of Professor Preston Maxwell in the Department of Gynecology at PUMC then. During this period, he was also Medical Advisor to the Ministries of Foreign Affairs and Transportation and Personal Physician to President of the Republic of China Li Yuanhong.[43] In Woo's research on the causes of osteomalacia, he came to the correct conclusion that it was a deficiency disease like rickets. He and his colleagues published several papers in medical journals. Despite this, one of his colleagues assessed him as follows: "Temperamentally he was no academic and was not interested in the critical analysis of laboratory data, but his priorities were practical, far-sighted and discriminating with a deep humanity and love of his fellow men." These comments turned out to be quite accurate. While at PUMC, Woo was particularly helpful to his Western colleagues, giving them advice on local customs and values, saving them from committing irrevocable mistakes, but he did not remain in academic medicine for long.[44]

Woo returned to Hong Kong in 1924 and established a highly successful private practice in his office in China Building and in his private Babington Hospital.[45] In 1928, he was elected President of the Hong Kong Branch of the British Medical Association. In the same year, he became the first Chinese elected as President of the China Medical Association[46] and the last president of that association, which amalgamated with the National Medical Association of China in 1932 to become the Chinese Medical Association. The China Medical Association was originally the Medical Missionary Society of Canton, founded in 1838 by medical missionaries.

Woo became a world-renowned expert in gynecology. He was the first to introduce radium for treating cancer of the cervix in Hong Kong, when the government was unable to provide such a service. He managed to obtain a supply of radium, hoping to relieve the suffering of these patients. Radium was very expensive then. One gram costs HK$230,000, and treatment for one patient required 50 mg, about HK$10,000. He generously shared his radium supply freely with Professor W. C. W. Nixon of the Department of Obstetrics and Gynecology, HKU.[47] He appealed to the people in Hong Kong over the radio to donate generously to the British Empire Cancer Fund for the purchase of equipment and radium for treating cancer.[48]

At the same time, he was involved in several community services. A devout Christian and a member of St. Paul's Church, he and another doctor started a free clinic on the Gospel Boat moored at Aberdeen in 1926. The Gospel Boat was organized by the Missionary Society of the Chinese Christian Council.Woo and his friend were the first to hold floating clinics for the boat people in Hong Kong. The government had motor launches to take medical officers to various places not accessible by land only in 1932. In 1930, the Chinese Christian Council moved the free clinic on the Gospel Boat to a clinic on land. It was so popular that Woo applied to the government to set up a public dispensary at Aberdeen for its residents.[49]

As an officer of St. John Ambulance Brigade, Woo helped establish 10 clinics in different parts of the New Territories in the 1930s.[50] Before then, the deprived people in the New Territories had no medical care. In the 1930s, two voluntary organizations, St. John Ambulance and the Medical Benevolent Society, began sending doctors and nurses to different parts of the New Territories to treat patients during weekends. Later, clinics were established with a nurse or a midwife stationed there throughout the week. To avoid duplication of services, the two voluntary organizations combined to form St. John Ambulance New Territories Medical Benevolent Society. They also ensured that there was no duplication of services with government clinics in the New Territories, so that there would be resources to open new clinics where there were none before.[51] Some of these clinics became regular government outpatient clinics after World War II.

Woo was concerned with opium addiction and actively campaigned against it. He sat on the board of many organizations and churches. He was President of Young Men Christian Association (YMCA) in 1935–1936 and Governor of South China District YMCA in 1936–1937. He was a charter member of the Rotary Club in 1930 and served as President in 1940–1941.[52]

In the 1930s, following its ambition to become a major world power but with inadequate natural resources, the Japanese Empire began its aggressive expansion. In 1931, Japan conquered Manchuria,[53] a place rich in minerals and lumber in the northwestern part of China. Since then, Japan continued to invade other parts of northern China. In 1932, Woo organized a relief team of Chinese doctors and nurses from Hong Kong to go to Shanghai to attend to the injured arising from the January 28 Incident when violence erupted between anti-Japanese and anti-Chinese groups in the Shanghai International Settlement.[54] When China finally declared war on Japan in 1937, Woo founded the International Medical Relief Committee and became its inaugural chairman.

During the Japanese Occupation, the Japanese seized Babington Hospital and accused Woo of being a British spy because of his close tie to Dr. Percy Selwyn Selwyn-Clarke, the Director of Medical Services.[55] It is unclear how long he was incarcerated. During the war, Woo and Dr. Tseung Fat-im provided a great deal of help to Tai Po Orphanage,[56] an Anglican-sponsored institution, which was dependent on donations. He also served as Medical Superintendent of Alice Memorial and Affiliated Hospitals during this most difficult period.[57] Over the years, he had kept in close contact with the hospital and was its consultant gynecological surgeon and a member of the executive committee of the hospital at one time.

After World War II, Woo resumed his private practice and his many community activities. He rebuilt Rotary Club in Hong Kong in 1945 and attempted to reestablish those in China, which was a great challenge.[58] He introduced Rotary Club to Macau, leading to the formation of Macau Rotary Club in 1947; he also organized another Rotary Club in Kowloon in 1948. He was the fourth member from the Hong Kong Rotary Club to serve as an officer of Rotary International.[59] In 1947, he toured the US to raise funds to establish the Department of Gynecology and Obstetrics at Lingnan University.[60]

Woo received many distinctions and appointments, including a fellowship of the Royal College of Surgeons in 1949, and an honorary fellowship of the International College of Surgeons, and an honorary visiting professorship of Lingnan University. He was a consultant to the Cancer Clinic in Macau, and a lecturer and examiner of the Medical Faculty at HKU. In 1956, Alice Ho Miu Ling Nethersole Hospital named an operating room after him in the new wing.[61] For his contributions to St. John Ambulance, Woo was appointed Commander of the Venerable Order of the Hospital of St. John of Jerusalem in 1949 and was awarded an OBE in 1954. He was one of the best-loved and best-known Chinese surgeons in East Asia.[62]

Dr. Woo Wai-tak, Arthur died in 1964 after a painful illness, leaving his wife, one son, and five daughters.[63] Professor W. C. W. Nixon had this to say about him: "His exuberance was infectious, and his ready smile brightened the burden of illness. The words of Tennyson, 'One only joy I know, the joy of life,' epitomized Arthur Woo's attitude to the world around him. He gave all he had to the succour of those less fortunate than he, and his marked success in the treatment of patients was due to the empathy he possessed to an unusual degree."[64]

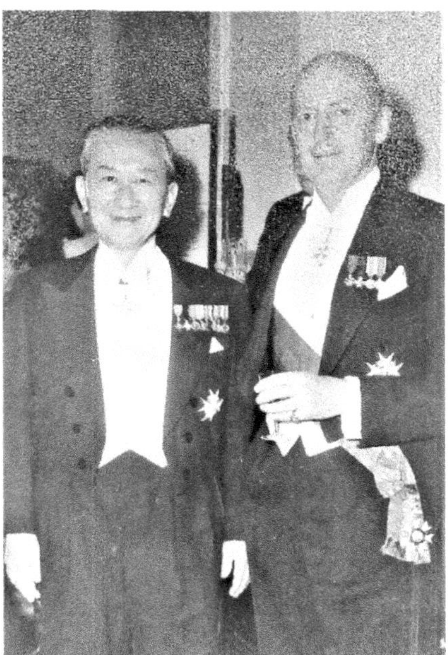

Figure 5.5 Dr. Arthur Woo and Governor A. Grantham
Source: HKMMS reproduced with permission

Tseung Fat-im 蔣法賢 (1903–1974)

MBBS, JP, OBE, LLD, KStJ

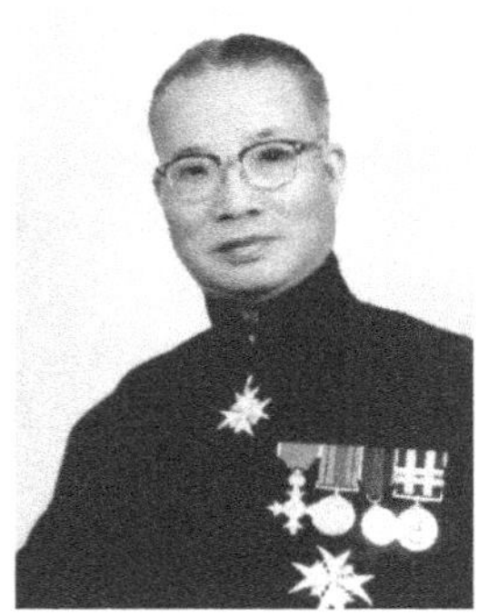

Figure 5.6 Dr. Tseung Fat-im

Image courtesy of United College, The Chinese University of Hong Kong

Dr. Tseung Fat-im was a private physician with specialization in diabetes and metabolism. An inspirational leader, he dedicated himself to advance not only medical but also educational and social services in the community.

Tseung was born in 1903 in Guangdong province. He attended Queen's College and entered the Faculty of Medicine at HKU. As a student, he distinguished himself by collecting a number of prizes and scholarships.[65] In his senior years, Tseung was a student of Professor John Anderson, who was appointed in 1923 as the founding chair to establish the Department of Medicine.[66] Tseung left behind something rather special to the Hong Kong Museum of Medical Sciences (HKMMS)—his two notebooks, one containing all the notes he took of Professor John Anderson's lectures and the other one of Professor C. Y. Wang's lectures, with beautiful illustrations.[67] These two notebooks, bearing the footprints of medical education and medical practice in the 1920s, were valuable acquisitions of the museum.[68] It is not surprising that Tseung was appointed clinical assistant to Professor Anderson's unit in Government Civil Hospital after he graduated with an MBBS degree in 1925. During the ensuing 18 months of training, Tseung carried out a special study on biochemistry and diabetes mellitus. The results were published in *Caduceus* in 1926.[69]

Although Tseung left for private practice after 1927, he remained active in the academic medical circle. He was at various times Honorary Treasurer of the Hong Kong University Medical Society, Vice-President of Hong Kong Chinese Medical Association, a Council Member of the British Medical Association, and Honorary Secretary and Treasurer of the National Medical Association of China Hong Kong Branch. He also served on the Hong Kong University Club and Hong Kong University Graduates' Association.[70] He was elected President of the Hong Kong University

Alumni Association in 1940, and a member of the Court, Council, and later Chairman of the Convocation of HKU for two successive terms between 1962 and 1968.[71]

Gradually, Tseung established a reputation as an excellent physician and a benefactor, devoted to the well-being of the community. In 1930, when the Medical Benevolent Society[72] was formed to establish free clinics in the New Territories for the poor, he was one of the founders and Honorary Secretary and Treasurer of the society until its amalgamation with St. John Ambulance Association. The amalgamation removed any duplication of provision of clinics, and new clinics were established in other parts of the New Territories without such a service instead.[73] The same year Tseung was appointed by the Hong Kong Government as a member of the Medical Board. It seems that the demand for his volunteering services was endless. From 1930 to 1934, he was an honorary lecturer to the nurses at Tung Wah Hospital, and he also financed a medical clinic under the auspices of the Chinese Buddhist's Association for a few years. Realizing the importance of public health education, he organized health campaigns and health education classes in conjunction with the YMCA and YWCA.

In 1934, he went on a world tour to update his medical knowledge, visiting prominent medical units in Europe and the US, and maternal and children's hospitals in London and Vienna. He also entered postgraduate study in Rotunda Hospital in Dublin. On his return, he went into partnership with Dr. Arthur W. Woo,[74] a prominent private doctor in Hong Kong. Later in life, Tseung was elected a Fellow of the Royal Society of Medicine and a Fellow of the Royal Society of Tropical Medicine and Hygiene, London.[75]

During the Second Sino-Japanese War, when Japanese troops marched southwards from Manchuria toward Shanghai, Tseung was also one of the organizers of Hong Kong Medical Relief Committee with Dr. Arthur Woo and served as its Honorable Secretary.[76] During Japanese Occupation, he remained in Hong Kong to serve the local population. In 1943, Tseung met Miss Tso Lai-ki, who was the daughter of Dr. Tso Seen-wan and working as an almoner[77] at Nethersole Hospital,[78] and they were married. Tso was a prominent barrister and a legislator, who was devoted to improving the health of the local Chinese and especially the health of women by introducing Western medicine. He was largely responsible for the founding of Wan Chai Maternity Hospital and Tsan Yuk Hospital

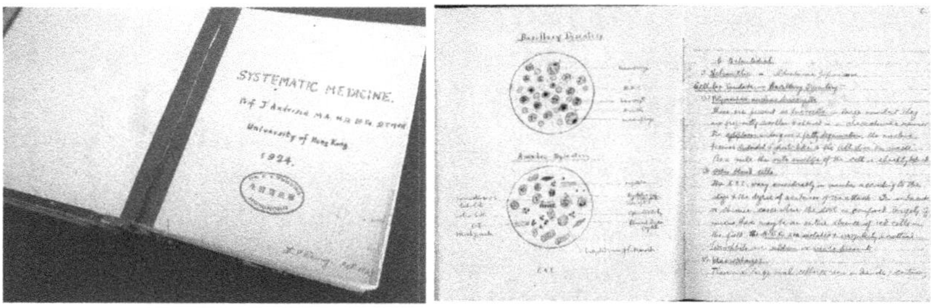

Figure: 5.7a and b Two notebooks of Dr. Tseung Fat-im
Source: HKMMS, reproduced with permission

(Chapter 6) to reduce the high maternal and infant mortality in Hong Kong.[79] Tseung and his father-in-law had much in common.

After World War II, Tseung's activities in the community became more numerous and widespread, mostly related to social welfare and education. He served as a member of the Sze Yap Commercial and Industrial Association, San Wui Commercial Society, and General Committee of the China Chamber of Commerce. He was Honorary Director of the Chung Sing Benevolent Society. Being a good friend of Bishop Ronald O. Hall of the Anglican Church, he was invited to be Assistant Secretary to Tai Po Rural Home and Orphanage, later renamed St. Christopher's Home. He served as the home's Council Chairman from 1964 to 1974. He was also Chairman of Boys' and Girls' Clubs Association of Hong Kong (1947–1950) and Chairman of Hong Kong Society for the Protection of Children (1950–1951). Tseung had been involved with the Rotary Club in Hong Kong since 1937 and was its President from 1947 to 1948. Later he served as an advisor to Rotary International and an officer of Rotary International. In 1954, Tseung was appointed Justice of the Peace.

Before World War II, there was no perceived demand for Hong Kong, a British Crown Colony, to provide its own system of university education in the Chinese language. There were two types of secondary schools in Hong Kong: Anglo-Chinese secondary schools, which prepared students for higher education in HKU and universities in other parts of the British Commonwealth and the US; and Chinese middle schools, which prepared students for universities in China. Due to the establishment of the People's Republic of China in 1949, many graduates from Chinese middle schools had no easy path to higher education although some students found their way to universities in China.[80] In the late 1950s, the government approved the founding of post-secondary colleges that were organized in Chinese rather than British curricula and staffed by teachers from universities in China. Of these, Chung Chi College, New Asia College, and United College were chosen.

Tseung was President of United College of Hong Kong and Chairman of the Board of Trustees. United College, located at 147 Caine Road, Hong Kong, had 600 students. It was established in 1956 by the amalgamation of students and staff from five private colleges in Guangzhou and nearby areas after they had moved to Hong Kong.[81] Tseung resigned in 1959, when the heads of the five schools tried to take control out of the hands of the Chairman of the Board of Trustees.[82]

Up to that time, the Hong Kong government agreed with the recommendations of the Keswick Committee,[83] that HKU should remain the sole institution of higher learning with degree-granting authority. By 1956, the attitude of the government had changed, and the possibility of a second university was entertained. Eventually, the three post-secondary colleges formed the Chinese University of Hong Kong (CUHK), inaugurated by Sir Robert Black, then Governor of Hong Kong, in 1963.[84]

Tseung's work with St. John Ambulance Brigade received recognition; he was admitted to the Most Venerable Order of the Hospital of St. John of Jerusalem as an Associate Officer in 1946 and was promoted to Associate Commander of the Order in 1952.[85] In 1969, he was conferred the degree of Doctor of Laws (*honoris causa*) by HKU.[86]

Dr. Tseung Fat-im passed away in 1974 at the age of 71 and was missed by all levels of community for his altruism, self-sacrifice, and devotion to the community by offering his services so freely to satisfy the medical, social, and educational needs of Hong Kong.

6. The Pioneer Women Doctors
Changing the Paradigm of Women's Medicine in Hong Kong

In England, women were denied access to medicine until the latter half of the nineteenth century. At the University of Edinburgh, although women finally gained admittance to clinical training, when they passed the examination, they were given a Certificate of Proficiency and not a medical degree as their male counterparts.[1] Elizabeth Garrett Anderson, the first women in Britain to be awarded a medical qualification in 1865, succeeded in her bid only after her father threatened to sue the Society of Apothecaries (later the British Medical Association). The society changed its regulations to bar further entry of women. In 1874, Anderson and her colleagues established the London School of Medicine for Women, to overcome the difficulties of gaining entrance to medicine in established schools. However, even after graduation, they encountered many obstacles.[2]

The Lancet constantly attacked the efforts of women to become doctors, and when the British Medical Association decided to exclude female practitioners in 1878, an editorial on 17 August of that year exposed the predominant male sexist view of the role of women:

> Again "the woman question" in relation to the practice of physic and surgery, is forced upon us by the wise decision of the British Medical Association to exclude female practitioners.... the gracelessness of the passion which a well-meaning but misguided young woman assumes when she undertakes the practical study of medicine, and waiving the question of female personal and social disabilities for the vocation of physician and surgeon, there is the all-important issue of natural and constitutional fitness.... the ministry of women is one of help and sympathy. The essential principle, the key-note of her work in the world is *aid*; to sustain, succour, revive and even sometimes shelter, man in the struggle and duty of life, is her

> peculiar function. The moment she affects the first or leading role in any vocation she is out of place … If women undertake the duties of physicians and surgeons, we shall presently feel the want of nurses….[3]

It was not until 1944 that the British government required that all schools receiving public funding should admit a reasonable proportion of female students. However, gaining a license to practice medicine did not mean smooth sailing thereafter; medical women had to fight an uphill battle to be treated as equals.[4]

In China, the issue was entirely different. It was whether women were able to have medical care. Chinese women then had virtually no legal rights and were relegated to an inferior role, confined in their households. Their social position was constricted by the Confucian concept of a woman's role in the family. When they were sick, they could be seen by a male doctor only in the company of a male relative. Apart from feeling the pulse, physical examination of other parts of the body was not possible. When medical missionaries arrived in China in the second half of the nineteenth century, they found that female Chinese patients could not be reached.[5] Female medical missionaries were added to the team to gain access behind closed doors. Since language was another major barrier, the missionaries began to train local Chinese girls in Western medicine so that they could use their skill to treat Chinese women. In 1879, Dr. John Kerr of Canton Hospital started training local girls. The first batch of students was girls from the nearby True Light Seminary.[6] When Kerr resigned from Canton Hospital in 1899 to start a Refuge for the Insane, the female students were left unattended. Dr. Mary Fulton, a medical missionary who came to Canton earlier in 1884, took over the responsibility for these students. She started a new school for young women in 1900, which was later renamed Hackett Medical College after its donor.[7]

In Hong Kong, the Chinese elite realized that only a woman doctor would be able to introduce Western medicine to Chinese women. When the new Alice Memorial Maternity Hospital in Hong Kong was planned, the Chinese elite donors demanded that a female doctor oversee the hospital. When the hospital was opened in 1904, Dr. Alice Sibree arrived from England to supervise it.[8] Although Dr. Sibree gained the trust of the Chinese women, she had a hard time working with Dr. R. M. Gibson, the Medical Superintendent of Alice Memorial Hospital, who held the prevalent negative view of women as doctors. Nevertheless, Sibree persevered until the end of her contract and started her own private practice. She was then able to introduce the Western method of delivery to Chinese women in Hong Kong by training Chinese midwives.

The first Chinese female doctors in Hong Kong were not trained by medical missionaries. They obtained their medical education on their own initiative at a time when few girls received education beyond the primary level. At the time of the opening of HKU in 1912, conservative climate prevailed, and it did not admit women. University regulations required that students should reside in hostels, but there was no female residence in the university. Request for admission of a girl as an external student had been declined. In January 1921, the new Vice-Chancellor Sir William Brunyate arrived. He was more sympathetic to women who wished to receive higher education. Tso Shuk-kei, daughter of Dr. Tso Seen-wan, a barrister trained in London, made an emotional appeal to Sir William during the speech day of St. Stephen Girls' School to allow admission of girls to HKU. The University Senate responded by allowing female students to attend lectures but not as registered students.[9] Tso herself was admitted later to the Faculty of Medicine but unfortunately died of cellulitis of the neck in 1928, before her final examination.[10]

The first female students were admitted to HKU in 1921, a decade after the university was inaugurated. That year, Rachel, daughter of Mr. Edward Alexander Irving, Director of Education, applied for admission and was at first refused by the University. Her father consulted the attorney-general, who found no legal ground in the University's regulations to reject her application. The Senate therefore resolved to admit Rachel to the third-year Arts Faculty, as she already had a Social Science Certificate at Bedford College, London University. Thus, in September 1921, three female students, Rachel Irving, Irene Ho Tung, and Lai Po-chuen, were admitted to HKU; the latter into the Faculty of Medicine. In the spring term of 1922, Eva Ho Tung was also enrolled in medicine.[11] The addition of two female medical students to the Faculty of Medicine, HKU, was a landmark event. The official publication of the HKU Medical Society, *Caduceus*, printed a clear message of welcome: "It is a pleasing fact that the University has now thrown open its doors to women.... It is difficult to exaggerate the important role medical women will play in China. To those who are acquainted with the susceptibilities of the average Chinese woman it is not strange that there should be such a widespread belief in the mission of the woman doctor in carrying the knowledge of scientific healing into the Chinese home."[12]

Although the pioneer Chinese women doctors were accepted by their male counterparts in the profession in Hong Kong, their experience with civil servants who determined the pay scale in government service was entirely different. The salary of Lai Po-chuen, who joined the government Medical and Health Services, illustrates gender discrimination in Hong Kong then. Although there appears to have been gender parity in pay for a short time in 1929, after the war female doctors and other female civil servants were paid about 80% of that of their male counterparts because of the recommendations of the 1947 Salaries Commission.[13] The rationale given was that a man needed to provide for his wife and children. This new policy was to be implemented in 1948, but two-thirds of the woman medical officers resigned in protest.[14] In contrast, in Britain, equal pay in civil service was accepted in principle after the Royal Commission on Equal Pay in 1946 and was phased in from 1955 for non-industrial workers.[15] The Hong Kong government did not follow suit. In 1959, another Salaries Commission revisited the issue in Hong Kong and maintained that woman civil servants should be paid at around 75% of the salary of their male counterparts. However, an exception was made for single female medical officers who had the same qualifications and worked similar hours as male doctors.[16] Married female medical officers would be employed as temporary staff since they were not considered "career" officers and paid 75% of the salaries of male officers.[17] The married female medical officers protested against such unfair treatment and formed an association to press their case. They took the case to the Secretary of State in Britain and caused a stir in Parliament.[18] Meanwhile, nurses, teachers, and other advocacy groups also petitioned the government for equal pay for women. The government finally agreed to implement a new policy of equal pay for female civil servants in phases with the year 1975 as the target endpoint.[19] For married female medical officers, the government agreed to start equal pay with male medical officers from 1 November 1969, but they were still employed as unpensionable staff with less vacation leave and fewer other fringe benefits.[20] Thus, after a decade of lobbying, married female medical officers still had not won the day. It would take another 10 years before they gained parity in salary and in fringe benefits with their male counterparts.[21]

Traditionally, most of the time men had their wives looking after their needs and their children at home so that they could concentrate on their work. A woman with a full-time job had the dual responsibility of her job and her family. It is difficult for women to combine a satisfactory family life and be able to devote themselves to their profession. At that time, women who took up the medical profession often had to sacrifice their personal life and happiness. Of the three pioneer female doctors in Hong Kong, only Alice Sibree was married. She did not have any children, which is usually the determining factor for a woman to give up her profession. Eva Ho Tung and Lai Po-chuen remained single. Eva waited for three years after she matriculated from Diocesan Girls' School before she was allowed into HKU. Having achieved their goal of becoming a doctor, it became much harder for them to give up their profession.

The first three female doctors in Hong Kong all specialized in obstetrics and gynecology and treated infants and children—specialties deemed socially acceptable for female doctors then. The work of these pioneer female doctors led to reduction in maternal and infant mortality, better trained midwives, and improved health of infants and children. They paved the way and set examples for future generations of women.

Alice Deborah Hickling (née Sibree) (1876–1928)

MBChB, LRCP, LRCS (Edin), LRFPS (Glas), MBE

Dr. Alice Deborah Sibree was a pioneer in maternal and infant health and changed the paradigm of maternal care in Hong Kong.

Sibree was born in 1876, daughter of the Rev. Dr. James Sibree, a missionary of the LMS in Madagascar. She received her medical education at the London School of Medicine for Women, and special training in obstetrics and gynecology at the Rotunda Lying-in Hospital in Dublin. After she became a licentiate of the Royal College of Physicians (LRCP) and the Royal College of Surgeons (LRCS), Edinburgh,[22] she joined the LMS. In 1904, she received instructions from the LMS to oversee the new Alice Memorial Maternity Hospital (AMMH) in Hong Kong.

In the nineteenth century, both infant mortality and maternal mortality were very high in Hong Kong.[23] At that time Chinese women would not see a Chinese male doctor let alone a foreign male doctor. Chinese women had their confinement at home carried out by traditional midwives (*wan pos*), who learned midwifery and deliveries from oral tradition and from attending childbirths with another *wan po*, who knew nothing about sepsis, one of the major causes of maternal deaths.[24] When the inquiry into high infant mortality in 1903 found that infection and malnutrition from poverty and lack of knowledge on feeding and hygiene were the underlying reasons, the government proposed education of mothers and training of midwives in Western methods of delivery. Since AMMH, which was built from donations of the Chinese elite in the community, was opening soon in 1904, the Colonial Administrator, Mr. Francis Henry May, later Governor, suggested training Chinese midwives to be carried out in this new hospital.[25]

When the LMS asked Dr. Ho Kai, who was responsible for raising funds to build the new confinement hospital, for more donations for the salary of a doctor for the hospital, Dr. Ho Kai and his friends insisted on having a woman doctor to care for Chinese women. This doctor should learn Cantonese—a dialect few foreigners could master readily—during the first year after arrival to be able to communicate with the locals. Unlike her male colleagues, Sibree became fluent in Cantonese within the first year. As a result, she was welcomed into the homes of rich and poor Chinese families alike to do her medical and missionary work.[26] She recommended formal training of midwives, which was a two-year course based on the British curriculum. The student midwives had to complete general nursing training before being admitted to this program. The first three student midwives she trained all passed the first government examination for midwives held in 1906 and received the certificate of qualification. As a result, the government began to send midwives to AMMH for training.[27] By 1907, three years into her contract, six trained midwives were employed by the CPD and government clinics, and she was appointed their supervisor. They attended 579 domiciliary confinements that year.[28]

Dr. Robert M. Gibson, Medical Superintendent of Alice Memorial Hospital and Nethersole Hospital, however, carried the prevailing sexist attitude of all male doctors at the time, that women should be nurses and not doctors.[29] He did not give Sibree any opportunity to attend general medical patients in Alice Memorial Hospital and outpatient clinics. Despite the difficulties with Gibson, Dr. Sibree's services were much sought after by Chinese women in the community.[30] Sibree initiated a health education program in the hospitals for mothers after delivery, on nutrition and general care of infants. At the end of her contract in 1909, she resigned from the LMS.[31]

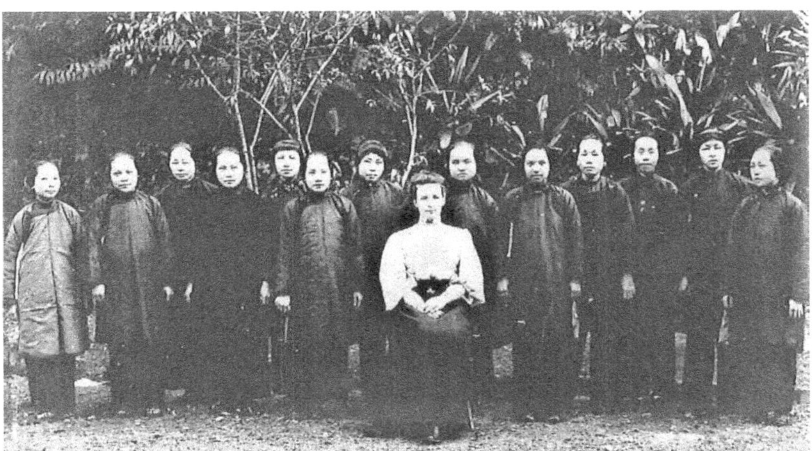

Figure 6.1 Dr. Alice Hickling and her student midwives, 1906
Image courtesy of Alice Ho Miu Ling Nethersole Charity Foundation

She returned to Hong Kong the following year, in 1910, and started her own private practice. She married Mr. C. C. Hickling, manager of Taikoo Sugar Refinery, and was known as Dr. Alice Hickling from then on. She proposed to the government that another maternity hospital be built in Hong Kong with midwifery training, as the six training places in AMMH were far from adequate. The proposal, however, was turned down because a nurses' training institute was being built next to the AMMH and Ho Miu Ling Hospital.[32] In 1914, Hickling was appointed to the Midwives Board.[33] As a member of the Midwives Board, she paid special attention to probation nurses and endeavored in every way to protect the interests of these young women, who, when qualified, had to compete with unqualified midwives in the colony.[34] She was reappointed Supervisor of Midwives in 1916. From 1918 to 1919, Dr. Hickling was Acting Medical Officer of Health[35] and was awarded an MBE in 1919 for her wartime services and received the decoration of Sister of the Order of St. John of Jerusalem.[36]

In 1919, Hickling worked with Dr. Tso Seen-wan, Chairman of Chinese Public Dispensary Committee, to convert the Eastern District Plague Hospital, which had hardly any plague patients, into a maternity hospital, Wan Chai Maternity Hospital. She became supervisor of the hospital at the invitation of Dr. Tso Seen-wan.[37] The hospital was an instant success, handling close to 200 patients during its first year. As discussed in Chapter 3, buoyed by the success of Wan Chai Maternity Hospital, the Chinese Public Dispensaries Committee asked the government to grant a piece of land for a larger venue in the more congested area of Sai Ying Pun, adjacent to the Western Chinese Public Dispensary.[38] The Registrar General enthusiastically supported this proposal, and after a successful fundraising campaign when Tso raised HK$20,000 from the local community, Tsan Yuk Hospital was built and opened on 17 October 1922 with a training school for midwives.[39] It had accommodation for 28 patients, and living quarters for nursing staff and six trainee midwives. All the hospital staff was Chinese except for Hickling, who was the supervisor. Tsan Yuk was the first hospital practicing Western medicine where the most senior staff—the doctor in charge, Dr. Chiu Hin-yeung, and the matron, Miss Leung Sheung-chi—were Chinese. By the end of its first year Tsan Yuk had handled 436 cases, and Wan Chai Maternity Hospital 814 cases, indicating that the Chinese community appreciated such services and that there was an increasing demand for them.[40] From 1923 to 1928, Hickling was Assistant Medical Officer in charge of all Chinese hospitals and CPD.[41]

Hickling established in Tsan Yuk an operating theater, a gynecology ward, and gynecology clinics. Because of her connection with Rotunda Hospital, she sent the matron, Miss Leung, to attend a course at Rotunda Hospital. On her return, Miss Leung reorganized Tsan Yuk and the teaching of midwifery, based on the principles at the Rotunda Hospital. The operating theater and labor ward were enlarged. The two smaller wards were changed into a waiting ward and a surgical ward. As a result, the number of admissions and operations in the hospital doubled.[42] It was due to Hickling's efforts that Professor Richard Tottenham, the founding professor of the Department of Obstetrics and Gynecology, transferred the department's clinical, teaching, and research activities to Tsan Yuk Hospital. Hickling placed 20 to 25 beds on the second floor of the hospital under the control of Tottenham, and obstetric cases occupied the first floor.[43] From 1926, medical students were able to do their obstetrical and gynecological clerkship in Tsan Yuk Hospital. As a result, the hospital became not only the training center for midwives but also for medical students and trainees in obstetrics and gynecology; in fact, the hospital was the cradle of all specialists in this discipline in Hong Kong. Its low maternal mortality set a benchmark for other maternity units in Hong Kong.

Hickling not only pioneered in women's medicine in Hong Kong but also founded the first "baby clinic" in Tsan Yuk Hospital, which was the forerunner of the Maternal and Child Health Center, to care for babies up to two years of age. Later, infant care centers were established at other maternity hospitals or hospitals with maternity units such as AMMH. Later, infant healthcare centers were formed outside hospitals in different districts in Hong Kong and Kowloon. In these centers, babies were weighed, given smallpox vaccination and anti-cholera inoculation, and mothers received health education.[44]

Dr. Alice Hickling died in Hong Kong in September 1928. In commemoration of her 25 years of service to education and medical and health of women and infants, a portrait was presented by the staff of past and present nurses of Tsan Yuk Hospital to be hung in the Nurses Dining Room in the hospital and unveiled by Lady Clementi in the presence of Dr. Tso Seen-wan and many dignitaries of Hong Kong in December 1929.[45]

Dr. Alice Hickling brought Western medicine and popularized it among Chinese women. She was also responsible for the training of generations of midwives, and established Tsan Yuk Hospital as a center where medical students and specialists in obstetrics and gynecology received training in Hong Kong. Professor Tottenham once said, "Dr. Hickling had the great gift of being able to get things done, a quality that is particularly rare in this Colony." Professor Gordon King believed that Tsan Yuk Hospital owed its existence to her: "I often think that the very existence of the Tsan Yuk Hospital is her true memorial." In the spirit of a true missionary, her tombstone bears the simple inscription:[46]

In loving memory of Alice D. Hickling

Born Nov. 18, 1876
Died Sept. 22, 1928

Jesus said:

"Let us go over unto the other side."

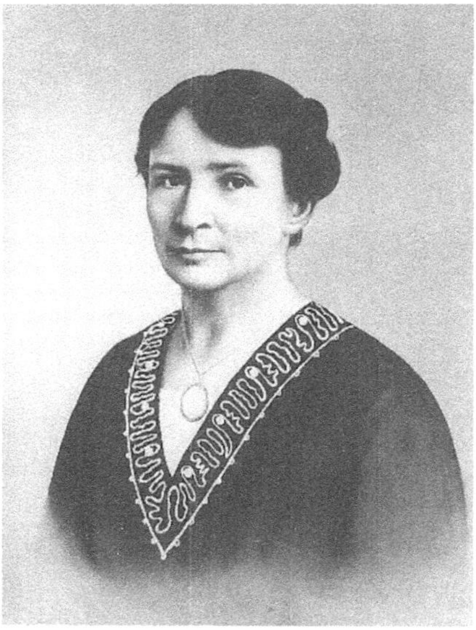

Figure 6.2 Portrait of Dr. Alice Hickling (née Sibree)
Source: HKMMS, reproduced with permission

Eva Ho Tung 何綺華 (1903–1993)

MBBS, LM, DTMH, DGO, MRCPI

Dr. Eva Ho Tung, born in July 1903, was the fourth daughter of Sir Robert and Clara Ho Tung. Sir Robert, a very successful businessman and philanthropist, was the first Chinese[47] to be allowed to live at the Peak. Although the family was living there, Eva was not permitted to enter the British school there. She received home education at first and in 1914, enrolled in Diocesan Girls' School at Kowloon. An excellent student, she won the Sir Frederick Lugard Scholarship after two years at DGS. She and her sister Irene, both passed the Senior Local Examination (matriculation examination at HKU) in 1918 but had to wait until the academic year 1921/1922 before they were permitted entry to HKU, as discussed.[48]

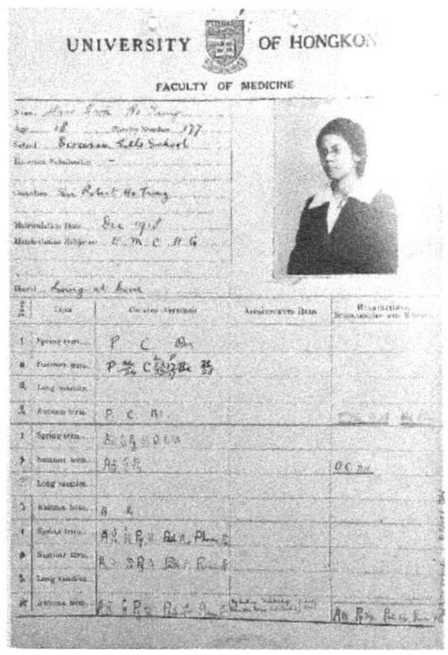

Figure 6.3 Student record at HKU of Eva Ho Tung
Image courtesy of University Archives, the University of Hong Kong

Eva Ho was admitted to the Faculty of Medicine, HKU, in the spring term of 1922. Although she was one term behind Lai Po-chuen (see below), she emerged as the first female medical graduate of HKU. A dedicated student, she was awarded half value (shared with another student) of both the Ng Li Hing and Chan Kai Ming scholarships for her stellar performance in anatomy and physiology during the third-year examinations.[49] She was also the only candidate who passed all the subjects in one sitting at the final MBBS examination. In December 1926 diet, the passing rate for part 1 of the final examination (surgery, obstetrics, and gynecology) was only 45.5% and it was even lower (28.6%) for part 2 (medicine and pathology).[50] The first female graduate in medicine from HKU, not surprisingly, drew the attention of the news media.[51]

Before World War II, medical graduates were not required to do internship before registration. Most graduates went directly into employment or into private practice. Only a few with academic aspiration were invited to join the university departments as House Physician or

House Surgeon. Eva Ho Tung chose to pursue her postgraduate studies in Britain. In her company was her sister Irene and Dr. Yeo Kok-cheang (Chapter 8), who had graduated in 1925. In London, both Eva Ho Tung and Yeo Kok-cheang obtained their Diploma in Tropical Medicine and Hygiene in 1928.[52] After this, she left for Dublin to continue her training in obstetrics and gynecology at the Rotunda Hospital and obtained the Diploma in Gynecology and Obstetrics (DGO).[53] *Caduceus* proudly reported that she was the first Chinese to obtain the MRCP (Ireland) qualification.[54] She then went to Vienna for further training in obstetrics before returning to London. It is unclear when she returned to Hong Kong, but there is a record that she joined the Department of Obstetrics and Gynecology in 1935.[55]

When Professor William Nixon founded the Eugenics League in 1936, Eva Ho Tung was invited to join the Executive Committee and the Medical Subcommittee of the league.[56] In April 1937, she was promoted to First Assistant to the professor of the department.[57] When Guangzhou fell to the Japanese in October 1938, she resigned to take part in war efforts against the Japanese in China, as did other medical graduates from HKU. She became a member of the China Defence League, which was started by Madame Soong Ching-ling, widow of Dr. Sun Yat-sen, and worked tirelessly for the organization in Hong Kong.[58] However, she preferred activities related to her profession, so later that year she left for Kweiyang (Guiyang) to join the Medical Relief Corps of the Chinese Red Cross under Dr. Robert Lim, a physiology professor at Peking Union Medical College.[59] She commanded a field unit to provide medical care and to perform anti-epidemic work.[60] In December 1941, she returned to celebrate her father's eightieth birthday. The Japanese attacked Hong Kong a few days after the celebration and prevented her return to Free China. For the brief period in Hong Kong, she volunteered at University Relief Hospital, which was under the charge of Professor Gordon King.[61] But she managed to escape into Free China and served her country until the end of the war. It must have required tremendous courage and utter devotion to treat the injured in the war zone for over four years—a very long time for a man, let alone for a woman.

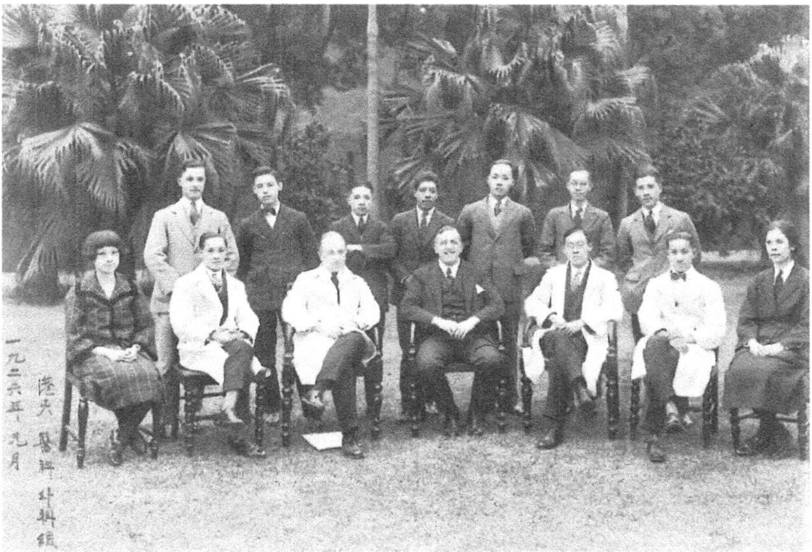

Figure 6.4 Dr. Eva Ho Tung (sitting, far right) and Dr. Lai Po-chuen (sitting, first left) with Professor K. H. Digby (sitting, center) during their surgical clerkship, 1926

Source: HKMMS, reproduced with permission, photograph was donated by the family of Dr. Ko King-fan

When she returned to Hong Kong after the war, she started her own practice in obstetrics and gynecology in Central District[62] and admitted her patients to Hong Kong Sanatorium and Hospital. Her practice was highly successful. In 1960, she was so busy that her health deteriorated. She closed her practice and moved to New York. After working for a while as a medical statistician, she retired.[63] She died in New York in 1993, at the age of 90.

She is remembered by her siblings and friends as a brilliant scholar, a courageous patriot, and a highly successful obstetrician.

Lai Po-chuen, Pauline 賴寶川 (1903–?)

OBE, MBBS

Unlike Eva Ho Tung, Dr. Lai Po-chuen was brought up in an ordinary family. Her father, a storekeeper of the Public Works Department, enabled the family to live in the government quarters in Wanchai.[64] She studied at Italian Convent School (known as Sacred Heart Canossian College today) and matriculated in 1921.[65] She entered HKU in the autumn term of 1921 at the age of 18—the first female medical student at HKU.[66]

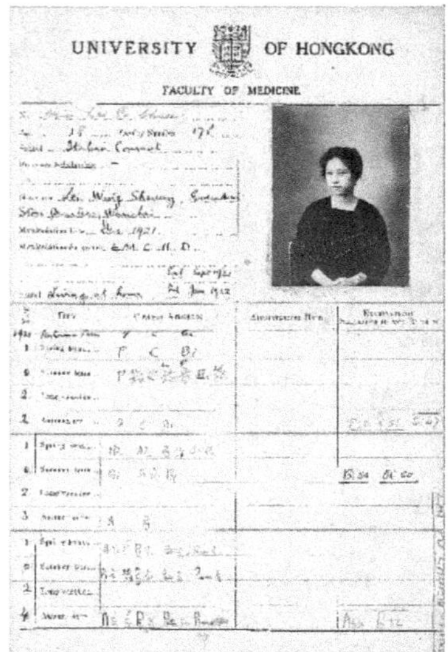
UNIVERSITY OF HONGKONG

FACULTY OF MEDICINE

Figure 6.5 Student record at HKU of Lai Po-chuen

Image courtesy of University Archives, the University of Hong Kong

Lai was a less brilliant student than Eva Ho Tung was. She had to take supplementary examinations in some subjects. For some reason (maybe ill health) she was absent from part 2 of her final examination in the summer of 1927 but was successful in passing both parts at the December diet that year.[67]

Lai joined the Government Medical Department as a Chinese Medical Officer on 1 June 1928. Her immediate posting was assistant to Dr. Alice Hickling, Assistant Medical Officer in charge of Chinese Hospitals and Chinese Public Dispensaries.[68] Lai likely worked at Tsan Yuk Hospital which belonged to the CPD system and received her postgraduate training there.[69] There was disparity in salary between gender and race. Her annual salary was only HK$1,800 in 1928.[70] Dr. Yeo Kok-cheang, who graduated in 1925 and was appointed Chinese Health Officer in December 1928 after overseas studies, received an annual salary of HK$3,420 because of his diploma, his seniority and was employed as an expatriate from England. However, in 1929, Lai's salary was adjusted to the same level as Yeo's even though Yeo was two years her senior and had a higher qualification. This was most unusual as, after the war, gender disparity in salary returned as Lai's salary was only about 75% of her male counterpart. There was also racial discrimination too. Dr. Agnes Dovey, a European officer, who was appointed Visiting Assistant Medical Officer to Chinese Hospital and Dispensary the same year, earned a much higher annual salary of HK$6,000.[71]

Lai, as a woman doctor, was posted at Tsan Yuk Hospital, which was also a teaching hospital of HKU. Based on her clinical work at Tsan Yuk Hospital, she co-authored a paper on the use of colonic ether as anesthetic agent for labor and gynecological operation in 1928.[72] She worked in Tsan Yuk Hospital until 1933.[73]

In 1939, Lai was appointed Secretary of the Midwives Board and Supervisor of Midwives and simultaneously Health Officer and Inspector of Schools.[74] The Midwives Board was created by the Midwives Ordinance 1910 to oversee the training and examination of midwives, their registration, and practices.[75] The Supervisor of Midwives was responsible for overseeing government midwives working in the dispensaries. This included inspection of their bags, records, quarters, and investigation of cases with puerperium complications and infant deaths.[76] Lai's obstetrical training in Tsan Yuk Hospital had prepared her well for such duties. Before World War II, the school health program had two parts: medical examination of school children and inspection of school environment, lighting, ventilation, space, and sanitation.[77] Lai was responsible for the medical examinations of school children.

Apart from her work in the Medical Department, Lai was active in voluntary organizations. The Anti-Tuberculosis Association was formed in 1940 with Dr. Selwyn-Clarke as its president. Lai was a member of the Council of the Anti-Tuberculosis Association, which was chaired by Mr. Lo Man-kam.[78] She was also an active member of the St. John Ambulance Association and Brigade as early as 1930 and gave lectures on home nursing in the Chinese Nursing Division of the Association.[79] She staffed a first aid post at Victoria Hospital for Women and Children on Barker Road during the Battle of Hong Kong. The hospital was directly hit by Japanese bombs. Her bravery was praised in a report of St. John Ambulance on the war time activities.[80] As Lady Divisional Surgeon, she was awarded Serving Sisters of the Most Venerable Order of Hospital of St. John of Jerusalem in 1946.[81]

After the capitulation of Hong Kong to the Japanese on Christmas Day 1941, Lai stayed on to help the humanitarian work organized by Dr. Selwyn-Clarke, who was Director of Medical Department before the war.

This included taking care of the dependents of internees or servicemen who died during the war and supplying necessary drugs and food items to the camps,[82] as well as the anti-tuberculosis work in two wards of French Hospital.[83] When Dr. Selwyn-Clarke was incarcerated, she carried on the humanitarian work in a clandestine manner with considerable risk to herself. For her invaluable work during the war time, she was awarded an OBE in 1946.[84]

After the war, Lai resumed duties as government medical officer in September 1945 and was in charge of Wanchai Health Center.[85] Established in 1932, the Wanchai Health Cente on Lockhart Road [86] housed the first of five government infant welfare centers or "baby clinics," which aimed at decreasing the high infant mortality rate. The Wanchai "Baby Clinic" proved highly popular and soon became overcrowded. It inspired two other baby clinics to be built: Lady Ho Tung Infant Welfare Center in Fanling in 1934, and Violet Peel Infant Welfare Center in Wanchai built by donations from the Chinese community in 1935.[87] Two other baby clinics were also founded in Kowloon and Sai Ying Pun before the war.[88]

Lai oversaw both the Infant Welfare Centers and the School Health Program in 1946.[89] In 1947, she was promoted to Lady Medical Officer, a post previously reserved for Europeans but opened to local Chinese after the war.[90] Lai left government service for private practice after two more years. In 1964, the Infant Welfare Centers were renamed Maternal and Child Health Centers to reflect the true nature of their work which included prenatal, neonatal, and gynecological problems of mothers, along with teaching mothers about caring for babies up to two years of age.[91]

It is unclear when Lai retired from private practice. In 1969, her practice was located at 796 Nathan Road.[92] Her younger sister, Lai Po-kan, who won the British Boxer Indemnity Scholarship in 1936 to study at Oxford, returned to Hong Kong in 1998 to take care of her.[93] Lai died shortly afterwards.

When Lai left the civil service in 1949, there were three other women medical officers and one assistant woman medical officer in the Government Medical Department. The starting salary for female medical officers was HK$860 per month while their male counterparts was HK$1,060. Female doctors were also at a disadvantage in career advancement. They were usually assigned to maternal and child, and school services, positions with limited prospect for promotion. Lai and Yeo Kok-cheang entered government service in the same year. Yeo was promoted to senior grade in 1939, after 11 years of service. In 1947, Yeo was promoted again to Deputy Director of Health Services,[94] and in 1952 he became the first Chinese to head the Medical Department. On the other hand, it was not until 1947, after about two decades in government service, that Lai Po-chuen became Medical Officer of School and Child Health.

Unlike pioneer woman doctors in nineteenth century England and the US, female pioneer doctors in Hong Kong seemed to be well accepted by their male colleagues. Dr. Eva Ho Tung moved up the academic ladder to be first assistant to the professor. But, in prewar Hong Kong, professorship was basically a European reserve. After World War II, people's attitude changed. Professor Daphne Chun was appointed to Chair of Obstetrics and Gynecology of the Faculty of Medicine, HKU, in 1957 despite some opposition.[95] But the issue of racial and gender discrimination in pay was not resolved until the 1970s while gender discrimination in education and in employment remained much longer.

In the twenty-first century, there are more women admitted to medical schools, and there are now even women doctors working in specialties such as surgery, including orthopedic, neurosurgery, or cardiac surgery, which used to be the domain of male doctors. No doubt, female doctors are in the mainstream now in the Western world.

7. The Wartime Heroes
Making a Difficult Choice in the Face of Adversity

The Japanese Army finally attacked Hong Kong on 8 December 1941, after halting its southern march for two years at the border at Shenzhen. After 17 days of ferocious fighting, Hong Kong surrendered and became an occupied territory until the end of war in August 1945. The war and Japanese Occupation shattered the medical and health infrastructure of the colony. But Hong Kong had been affected much earlier, when Japan invaded and occupied Manchuria in 1931 and then annexed more land in northern China in the 1930s. One of the most obvious effects was the influx of refugees from the mainland. The population in Hong Kong was around 850,000 in 1931, rising to around 1.82 million in 1941. The climb in population was particularly steep after China declared war on Japan in 1937. As the Japanese Army swept southward taking over the coastal areas, it brought a surge of about 740,000 refugees to Hong Kong. This massive influx overwhelmed the already congested housing, resulting in more overcrowded and unsanitary living conditions. The deterioration in housing aggravated existing diseases such as tuberculosis and other respiratory infections. As well, the refugees brought in cholera and smallpox, posing a serious threat of epidemics of these diseases in the colony.

In the late 1930s, the medical and health services in Hong Kong were relatively well developed. The medical establishment, consisting of hospitals and clinics provided by the government and charitable organizations, was traditionally concentrated more on Hong Kong Island, as it was acquired first as a colony in 1842, whereas Kowloon was ceded in 1860 and the New Territories leased in 1898. The population in Kowloon had been rising rapidly since the turn of the century, reaching 120,000 in 1921. A new hospital, Kowloon Hospital, was opened in 1925 to serve the population in Kowloon and the New Territories. The influx of immigrants and refugees in the 1930s further increased the population in Kowloon to a remarkable level at 400,000 in 1940. Although the new state-of-the art

Queen Mary Hospital was completed in 1937, it did not help the marked increase in population between 1938 and 1941. The whole medical system was bursting at the seams.

After Hong Kong surrendered to the Japanese, those who took part in the resistance became prisoners of war (POWs) and interned at Sham Shui Po Camp and Argyle Street Camp. Surprised to find so many foreign civilians in Hong Kong, the Japanese initially did not know what to do with them. In early January 1942, the Japanese rounded up all foreign civilians who could be found, around 1,000, and assembled them at the parade ground, now Cheung Kong Center. They were then taken to several old hotels located along the waterfront of Des Voeux Road Central, where they were accommodated in filthy conditions, up to 10 in a room, for 15 days until the Japanese authorities decided to place all of them in Stanley Internment Camp.[1] There were, however, exceptions.

Three British physicians, who followed their conscience, chose different routes. Dr. Percy Selwyn Selwyn-Clarke, Director of Medical Services of the British colonial administration, felt that he would be more useful outside the camp. He obtained permission from the Colonial Secretary, Mr. F. C. Gimson, to work with the Japanese, to safeguard public health and sanitary conditions in Hong Kong and to secure the scarce food and medication supply to the civilian internees and POWs until he was arrested by the Japanese, on suspicion he was a spy.[2] Dr. Lindsay Ride did not agree with Dr. Selwyn-Clarke. He and three others escaped from Sham Shiu Po Camp in January 1942 on a sampan to the mainland and encouraged others to do so.[3] Dr. Gordon King remained outside to take care of patients in University Relief Hospital on the campus. He secretly left for Free China just before he was interned at Stanley Camp.[4]

All three of them served differently, and all contributed to war efforts and to the people in Hong Kong. They could be considered our "wartime heroes," and their stories are presented in this chapter.

Percy Selwyn Selwyn-Clarke 司徒永覺 (1897–1976)

KBE, CMG, MC, C St J, MD, BS, FRCP, MRCS, DPH, DTM&H, Bar.-at-Law

Sir Percy Selwyn Selwyn-Clarke was born in 1897 in London with the name Percy Seibourne Clarke. He graduated from St. Bartholomew Hospital Medical School in 1916 and joined the army as a medical officer during World War I. He changed his name by deed poll to Selwyn Selwyn-Clarke because there were too many Clarkes in his division. After World War I, he entered Colonial Medical Service and was posted to West African Medical Service in Gold Coast in October 1919, marking the beginning of his lifetime service in public health. He took leave in 1923 to study law in London and was called to the bar on 28 January 1929, even though he never practiced law. On his return to Gold Coast, he was promoted to Senior Health Officer in 1924 and Assistant Director of Health in 1929. Between 1930 and 1932, he was seconded to Malaya as Chief Health Officer. He then returned as Assistant Director of Medical Service and the Gold Coast Central Council Branch of the British Red Cross Society. In 1935, he married Hilda Alice Browning before leaving for his next posting to Nigeria the following year. They returned to England for the birth of their only child, Mary, in September 1936.[5]

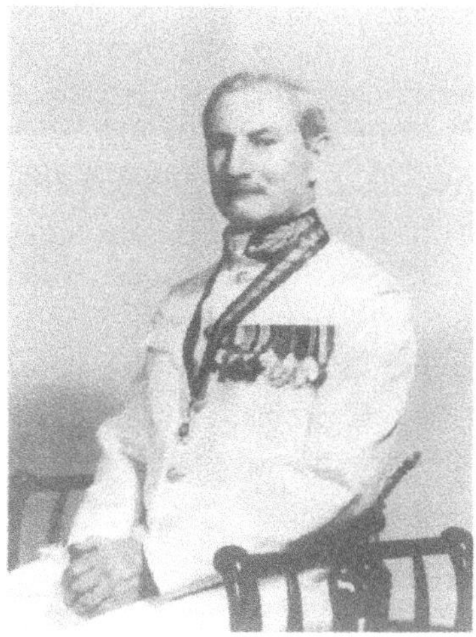

Figure 7.1 Dr. Percy Selwyn Selwyn-Clarke

Source: Mervyn Horder, "The Hard Boiled Saint: Selwyn-Clarke in Hong Kong," *BMJ*, 1995 Aug 19; 311 (7003): 492, via National Library of Medicine, National Institutes of Health, US, accessed on 2 February 2024, https://www.ncbi.nlm.nih.gov/pmc/articles/PMC2550548/?page=1.

When Dr. Selwyn-Clarke arrived in Hong Kong in March 1938 to head the Medical Department, he faced a number of challenges. In his speech to the Legislative Council on 13 October 1938, Governor Sir Geoffry Northcote highlighted four main issues facing Hong Kong: malnutrition, crowded unsanitary housing, inadequate infant welfare, and the threat of infectious diseases such as smallpox and cholera. These issues were, of course, interrelated and needed to be tackled to prevent the major prevalent infectious diseases. All these, however, were the result of the massive influx of refugees to Hong Kong.[6] In addition, the Medical Department was tasked to review and improve the hospital system.[7]

Dr. Selwyn-Clarke chaired the Technical Committee for the Reorganization and Improvement of Official Hospital and Clinical Facilities. At that time, the local medical facilities had been inundated by this sudden influx of people. He observed that in Tung Wa hospital: ".... it was a common sight for patients to be nursed on the floor and veranda of hospital wards and over a third shared beds with other patients."[8] Although the committee was asked to look into use of public hospitals, it actually reviewed the whole healthcare infrastructure including hospital, clinics, and laboratories provided by both government and non-government sectors. The recommendations were ambitious: more hospitals, polyclinics, and laboratories to be built, financial resources permitting. The proposed new hospital to serve the needs of the large population in Kowloon and other improvements did not happen until decades after World War II.

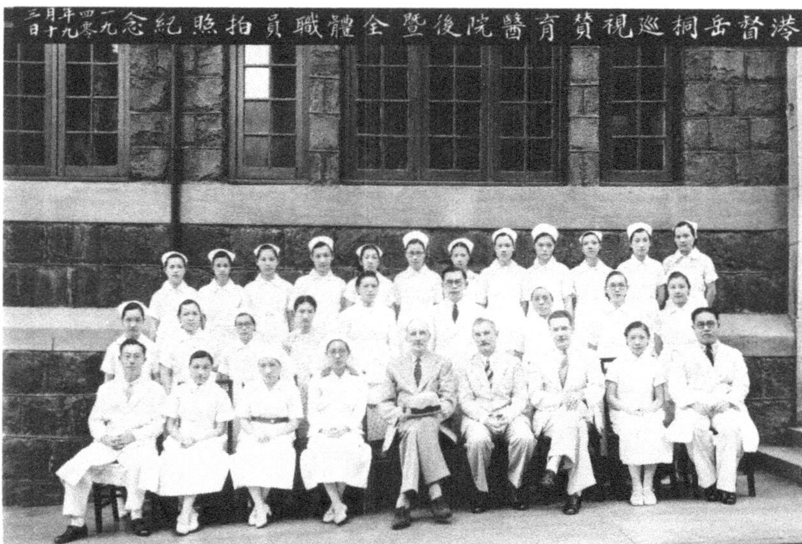
港督岳桐巡視贊育醫院後暨全體職員拍照紀念
一九四零年九月十三日

Figure 7.2 Dr. Selwyn-Clarke (front, R4), Dr. Gordan King (front, R3), Acting Governor Norton (sitting, center) and staff of Tsan Yuk Hospital in front of Old Tsan Yuk Hospital, 1940

Source: HKMMS, reproduced with permission, photograph donated by Professor Gordon King

Meanwhile, Dr. Selwyn-Clarke tackled the widespread problem of tuberculosis and beriberi. He became the founding president of the Hong Kong Anti-Tuberculosis Association in 1940, an important voluntary organization to combat the scourge. The association ran education campaigns for the public, such as anti-spitting, and raised funds to operate TB clinics and to build a sanatorium.[9] Mr. Lo Man-kam, Senior Chinese Member of the Legislative Council, commented that "it was due to his (Selwyn-Clarke) ... fervour, zeal, the indomitable spirit of persistence and insistence ... before any real or substantial progress could be made."[10] In addition to deficiency diseases, poor nutrition also increased the prevalence of tuberculosis. Selwyn-Clarke tried to lower the price of food so that the poor could afford better nutrition. For example, he created the Equitable Rice Sales Committee to control price of rice and to promote consumption of "red rice" to prevent beriberi.[11] In public education materials including film shows he emphasized soya bean as a good source of inexpensive and valuable protein.[12]

After the fall of Guangzhou, the Japanese Army continued to march south. Since Japan was not at war with Britain, its army paused at the border at Shenzhen. The British government, in preparation for possible invasion by Japanese troops, ordered the Hong Kong government to organize its own defence with a target of surviving a siege of 130 days. So, in addition to maintaining the daily operation of the Medical and Health Services, Selwyn-Clarke transformed the existing hospitals into casualty clearing hospitals. He also created relief hospitals and about 20 first-aid posts in places like schools.[13] Meanwhile, he prepared enough drugs and medical supplies that could last 130 days of siege. He included soya beans in food stores against the protests of his Chinese colleagues, who did not understand its value.[14] By July 1940, the government ordered the evacuation of British women and children from Hong Kong, believing that war was imminent.

On 8 December 1941, the long-dreaded invasion of Hong Kong by Japan began simultaneously as it bombed Pearl Harbour. After 17 days of fierce resistance by the British Army and the Hong Kong Voluntary Defence Corps, the Hong Kong government surrendered on Christmas Day. Throughout the battle, Selwyn-Clarke moved between hospitals, first-aid posts, and areas of heavy casualties. In the immediate aftermath of the surrender, there was no water or electricity because the water mains and power stations were hit and destroyed in a number of areas.

Accumulation of refuse and human waste that had not been collected created serious threats to public health.[15] Selwyn-Clarke did something unusual. After seeking the consent of the Colonial Secretary Mr. F. C. Gimson, who was already interned,[16] Selwyn-Clarke proposed to the Japanese military government to allow him to stay on so that he could direct his staff to maintain the essential services to prevent epidemics and to lessen suffering. For fear of infectious diseases outbreaks, the Japanese authorities agreed reluctantly and appointed him as "adviser."

Selwyn-Clarke negotiated with Japanese authorities to keep the hospitals open. He helped secure food and drugs for these hospitals even when the Japanese gradually took over supervision. He also opened two TB wards in the French hospital. In autumn of 1942, he was able to persuade the Japanese to reopen many of the public dispensaries.[17] In the meantime, he was running the necessary sanitary services with only a skeleton staff for collecting and disposing of refuse and human waste, burying the dead, and securing a clean water supply.

He took it upon himself to look after those interned in civilian and POW camps and their dependents outside who had no support. An informal welfare committee was formed, and with donations from people he was able to provide additional food and medical supplies to those interned. When diphtheria broke out in the Sham Shui Po POW camp, he was able to "smuggle" some anti-toxin to the camp doctors and saved a few lives.[18] His humanitarian work and its network drew the attention of the Kempeitai, the military police arm of the Imperial Japanese Army that also served as a secret police force. Selwyn-Clarke was arrested in May 1943 for alleged spying activities, interrogated, and tortured. This left him with permanent injuries to the spine and left leg, and he had to walk with aid afterwards. On 8 December 1944 he was released from Stanley Prison to Ma Tau Wai Camp, where he stayed until the Japanese surrender in August 1945.

After his arrest, the supply network that Selwyn-Clarke set up continued to function with the help of volunteers like Dr. Lai Po-chuen, a former Chinese Lady Medical Officer.[19] His relief work had a great effect on many people. Mothers of babies and small children, in or outside the camp, were particularly grateful to him for the supply of milk and other foods.[20] His resourcefulness and kindness earned him the name "hard-boiled saint" from his supporters.[21]

When the Japanese surrendered, Selwyn-Clarke left Ma Tau Wai Camp immediately and called back all the old staff to resume providing sanitary services as soon as possible, to prevent epidemics. Under his leadership, the Medical Department was restored soon after the British resumed control of the government. Despite his ordeal under the Japanese Kempeitai, he refused to act as a witness in the War Crimes Tribunal.[22] A true humanitarian, he was known to use his own money to buy each Japanese POW under his supervision a toothbrush. In 1947, he left Hong Kong to become the Governor of Seychelles. He was the first officer in medicine to be promoted to governorship by the Colonial Office.[23] At the farewell party given by Tung Wa Group of Hospitals, the Chairman of the Hospital Board said: "It owes much to his wise guidance that the Tung Wa Group of Hospitals has developed to be a well-organised and modern-equipped institution on scientific basis."[24] When the new nurses' quarter of Kwong Wah Hospital was opened in 1952, it was named after him to commemorate his guidance given to the Tung Wah Medical Committee during his time as Head of the Medical Department.[25]

As Governor of Seychelles, Selwyn-Clarke introduced progressive reforms and was dubbed "socialist governor" by people who were more conservative. Knighted in 1951, Sir Percy Selwyn Selwyn-Clarke returned to England and worked as Principal Medical Officer of the Ministry of Health for another five years before retirement. But he continued to be active in medical and other organizations as a volunteer afterwards.[26] He died in 1976, and a memorial service was held at St. John's Cathedral.[27]

Sir Percy Selwyne Selwyn-Clarke deserves our respect and admiration for working with the Japanese after Hong Kong surrendered in 1941, at the risk of implicating himself as a collaborator with the enemy. His selfless action also led to his imprisonment, torture, and permanent disability.

Lindsay Tasman Ride 賴廉士 (1898–1977)

CBE Mil, ED, MD, MRCS, LRCP, Hon LLD Toronto, Melbourne, London, HK

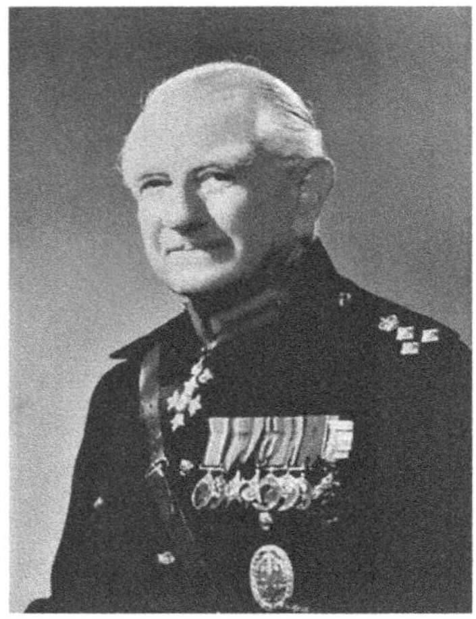

Figure 7.3 Professor Sir Lindsay Ride, Dean, Faculty of Medicine, 1930–1932; 1935–1939; 1939, Vice-Chancellor of HKU, 1949–1964

Image courtesy of Elizabeth Ride Archive

Professor Sir Lindsay Ride was born in Australia in 1898 into a Presbyterian family, and his father was a missionary. He was awarded a scholarship to Scotch College, Melbourne, where he discovered his talent in sports. In 1917, he enlisted in the Australian Imperial Force, and fought on the Western Front in World War I in early 1918. He was discharged in 1919, after being wounded on two occasions. After the war, he started medical studies at the University of Melbourne. Elected as a Rhodes Scholar in 1922, he continued his studies in England. At New College, Oxford, he obtained a BA in Physiology in 1924, and an MA and a BMBCh in 1927, while excelling in various sports such as rowing, cricket, and rugby. After clinical training at Guy's Hospital, Ride became a MRCS and a LRCP in England.[28] As a junior registrar of Sir Charles Sherrington, who later won the Nobel Prize in physiology, Ride was initiated into the world of medical research.[29]

Ride was appointed Professor of Physiology at HKU in 1928, at the age of 30. He succeeded Professor H. G. Earle, who joined the newly established Lester Institute in Shanghai. Genetics was Ride's main research interest. In the early 1930s, he received a grant from the Rockefeller Foundation for genetics research in Borneo. In 1936, he was awarded Doctor of Medicine from Oxford University and the title of his thesis was "The Relation of Human Genetics to Clinical Medicine." Two years later, he published a textbook in Bristol, England, entitled *Genetics and the Clinician*, based on his thesis. At HKU, he collaborated with clinical colleagues in studies of cholera[30] and beriberi in pregnancy.[31] For many years, Ride was the editor of *Caduceus*, the academic journal of the HKU Medical Society, and published frequently in this journal and in international ones.

He held the deanship in 1930–1932 and 1935–1939, when the Faculty of Medicine, HKU, was considered a small but important center for medical research in China.[32] He believed that in order to stay competitive in China and in East Asia, it was important for the HKU Medical Faculty to develop postgraduate training and to set up a department of public health.[33] However, at that time there was a debate on the position of the university and the Faculty of Medicine because the university was in financial trouble again. In 1911, Governor Lugard inaugurated HKU as a university for Hong Kong and China, but in the 1930s, students from the mainland were dwindling because a number of universities had been founded in China. However, there were many students from other regions in East Asia, such as Straits Settlements, Federated Malay States, Thailand, and Indonesia, attending HKU. Most people in Hong Kong were concerned with Governor Lugard's wider aims of the university and opposed further subsidies to the university on the ground that Hong Kong had no need of such an expensive establishment.[34] Ride, like Governor Lugard, had long advocated that the university open its doors to China and other areas in East Asia, so that these countries could be exposed to British culture. Thus, the medical school should embrace a wider calling instead of decreasing the budget and reducing the output of graduates.[35] In the same vein, he also argued for more funding to support research in the university to make it more competitive and be worthy of its name.

A soldier at heart, in 1931, Ride joined the Hong Kong Volunteer Defence Corps as Chief Medical Officer at first a lieutenant, but he rose rapidly in rank. In 1941, he was appointed Commandant of the Field Ambulance Unit during the Battle of Hong Kong and had many medical students serving under him. The unit under his command was praised for its success in carrying about 75% of the seriously wounded to hospitals.[36] After Hong Kong capitulated on Christmas Day 1941, Ride was sent to the POW camp at Sham Shui Po. The living conditions in the camp were appalling, and there was not much he could do under the Japanese. Unlike Dr. Selwyn-Clarke, who chose to stay outside the camp to help maintain public health services, Ride called on the internees to escape to aid the war effort. He and three others were successful in escaping to Free China on 9 January 1942. In July 1942, he smuggled a letter to Sloss, Vice-Chancellor of HKU, and internees in Stanley, in which he wrote: "Every doctor available should come and leave the camp medical work to Japanese helpers like our friend Percy."[37] Percy was obviously Selwyn-Clarke, whose action he disapproved of.

Once in Free China, Ride obtained permission from the British military authority, MI9, to create the British Army Aid Group (BAAG) under his command to aid in the liberation of Hong Kong. One of the specific tasks of BAAG was to aid allied personnel (POWs, civilian internees, and pilots who were forced to land) to escape or evade the Japanese. It was estimated that at least 800 Chinese political figures, non-Chinese soldiers, and civilians, and around 100 British, American Air Force personnel, and Indian soldiers were escorted to Free China.[38] BAAG helped people who stayed in Hong Kong by smuggling the much-needed medicine and food supplies to them. The second important role of BAAG was to gather military information to aid the war efforts in South China. BAAG had the cooperation of the East River Column, which was organized by the Chinese Communist Party, and other guerrilla groups to maintain an open route where its agents could gather and disseminate information. Although BAAG was disbanded in December 1945,[39] Ride's association with the military continued after the war, and he was appointed Commandant of the Hong Kong Volunteer Defence Force. For his war efforts, he was awarded a Commander of the Order of the British Empire (CBE MIL) in 1944 and Efficiency Decoration (ED) in 1948.

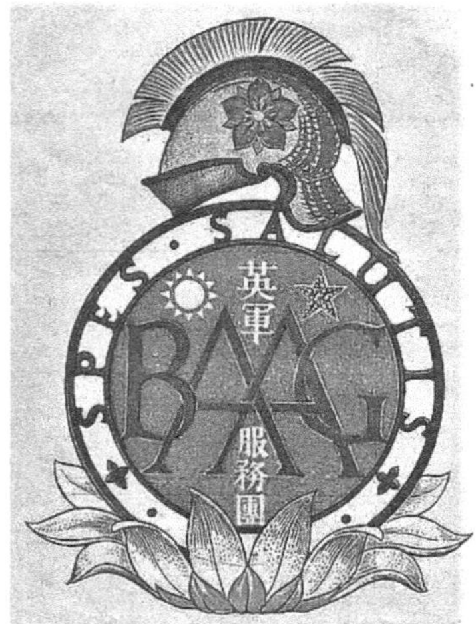

Figure 7.4a BAAG Crest

Source: Elizabeth Ride Archive at https://www.elizabethridearchive.com/, photos reproduced with permission

After the war, Ride helped restore HKU and became its Vice-Chancellor in 1949, to succeed Dr. Duncan Sloss. During his administration (1949–1964), the university grew, trebling the number of students, and 22 new buildings were added. In the Faculty of Medicine, in 1958, a new Pathology Building was opened next to Queen Mary Hospital. In 1964, the preclinical departments were moved from the main campus to the new Li Shu Fan Building on Sassoon Road. His other achievements included the addition of the following new structures: the School of Architecture, the Department for Extramural Studies, the Student and

Staff Health Service, and the University Press. He had laid the foundation for a much larger university by the time of his retirement.[40] As a renowned university educator, honorary degrees of LLD were conferred on him by the universities of Hong Kong, London, and Toronto. He became a Knight Bachelor in 1962 for his public services.

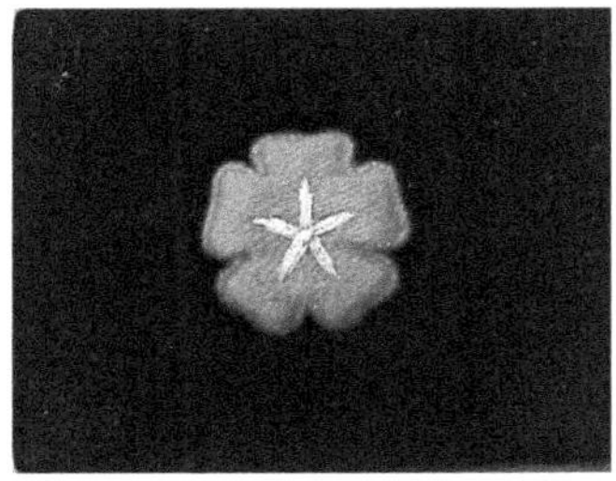

Figure 7.4b BAAG Shoulder Patch

Source: Elizabeth Ride Archive at https://www.elizabethridearchive.com/, photos reproduced with permission

Professor Sir Lindsay Tasman Ride remained in Hong Kong after retirement in 1964 to pursue his other interests. As a historian, he contributed to the scholarship of early missionaries in China, including Robert Morrison and James Legge. Ride and his wife spent many hours restoring and researching the history of the Protestant Cemetery in Macau. Ride was also was a staunch supporter of the Hong Kong Branch of the Royal Asiatic Society and served as its president for a number of years. The society has a Sir Lindsay and Lady Ride Memorial Fund, which subsidizes the publication of serious works on Hong Kong history, society, and culture which would otherwise not be possible, as they are usually not commercially viable.[41] A music lover, Ride was President of the Hong Kong Singers and Chairman of the Hong Kong Musical Society for many years. He had been a good sportsman from high school and represented Hong Kong in rugby and cricket. It is befitting that there is a Lindsay Ride Sport Center at the University campus in his memory. He died in Hong Kong on 17 October 1977 and was survived by his wife and four children from his first marriage.

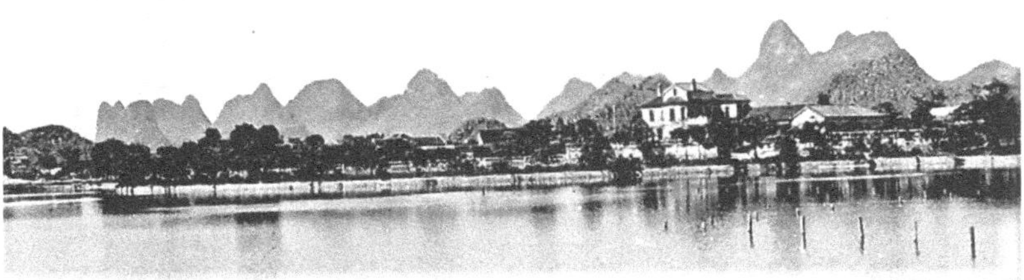

Figure 7.4c BAAG headquarter at West Lake, Guilin

Source: Elizabeth Ride Archive at https://www.elizabethridearchive.com/, photos reproduced with permission

Gordon King 王國棟 (1900–1991)

OBE, MD (UWA), LLD (HKU), FRCS, FRCOG, FRACS

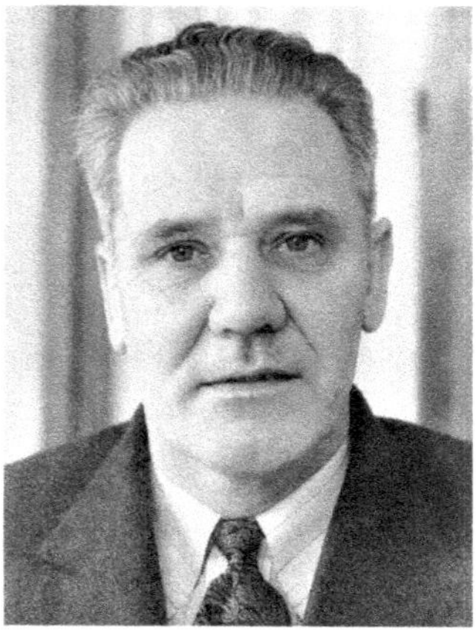

Figure 7.5 Professor Gordon King
Source: HKMMS, reproduced with permission

Professor Gordon King was born in 1900, the son of a Baptist minister. He graduated from London Hospital Medical College in 1924 and was elected a Fellow of the Royal College of Surgeons in 1926. He came to China in 1927 as a medical missionary of the Baptist Missionary Society and worked under Professor J. Preston Maxwell in the Obstetric Department of Peking Union Medical College, which was considered the mecca for that discipline in China.[42] In the same year, he married Mary Ellison, a fellow medical missionary. In 1931, he was appointed Professor and Head of the Department of Obstetrics and Gynecology at Cheeloo University, a Christian institution in Shandong. Due to the invasion of China by Japan in 1937, he left Cheeloo University.[43] His connections in China proved to be a great asset during the war years, as discussed later.

In 1938, King succeeded Professor William Nixon as Professor of the Department of Obstetrics and Gynecology at HKU. He was also appointed Dean of the Faculty of Medicine at HKU in 1940 and Medical Superintendent of University Relief Hospital at the campus main building, should war break out.[44] After the fall of Hong Kong, King secretly left for Free China in February 1942 with a guide introduced by Dr. Daphne Chun, just before he was sent to Stanley Camp. He explained after the war that there were three main reasons for the decision: 1) his experience in Cheeloo University under Japanese Occupation in 1937; 2) his ability to help HKU students who had left for Free China; and 3) the personal abuses he received from the Japanese Kempeitai at University Relief Hospital.[45] After a long journey in the mainland, he arrived at Chongqing in April 1942. On his way, he met groups of HKU students who encountered various difficulties, as many traveled to China for the first time. He decided to stay in China to help the HKU students who had now become refugees in China.[46]

There were two main tasks at hand: finding places for HKU students in Chinese universities and getting financial support from the British government. After discussion with the British Ambassador to China, a University Relief Work subsection was created under the Hong Kong Refugee Relief Bureau in Kukong (now Shaoguan), and a University Relief Fund was set up to provide assistance to the students. King secured agreement from the Chinese Minister for Education to allow HKU students to join any of the national universities of China, which were, fortunately, free of charge. A Hong Kong University Relief Committee with representatives from HKU (Gordon King), the British Embassy, the Ministry of Education, and other relevant Chinese organizations was formed to oversee the relief work. Although he was appointed Visiting Professor of Obstetrics and Gynecology at National Shanghai Medical College at Koloshan (Geleshan, Sichuan), his main preoccupation was looking after HKU students. Eventually he provided relief and placement for 346 students, which was more than half the total student body of HKU. He placed 115 medical students in eight universities to continue their studies.[47] After this, there was one more hurdle to overcome: to obtain recognition by the General Medical Council in England for the years of training in China. King started the negotiation in late 1942, and a favorable reply was received in June 1944. Students who had already completed two years or more of study in Hong Kong and had completed training and passed the required examination in one of these recognized universities in China would be eligible for registration with the GMC.[48]

In March 1945, King became a Commissioned Officer of the Royal Army Medical Corp. After the surrender of Japan, he returned to Hong Kong and became Assistant Director of Medical Services under the temporary military government of Rear-Admiral Harcourt. His main responsibility was to rehabilitate and reorganize government hospitals and clinics. His efforts in helping wartime students in China were repaid amply by having these new graduates from Free China to staff the Medical Department in Hong Kong after the war. A Medical Degrees Emergency Committee was formed by an Order in Council to determine eligibility of these wartime students.[49] Among the 63 wartime students who received a medical degree under the Medical Degrees Emergency Committee included Dr. Gerald Choa, who later became a distinguished doctor and contributed enormously to medical development and advances in Hong Kong. Altogether 97 wartime students who had studied in China obtained their medical degrees from HKU. In 1951, grateful wartime students gathered to honor their professor by donating a sum of money to the university to create the annual Gordon King Prize for Obstetrics and Gynecology.[50]

There was considerable delay in the opening of the university (see Chapter 9). When it finally reopened officially in 1948, King worked hard to restore the dilapidated HKU campus as a member of the Committee on the Reopening of the University initially and later the University Interim Committee.[51] In the same year, about 40 first year student entered the Faculty of Medicine.[52] As Dean of the Medical Faculty (1940–1949; 1951–1954), he was busy in rebuilding the faculty in several areas: 1) to reestablish the Pathology Department and to modernize the curriculum by the addition of bacteriology and parasitology; 2) to increase the facilities for clinical teaching, as Queen Mary Hospital was too small for the increasing intake of medical students; 3) to establish a new department of social medicine; and 4) to reintroduce short-course postgraduate studies.[53]

Under his leadership, clinical service at Tsan Yuk Hospital showed significant improvement. For example, maternal mortality at the hospital fell from 5.02/1,000 (1927–1941) to 0.89/1,000 (1945–1954), which was comparable to that of major maternity hospitals in other parts of the world.[54] Since the hospital, with only 85 beds, was too small for increasing demand from the postwar baby boom, King advocated for a bigger and better equipped maternity hospital. A new Tsan Yuk Hospital, with 200 beds, was built and opened in 1955, a most welcome addition to the obstetrics service. As a result, the department was recognized by the Royal College of Obstetricians and Gynecologists as a training center. King also encouraged his staff to conduct research. He himself was famous for the studies of molar pregnancies and the relationship between beriberi and toxemia of pregnancy.

Apart from academic work, King, as President of the Eugenics League, advocated and promoted the provision of facilities for scientific contraception so that married people could space or limit their families. Smaller families produce healthier and stronger children.[55] The league, as the pioneer in the field of family planning in Hong Kong, had been successful in introducing contraception in postnatal clinics. In 1950, the Eugenics League was reconstituted and renamed more appropriately The Family Planning Association of Hong Kong (FPA), with King as the chairman.[56] As the crude birth rate had risen rapidly from 20.1 to 34.2 per 1,000 from 1946 to 1961,[57] family planning became an important service to the community. In addition to birth control, the association offered counselling on infertility.

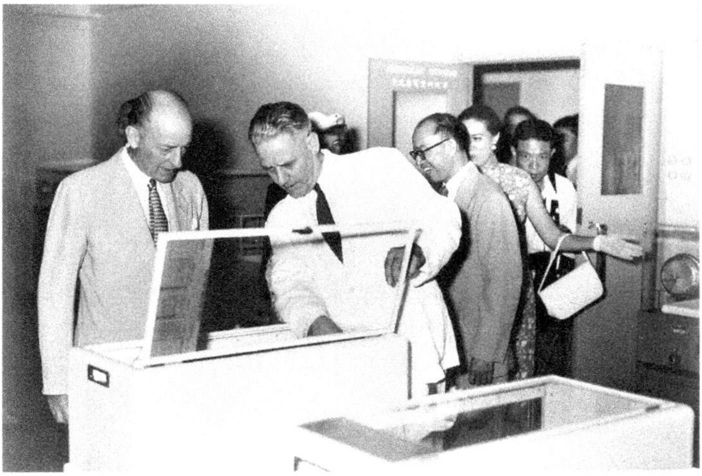

Figure 7.6 Professor Gordan King and Governor A. Grantham at premature baby nursery of new Tsan Yuk Hospital, Dr. and Mrs. K. C. Yeo next to King

Source: HKMMS, reproduced with permission

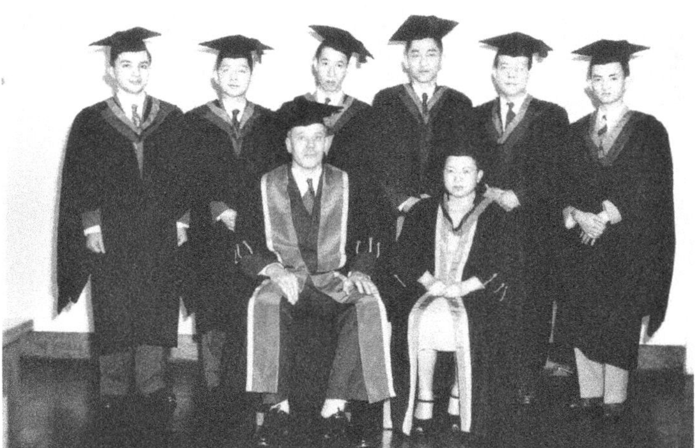

Figure 7.7 Professor Gordon King with Dr. Daphne Chun and 1951 graduates

Source: HKMMS, reproduced with permission, photograph donated by Dr. Joseph Pan

In 1956, King resigned from HKU to take up the deanship of the new medical school of the University of Western Australia (UWA). As consultant in obstetrics at Royal Perth Hospital, he published many research papers related to containment of maternal and perinatal mortality, and early diagnosis of cervical cancer. Retiring from UWA in 1965, Professor King was invited by the government of Kenya to help establish a medical school at University College, Nairobi, and he became Dean of the Faculty of Medicine (1967–1969).[58] His tie to the FPA in Hong Kong was renewed when he became its first full-time Director (1972–1973).[59] For his contribution to medical education, he was awarded an OBE (1954), MD (UWA, 1971), and LLD (HKU, 1973).

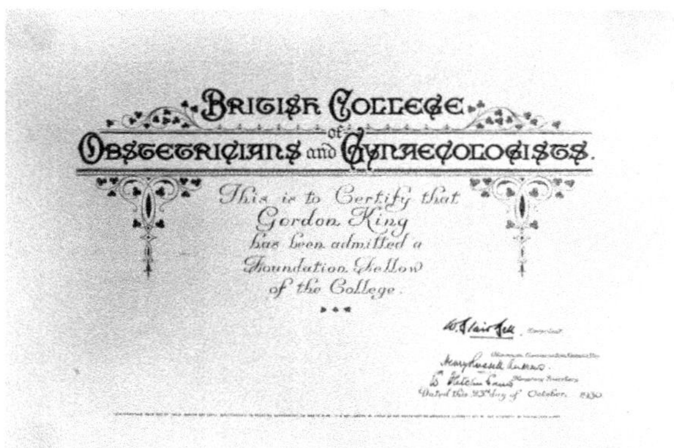

Figure 7.8 Professor Gordon King, Foundation Fellow of the College of Obstetricians and Gynecologists, 1930
Source: HKMMS, reproduced with permission

Professor Gordon King passed away in October 1991, in Perth, Western Australia. He was survived by his second wife (Chiu Bek-to) and three daughters from his first marriage. In addition to the Gordon King Prize of HKU Medical Faculty, the Hong Kong Museum of Medical Sciences has a lecture room named after him.

8. Government Public Health Experts Modernizing the Healthcare System

Hong Kong after liberation in August 1945 became a magnet for epidemics. There were problems with backup sewers, refuse, and night soil collection and disposal. The city was infested with rats, and flies and mosquitoes proliferated. Many houses had been destroyed, and the existing ones fell into disrepair due to lack of building supplies, so a housing crisis ensued. The situation worsened as residents streamed back from mainland China. All the conditions were in place for major outbreaks of infectious diseases.

As expected, in 1946, enteric fever and dysentery were prevalent, and about half to one-third of the cases died. The dreaded cholera epidemic arrived that summer, killing half of the 514 people infected, and the smallpox epidemic hit even harder that winter, killing two-thirds of the almost 2,000 people infected. Malaria, which had been almost wiped out before the war, returned with a vengeance, some 2,400 reported cases in 1946. Tuberculosis claimed the lives of thousands.[1] Over the next two decades, infection and infectious diseases would account for at least 60% of all deaths in Hong Kong.

After the Japanese surrendered, Dr. Percy Selwyn-Clarke left Ma Tau Wai Camp immediately and returned to work. He called back many of the old staff of the Medical Department and began rebuilding the department. His priorities were to reopen the hospitals and clinics, restore regular sanitary services, and mount an intensive anti-epidemic campaign to forestall future outbreaks.[2] In 1947, Selwyn-Clarke was promoted to become the Governor of Seychelles. Dr. Isaac Newton was appointed the next Director of Medical Department until 1951.[3]

In 1950, Hong Kong's main source of revenue from the fragile recovering entrepôt trade was shattered by a United Nations embargo against China when the Korean War broke out. Due to a meager budget during the postwar period, the Medical Department decided to concentrate on public health and prevention of infectious diseases such as cholera, smallpox, and tuberculosis, which were major killers at the time.

In the late 1950s, Hong Kong was transformed from an entrepôt into a major manufacturing center, and its economy improved and more funding became available for medical services. In 1964, the government issued a White Paper on the Development of Medical Services for the next 10 years.[4] Because infectious diseases were under control, more resources were placed in curative care. In addition to building a number of clinics to expand outpatient services, the number of hospital beds was to increase to a target of 4.25 / 1,000 population by 1974. Having reached the target in 1974, another White Paper on the Further Development of Medical and Health Services was published, aiming at further increasing the number of hospital beds to 5.5 / 1,000 in the following 10 years.[5] As the population of Hong Kong increased rapidly, there was a shortage of doctors. In 1959, there was only 0.36 doctors / 1,000 population, when 2.5 / 1,000 was recommended. Out of 700 positions in the Medical and Health Department, more than 100 were unfilled. Although the total number of medical student enrollments in the Faculty of Medicine, HKU, had increased from around 50 in the 1950s to 150 per year by 1972, due to the dramatic increase in the population, the number of doctors / 1,000 only increased marginally.[6] As a result, the government decided to establish another medical school in the Chinese University of Hong Kong. Thus, the decades covering 1970 to the 1990s were a golden period of medical services expansion and hospital building. Yet the transitional period was full of problems.

In the 1970s, the medical scene in Hong Kong began to change. As the standard of living improved, the people in Hong Kong began to adopt a Western diet and a Western style of living, which were conducive to developing chronic noncommunicative diseases such as stroke, ischemic heart disease, diabetes, hypertension, and cancer. These diseases were becoming the major causes of morbidity and mortality from the 1970s onward. The Hong Kong population was also aging, increasing the risk of chronic noncommunicable diseases.

At the same time, the traditional general practice had given way to highly specialized medicine in a high-technology and hospital-based system, which proved much costlier. However, studies have shown that healthcare systems that rely on primary care produced better health outcomes, reduced disease mortality, and resulted in higher patient satisfaction and lower healthcare costs. In 1981, the World Health

Organization promoted the primary healthcare approach as the key to achieving the goal of "Health for All" by the year 2000.[7] In Hong Kong in the 1980s, there were hardly any trained primary healthcare doctors. A stronger primary care system was badly needed to strengthen prevention and management of chronic diseases and supportive care for elderly people.

This chapter describes three distinguished physicians in the government services. The first two were appointed Director of Medical and Health Services during the first two phases of medical development in Hong Kong: Dr. Yeo Kok-cheang (Director 1952–1957), who valiantly fought against infectious diseases; and Dr. Gerald Choa (Director 1970–1976), who efficiently managed the myriad of difficulties associated with lack of medical care while awaiting new facilities being built in a rapidly growing population. The third one, Dr. Lee Shiu-hung (Director 1989–1994), was appointed Director of the Department of Health after the Medical and Health Department was split into the Department of Health and the Hospital Authority and there was a demand for primary care reform. These physicians successfully overcame the challenges and difficulties they encountered during their tenure and advanced medical services in Hong Kong. They were appreciated and honored by the people.

Yeo Kok-cheang 楊國璋 (1903–2004)

MBBS, MD, DPH, DTM&H, CMG

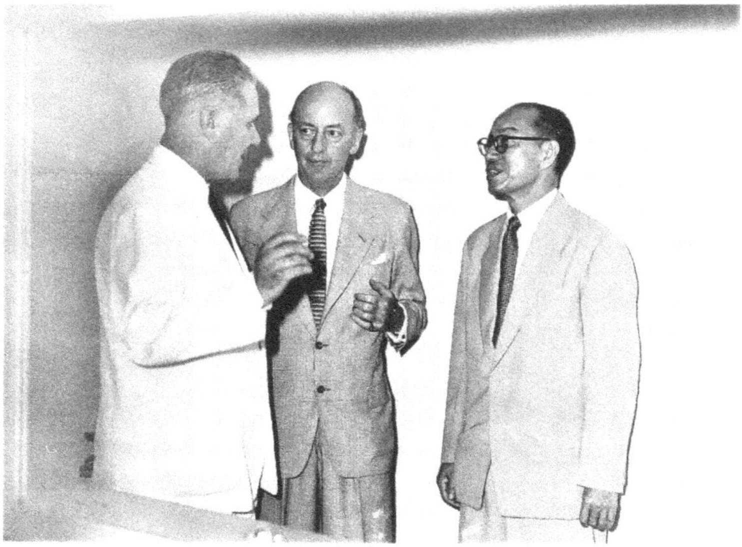

Figure 8.1 Dr. Yeo Kok-cheang (right) and Governor Grantham (center) and Professor Gordon King (left) at the opening of Tsan Yuk Hospital in 1955

Source: HKMMS, reproduced with permission

Dr Yeo Kok-cheang served the Medical Department of Hong Kong for 30 years. During World War II, he placed the good of the community before his personal welfare by remaining in Hong Kong. After the war, he led the fight against infectious diseases in Hong Kong, especially tuberculosis.

Yeo was born in 1903, in Penang, Malaya. He had a happy childhood. Because his father retired early, he was left with the responsibility of educating his younger brothers and sisters (eight altogether) after his graduation. After completing secondary school, Yeo studied medicine at HKU and obtained his MBBS in 1925. To further his education, he left for the UK to study public health in Cambridge and was successful in obtaining the Diploma in Public Health (DPH) with distinction. He also obtained the Diploma in Tropical Medicine and Hygiene (DTM&H) in Liverpool. He then applied for a position in the Government Medical Department in Hong Kong in 1928. Because he applied in the UK, he was given the terms of an expatriate. When the Colonial Office discovered its mistake, it kept its word and did not go back on the contract.[8] In 1930, he also completed his MD degree in state medicine in HKU. By 1939, he was promoted to Chinese Health Officer, Senior Grade.[9] He was married to Florence Ho Tung,[10] and they had three children, all born before World War II.

After Hong Kong's surrender to the Japanese, Yeo intended to escape to Free China, as did many doctors. However, Dr. Percy Selwyn-Clarke, Director of Medical Services, appealed to him to stay. When Selwyn-Clarke decided to work with the Japanese to maintain public health and prevent epidemics, he had anticipated his own imprisonment any time. Yeo was the Chinese Health Officer he trusted most and had the experience and knowledge to fight against infectious diseases in Hong Kong. Selwyn-Clarke implored Yeo to stay in Hong Kong for the people and all the internees in camps. It was a fateful decision that Yeo made. In 1943, Selwyn-Clarke was arrested, tortured, and sent to prison for spying. Yeo, too, was detained and placed in solitary confinement and interrogated day after day. He was finally released after two months. During his imprisonment, Yeo turned to Christianity and became a staunch Christian, together with the rest of the family. After his release from prison, Yeo continued to maintain public health in Hong Kong, working in the Bacteriological Institute. He was paid only by a small sack of rice for a family of five for the duration of Japanese Occupation. The family survived through the ingenuity and hard work of his wife who grew vegetables and sweet potatoes in the garden of their rented bungalow at Pokfulam.[11]

It was during the postwar era that Yeo demonstrated his remarkable skill as an administrator and a leader. As explained, during this period, the Medical Department used its meager budget wisely on preventive care, to counter the high incidence and death from infectious diseases rather than on curative care. The Medical Department organized several prevention programs against infectious diseases, starting early in 1946. The anti-malaria program, which had been completely dismantled during Japanese Occupation, resulting in a high malaria rate, was reconstituted. The Maternal and Child Health Centers (MCHC) were established in the same year to replace the Infant Health Centers to deal with the high maternal and infant mortality.[12] In 1947, Yeo became Deputy Director of Health of the Medical Department and Health Advisor to the Urban Council and was responsible for implementing preventive measures against infectious diseases. The department mounted a smallpox vaccination campaign in 1947, as refugees brought in cases of smallpox. Over one million residents were vaccinated every year for several years. As a result of this campaign, Hong Kong recorded its last few cases of smallpox in 1952.[13] Every year before the summer months, the department began a city-wide anti-cholera inoculation campaign and education program[14] and imposed strict quarantine measures every year to prevent a severe outbreak of cholera.[15] The Tuberculosis Service, was formed in 1947, to control the mounting number of new cases and deaths from tuberculosis.[16]

In 1950, Yeo was promoted to Deputy Director of Medical and Health Services, and in 1952, Director—the first Chinese to be appointed Director of Medical and Health Services.[17] He continued with the same policies for prevention of infectious diseases as before. In addition, he proposed compulsory treatment for individuals with venereal diseases, to counter the high incidence after the war. The Venereal Disease Ordinance, 1951 was passed, providing free consultation and treatment for individuals with venereal diseases.[18] In addition, all pregnant women were screened for syphilis; as a result, congenital syphilis almost disappeared after several years. He also started the combined immunization against diphtheria, whooping cough, and tetanus by trained staff in the MCHCs. By the 1970s, these three infectious diseases had virtually disappeared from Hong Kong.[19]

The other significant program that he initiated was BCG vaccination in 1952. After the war, the incidence of tuberculosis was high. In children, tuberculous meningitis accounted for 22% of tuberculosis deaths in 1948. When Yeo took over as Director, one of the important programs of the Government Tuberculosis Service was BCG vaccination. There were three teams for BCG vaccination with staff trained by the WHO, and they were sent to schools to vaccinate all school children who were tuberculin negative. By the late 1960s, the coverage of newborns and children reached 95%. Deaths from tuberculous meningitis were reduced drastically.[20] In the early 1950s, effective drugs for treatment of tuberculosis had yet to be widely available. As treatment involved surgical procedures and some patients were rather sick, hospital beds were necessary. Yeo helped the Hong Kong Anti-Tuberculosis Association, a NGO, to raise funds for a new hospital (Grantham Hospital) for tuberculosis patients.[21] When effective anti-TB drugs became more readily available, treatment could be carried out as outpatients. More TB clinics were added to meet the needs.[22] The death rate of TB declined from 208/100,000 in 1951 to 97/100,000 in 1957 when Yeo retired. The notification rate of TB dropped from 689 to 499/100,000 during the same period.[23]

Patients with leprosy had been outcasts of society even though the disease was not very infectious and effective drugs were available. Yeo helped the Mission to Lepers Hong Kong Auxiliary, a NGO, to found the leper colony on Hay Ling Chau, a small island off Lantau Island, and to build a hospital on the island. In the 1960s, there were 540 patients in the hospital, the highest number recorded. Yeo also helped raising funds for the operation of the colony on the island.[24]

As the 1950s wore on, Hong Kong's economy improved, and more resources became available to the Medical Department. Yeo not only improved the existing outpatient facilities by renovating and expanding them but also added a few new ones including: the Wan Chai Tuberculosis Clinic and Dental Clinic on Hong Kong Island, Shek Kip Mei Clinic in Kowloon, and Tsuen Wan Clinic, Sai Kung Clinic, North Lamma Island Clinic, and Silver Mine Bay Clinic in the New Territories.[25] Under his influence, Tung Wah Hospital also opened a new annex to expand its outpatient department in 1956.[26] A few urgently required hospitals were built either by the government or by NGOs: Tsan Yuk Hospital, Duchess of Kent Children's Hospital for Rehabilitation of Disabled Children, Grantham Hospital, and the Leprosarium in Hay Ling Chau, as mentioned. At the same time, a new hospital, Castle Peak Hospital, for psychiatric patients and a new general hospital, Queen Elizabeth Hospital, in Kowloon were planned.

Yeo opened Lewis Laboratory, the first specialized laboratory for cardio-respiratory diseases at the University Medical Unit, Queen Mary Hospital, in Hong Kong.[27] He established the position of a specialist anesthetist, paving the way for the growth of anesthesia and the development of that specialty locally.[28]

As an official member of the Legislative Council, Yeo proposed amendments to various medical ordinances such as An Ordinance to Repeal, and to Re-enact with Amendments, the Medical Registration Ordinance, Chapter 161, and to replace the Medical Board with a Medical Council.[29] He also proposed a bill to amend Chapter 164 for the Registration of Nurses, to change the requirement of nurses trained outside the colony and to provide appeals by nurses of decisions of the

Nursing Board to be heard by a judge of the Supreme Court.[30] Thus he made the law more equitable for the nursing profession.

As Director of Medical and Health services, Yeo was also appointed Professor of Social Medicine (part-time), HKU, a position which he retained until his retirement despite his very busy schedule as Director of Medical and Health Services.

In January 1956, Yeo was awarded CMG. There was great jubilation in the Chinese community because he was the first Chinese civil servant to be decorated for his dedication and achievements. He was made an Honorary Member of British Red Cross Society and honored by Tung Wah Hospital Board of Directors with a wing of the hospital named after him, the "Yeo Wing," in 1958. A hall of Tung Wah Eastern Hospital Nurses Residence was also dedicated to him, and Hong Kong Dental Society (renamed later Hong Kong Dental Association) elected him an Honorary Member of the Society.[31]

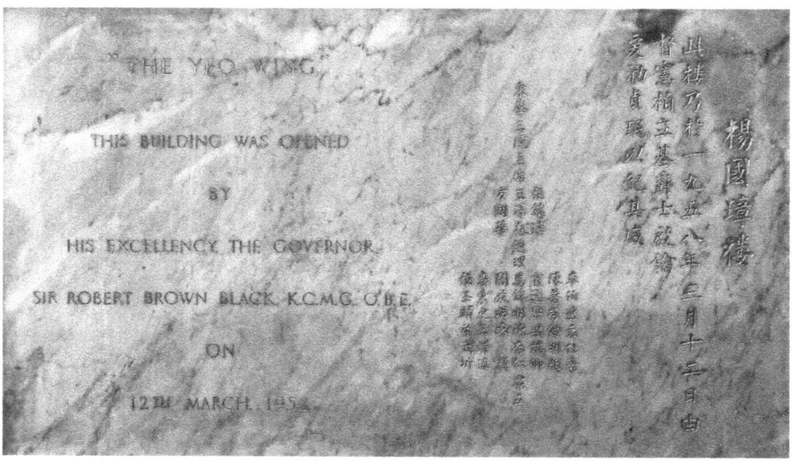
"THE YEO WING"
THIS BUILDING WAS OPENED
BY
HIS EXCELLENCY THE GOVERNOR
SIR ROBERT BROWN BLACK, K.C.M.G. O.B.E.
ON
楊國璋樓

Figure 8.2 Plaque outside Yeo Wing in Tung Wah Hospital named after Dr. Yeo Kok-cheang

Photo taken by Wong Tai-wai

Toward 1956, Dr. Yeo Kok-cheang made the heart-wrenching decision to spend more time with his family. He retired to England with his family in 1957 and became a senior hospital medical officer in psychiatry in St. Ebbas Hospital, Epsom, Surrey, England, where he served for 10 years. He died in 2004, at the age of 101.[32] Many in the Medical and Health Department felt that Dr. Yeo's success was due to his skilled administration. He was described by his deputy as "a leader who has been long the guide of our destiny, a leader we all respect for his humble sincerity of purpose, his courage and devotion to duty, his fairness and loyalty to his staff, his unassuming painstaking and conscientious leadership."[33]

Gerald Hugh Choa 蔡永業 (1921–2001)

CBE, MD Cheeloo, MB BS Hong Kong, DTM&H, MRCP, MD Hong Kong, FRCP, FRCP Edin, FFCM, FHKCP, FHKAM, Hon LLD

Professor Gerald Hugh Choa was a distinguished Director of Medical and Health Services (Director, 1970–1976), the founding Dean of the Faculty of Medicine at the Chinese University of Hong Kong and an eminent historian and author.

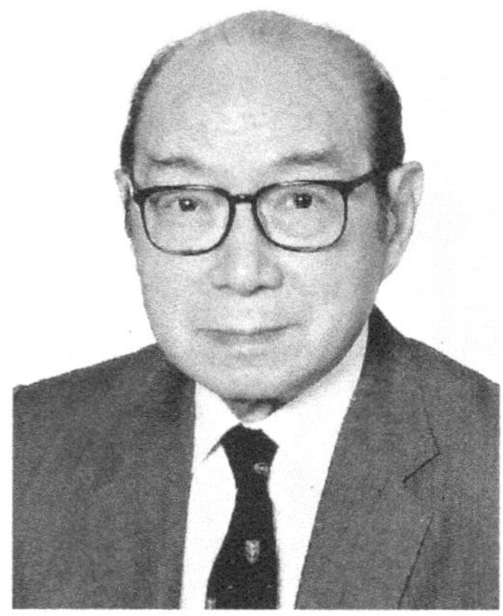

Figure 8.3 Professor Gerald Choa
Image courtesy of CUHK

Born into a prominent family in Hong Kong, Choa's lineage could be traced 200 years to Malacca, where his ancestor migrated from the province of Fujian, China. Over the years the family became highly successful in business and in real estate. It was Choa's grandfather who, after completing his education in Singapore, decided to move to Hong Kong. He too became a successful businessman.[34]

After attending Wah Yan, a Catholic secondary school in Hong Kong, Choa entered HKU for his medical education. During World War II, he was able to continue his medical studies at Cheeloo University, where he obtained his MD in 1945. In 1946, he was also awarded an MBBS by HKU. Choa pursued postgraduate training at University of Liverpool and University of Birmingham and Queen Square, London. He obtained a DTM&H and became a member of the Royal College of Physicians (MRCP) before returning to Hong Kong in 1952, when he was appointed Lecturer in the Department of Medicine, HKU.[35]

Professor Sir David Todd was a student of Choa when Choa returned from England. Todd wrote, "… when it came to physical examination, nothing we did was right, and we were certainly put in our place. What a fierce teacher, we thought. But initial impressions can be very wrong and behind that stern exterior was kindness itself. He was a superb clinician and erudite teacher, particularly in cardiology and neurology. Impeccably dressed, he was very much the gentleman physician."[36]

In 1956, Choa became the first Chinese to be appointed by the government as Specialist in Medicine at Queen Mary Hospital; in 1963, he was promoted to Senior Specialist. During this period, he remained active in academic pursuits, teaching students and trainees and engaging in research work. He published studies in hemolytic anemia in typhoid fever and neuroparalytic accidents of anti-rabies vaccination.[37] Dr. Arthur Van Langenberg, one of his trainees in the 1960s, wrote:

> I was a great admirer of the chief, Dr. Gerald Choa, a consummate gentleman, wise and expert in every branch of internal medicine: in short, the ideal general physician, into whose hands I would willingly place my life, if illness should strike. Dr. Choa ran the unit with cool efficiency ... never a raised voice was heard from Dr. Choa, although it was perfectly clear he did not suffer fool gladly.[38]

In 1967, Choa made a surprise move, leaving clinical medicine to become an administrator in the Government Medical and Health Department. There he rose rapidly in ranks and, in 1970, he was appointed Director of Medical and Health Services,[39] a post which he held until 1976.

While serving as the Deputy Director of Medical and Health services, Choa was partly responsible for the successful establishment of Estate Clinics, where doctors could practice in low-cost housing estates to deliver medical services inexpensively to the residents living in the estates. The doctors formed the Low-Cost Clinic Association of Registered Doctors (renamed Public Housing Estate Clinic Association of Registered Doctors), getting excellent advice from Choa in their negotiation with housing estates to make this valuable program possible.[40]

In the early 1970s, the general health of the population had improved: life expectancy had increased, maternal and infant mortality and crude death rates had fallen, and TB notification had declined, as did the other infectious diseases.[41] But there were many problems that required attention.

Firstly, family planning up to then had been carried out by a voluntary organization—the Family Planning Association—which operated a total of 32 clinics in 1973. It was highly successful in helping reduce the birth rate. It was only logical that the government should take over the responsibility of family planning, an important program for Hong Kong. In 1974, the government amalgamated all the clinics of the Family Planning Association with Maternal and Child Health Centers and named the newly expanded entity the Family Health Service, offering a comprehensive program.[42]

Secondly, drug addiction was a major problem in Hong Kong then. In the 1960s, the government established several treatment centers for drug addicts: Tai Tam Gap Correctional Institution,[43] Castle Peak Hospital,[44] and later Shek Kwu Chau Treatment Center.[45] However, the relapse rate for drug addiction was very high. Choa promoted Methadone Detox and Maintenance Program, which would allow drug abusers to keep gainful employment. After a successful pilot study, he organized a territory-wide program,[46] which remains an important part of the anti-drug addiction program today. Choa called on employers to hire reformed and cured drug abusers as a useful first step in their rehabilitation.[47]

Thirdly, the rising incidence of mental illness and the inadequate number of beds for these patients were problematic. The policy of rehabilitation and treatment of these patients as outpatients was met with resistance from the public, who refused to have half-way houses built in their neighborhoods. Choa planned for another psychiatric hospital to be built[48] and at the same time urged people to help rehabilitation by not rejecting patients with mental problems.[49]

Fourthly, the overcrowding of public hospitals and staffing problems were difficult to solve. The public hospitals were packed with camp beds, and staff morale was low.[50] By the 1970s, the population of Hong Kong had risen to around 4 million. Even though the number of hospital beds had reached the target of 4.25/1,000 in 1973, as recommended by the 1964 White Paper on the "Development of Medical Services in Hong Kong,"[51] the hospitals remained grossly overcrowded because of the rapidly rising population. Although the 1974 White Paper, "The Further Development of Medical and Health Services in Hong Kong," recommended increasing hospital beds to 5.5 beds/1,000 by the end of the next decade,[52] it would be necessary to relieve hospital congestion in the interim. Choa proposed the following plans to help the situation in major hospitals:[53] 1) to increase the fees of public hospitals from $2 to $3 a day while bringing down the fees of the government-subvented hospitals. This would likely provide accommodation in subvented hospitals for patients in the convalescent phase,[54] leaving the beds in public hospitals for acutely ill patients; 2) to divide Hong Kong into five regions for delivery of medical services. Each region would have one acute hospital for specialized care, and several smaller hospitals and clinics to provide basic services; and 3) to provide community nursing care for those who no longer required hospital care but had difficulty attending clinics for follow-up. Community nursing care would help prevent disease relapse by providing qualified domiciliary nursing care for discharged patients.[55] The shortage of staff and poor staff morale from overwork had to be solved. Unfortunately, there was only one long-term solution as proposed in the 1974 White Paper: the establishment of a second medical school and another nursing school to address the troublingly low doctor–population ratio (0.5 / 1,000) and nurse–population ratio (1.3 / 1,000) then.[56]

Choa also dealt decisively with complaints from patients of the practice of "payment" (bribery) for use of bedpans, and the filling of thermos, by implementing disciplinary action against any government hospital staff member found guilty of corruption or rudeness.[57] This was supported by the establishment of the Independent Commission Against Corruption (ICAC) in 1974.

Choa retired from the Medical and Health Department in 1976 after six years as director.[58] During his term, he also chaired the Action Committee Against Narcotics and served on the Legislative and Executive Councils as well as acting as the chair of many professional and charitable organizations. For his distinguished career in civil service, he was awarded CBE in 1972.[59] However, he reached the peak of his career only after his first retirement.

In 1977, Choa accepted a new challenge to become the founding Dean of the new Faculty of Medicine at CUHK. He was later appointed Professor of Administrative Medicine and Pro-Vice-Chancellor of the University.[60] Choa led the planning of the teaching hospital, the curriculum, and recruitment of teaching and research staff. It was no easy task to plan a new faculty and a new teaching hospital simultaneously. The first class of 60 medical undergraduates, admitted in September 1981, would commence clinical training in July 1983. Prince of Wales Hospital in Shatin was expected to be fully built and equipped with modern facilities in just 24 months. For reasons beyond the contractor's control, the completion date of the hospital had to be delayed by a year. An alternative plan had to be devised.[61] Fortunately, Dr. Edward Paterson of United Christian Hospital generously made its training facilities and patients available for clinical teaching, and some classes were conducted at Kowloon Hospital.[62] It was only the strong leadership of Choa, with his no-nonsense approach to the myriad of problems encountered by the medical school and the university that the first class of students were conferred their MBChB degrees in 1986. Choa retired in 1987 and was awarded an honorary LLD by CUHK for his invaluable contribution to the founding of its medical school.[63]

After his second retirement, Choa did not cease to work but remained honorary adviser to the Vice-Chancellor of CUHK and took up part-time clinical practice. He did indulge his passion for history during his spare time. He published a book on the history of Protestant medical missionaries in China, "Heal the Sick" Was Their Motto, in 1990.[64] A second book The Life and Times of Sir Kai Ho Kai, was published in 2000.[65] The latter is a fascinating story of Dr. Ho Kai, an important figure whose life epitomized the westernized Chinese elite during that era. Ho Kai played a vital role in establishing Alice Memorial and Affiliated Hospitals and Hong Kong College of Medicine (Chapter 3). This book is a rich source of reference materials for researchers in the history of medical development and medical education in Hong Kong. Due to his interest in history, Choa became the founding chairman of Hong Kong Museum of Medical Sciences Society. He was also the founding Vice-President of Hong Kong College of Physicians and the founding Fellow of Hong Kong Academy of Medicine. He was made an honorary Fellow of HKU in 1995.[66]

An erudite teacher, an academic, a brilliant administrator, a distinguished historian, and a humanitarian, Professor Gerald Choa will long be remembered as a renaissance man and honored by students of the Medical School of CUHK, his colleagues and friends, for his leadership and dedication to his profession and to public service.

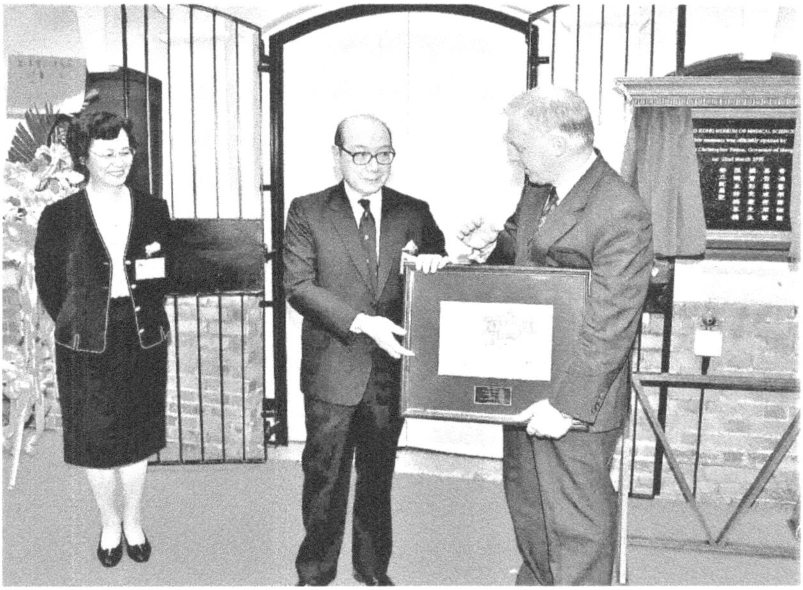

Figure 8.4 Professor Gerald Choa presenting a picture of the HKMMS building to Governor Chris Patten who officiated the opening ceremony of the museum. Professor Faith Ho standing on the left, 1996.

Source: HKMMS, reproduced with permission

Lee Shiu-hung 李紹鴻 (1933–2014)

SBS, ISO, MBBS, MD, DPH, DIH, FRCP, FFPH, FAFOM, AFOM, FFOM, FRACMA (Aust) , FHKAM (CM), Hon FHKCCM, JP

Professor Lee Shiu-hung was the first director of Department of Health (1989–1994) in Hong Kong after the Medical and Health Department reorganized in 1989 to become two institutions: the Department of Health and the Hospital Services Department. He contributed greatly to Hong Kong's public health by establishing the first school of public health in Hong Kong and in promoting public health and health education in the community.

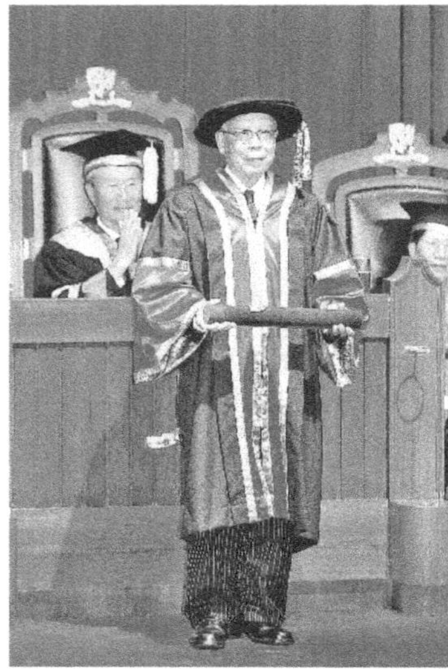

Figure 8.5 Professor Lee Shiu-hung, awarded Honorary Fellowship by CUHK, 2009
Image courtesy of CUHK

Lee was born in Guangdong province, the son of a merchant. The family migrated to Hong Kong during World War II. After graduating from St. Stephen's College, he entered the Faculty of Medicine, HKU and obtained his MBBS in 1958. He furthered his studies in Singapore and at the London School of Hygiene and Tropical Medicine in the UK, obtaining a DPH in 1963. In 1969, he was awarded a Diploma of Industrial Hygiene (DIH) and in 1991, he received his MD degree from HKU. Over the course of his career, he gathered professional qualifications in several specialties in medicine: community medicine, occupational medicine, public health, and medical administration.[67]

In 1960, Lee joined the Medical and Health Department as a health officer and, in 1989, he was promoted to Director of Health. Between 1960 and 1989, he served in different services of the Medical and Health Department, including health planning and administration, management of medical and health services, health education, occupational and environmental health, and infectious diseases control. Although infectious diseases as a cause of death in Hong Kong had dropped markedly by 1960, preventive measures had to be in place to prevent their recurrence. Lee was tireless in combating the recurrence of such diseases and personally led medical and nursing teams to various communities for immunization campaigns.[68] He relished the role he played during the cholera epidemic of 1962,[69] when he carried out investigations to trace the source of infection in the community.

In the late 1960s and 1970s, Hong Kong rapidly transformed into a regional manufacturing center. The incidence of a few occupational diseases in Hong Kong, such as silicosis, and decompression sickness, increased. Because of this, Lee went to update his knowledge in occupational diseases and received a Diploma of Industrial Health in 1969 and a fellowship in occupational medicine from the American College of Occupational Medicine in 1984,[70] showing how eager he was to learn more to serve the community.

As noted, the WHO promoted the primary healthcare approach as key to achieving the goal of "Health for All" by the year 2000. The government formed the Working Party on Primary Health Care in 1989, the year when Lee was promoted to Director of Health.[71] When the report of the Working Party was published the following year with a large number of recommendations,[72] Lee did his best to remedy the deficiencies identified by the Working Party and placed 68% of the budget of the Department of Health to primary care services.[73] Unfortunately at that time the public healthcare system was undergoing a drastic change, splitting into the Hospital Authority and Department of Health. The Hospital Authority took the lion's share of the budget (about 90%) each year. Because of budget constraints, the reforms carried out by Lee were limited. Critics of healthcare policy also found the exercise related to primary care inconsequential, noting that the recommendations were hardly implemented in the private sector, which is responsible for 80% of primary care.[74] Because of this, Lee had his plans mapped out after his retirement.

In 1994, Lee entered his second career after retiring from the civil service. He was appointed Professor of Community Medicine and Chairman of the Department of Community and Family Medicine at CUHK. He hoped to train family medicine doctors in community health who would practice preventive medicine in their career, especially in early detection and management of chronic noncommunicable diseases and cancer. Lee realized the importance of training public health professionals locally, which was lacking in Hong Kong. He became the chief advocate for the establishment of a school of public health at CUHK. In 2001, the School of Public Health was established at CUHK, and Lee was the founding director.[75] In 2009, the Departments of Community Medicine, Family Medicine, and the School of Public Health at CUHK were combined into one school: The Jockey Club School of Public Health and Primary Care.[76] Lee also pioneered in developing the Center for Health Education and Health Promotion in the Jockey Club School of Public Health, training primary and secondary school teachers on health education and in promoting healthy school projects. He became Chairman of the Healthy Schools Program, and at the same time Chairman of the University Health Services Committee and Chairman of the Advisory Committee on Health Promotion and Protection, to promote health and hygiene work on the CUHK campus.[77]

He retired the second time from CUHK in 2001, and the university bestowed on him the title of Emeritus Professor in Community Medicine and appointed him an Honorary Advisor of the School of Public Health, Honorary Advisor of External Affairs of Institute of Chinese Medicine, and a Senior College Tutor at Chung Chi College. In addition to the School of Public Health in CUHK, Lee founded the Hong Kong Society of Infectious Diseases and the Hong Kong Epidemiological Association.[78]

Lee's second retirement did not leave him less busy. He was a staunch supporter of the Healthy Cities Project, which was proposed by the WHO, to continually improve the physical and social environments in a city and expand the community resources to enable people to support each other in performing all the functions of life.[79] Through his promotion, Tseung Kwan O, Wan Chai, Central and Western District, Kwai Tsing, and Tsuen Wan were included in the Healthy Cities Project.[80]

Lee served on a number of committees: Chairman of the Hong Kong Council on Smoking and Health, Action Committee Against Narcotics, and Occupational Deafness Compensation Board. He was a member of the Scientific Committee on AIDS and Vice-President of the Hong Kong Tuberculosis, Chest, and Heart Diseases Association (previously Hong Kong Anti-Tuberculosis Association). As he was constantly promoting public health not only in Hong Kong but also around the world, he was honored in Hong Kong and overseas. In Hong Kong, he received several awards including Justice of the Peace, the Silver Bauhinia Star, Honorary Fellowship of CUHK and Hong Kong Academy of Medicine. Outside of Hong Kong, he received the WHO Medal from the Western Pacific Regional Office in 1988, and awards from the Asia Pacific Association for Control of Tobacco in 2007, and Alliance on Healthy Cities in 2010.[81]

A family man, happily married with four children, Lee enjoyed family life and family gatherings and spending time with his children and grandchildren. He loved swimming, tennis, singing, listening to music, dancing, photography, and traveling. It is hard to imagine that he would be able to find time for all these activities with his numerous commitments even after retirement. He passed away in 2014 and was missed by his family, colleagues, and friends around the world.[82]

A letter to the Editor of the Hong Kong Medical Journal in April 2014 gives us the circumstances of Professor Lee Shiu-hung's death and allows us a glimpse of his utter devotion to society. He was a Guest of Honor of the Annual Winter Charity Dinner sponsored by "Love U All Charitable Foundation" on 6 January 2014. Halfway through the dinner, Professor Lee offered impromptu entertainment and sang a Xinjiang folk song. After singing the top notes at the end, he went back to his seat. Five minutes later he fell on the carpeted floor and rapidly lapsed into a deep coma and died peacefully. He died befitting the title of a true "Doctor for Society."[83]

9. Government Specialists
Developing New Branches of Medicine

Ever since the founding in 1911, HKU did not have a hospital for the Faculty of Medicine. Clinical teaching was carried out by private practitioners initially at Alice Memorial and Affiliated Hospitals and in 1914, at Government Civil Hospital, which was more spacious. When the university clinical departments were established in 1923, each department was assigned a certain number of hospital beds for teaching in Government Civil Hospital which had 212 beds. Forty-two beds and four cots were assigned to the University Medical Unit[1] and about 50 to the University Surgical Unit. The University Obstetrics and Gynecology Unit was assigned 25 beds in a bungalow at Government Civil Hospital. But Professor Tottenham found that the operating theatre was always used by Surgery, and the bungalow was small. He transferred his teaching unit to Tsan Yuk Hospital, which was more spacious and had a gynecology ward with 20 to 22 beds, an obstetrics ward, and an operating theatre[2] (Chapter 6). The Government Medical Department had the control of all the beds in Government Civil Hospital, and the government medical officers who were not regarded as specialists had the use of the remaining beds after about half of them had been assigned to the university units.

During Sir Richard Needham's visit on behalf of the General Medical Council in 1933, among other things, he recommended a closer collaboration between HKU and the government staff.[3] Over the years, the government medical officers took an active role in teaching medical students. In 1937, the new Queen Mary Hospital was built. All staff and patients from Government Civil Hospital moved to the new hospital. There were 546 beds at the Queen Mary Hospital, 170 of which were assigned to HKU.[4]

After World War II, some of the medical officers in the Government Medical and Health Department became specialists too. As a result, in teaching hospitals, there were the government surgical, medical, and obstetrics and gynecology units, and each one was headed by a government specialist just like their university counterparts. In 1989, when the public healthcare system was divided into two institutions, the Hospital Authority and the Department of Health, in teaching hospitals such as Queen Mary Hospital, Prince of Wales Hospital and others, the government and the university units were combined to form one unit of each basic branch of medicine: medicine, surgery, orthopedics, pediatrics, and obstetrics and gynecology for administration, clinical service, and teaching. Full integration of these units occurred in 1995/1996 and greatly simplified the management in the hospital. Teaching is now carried out by all university and government staff in these hospitals.

During the first few decades after World War II, in teaching hospitals, specialties that required expensive equipment, such as radiology and radiotherapy, were developed by the government only. The government was also responsible for certain branches of medicine such as mental illness, tuberculosis, and anesthesia. Some NGOs were devoted to patients of diseases that required long term care such as tuberculosis and leprosy. Medical students were taught tuberculosis by the Columban Sisters at Ruttonjee Hospital and leprosy by the staff at Hay Ling Chau Leprosarium. The Leprosarium was opened in 1951 to accommodate about 500 lepers and closed in 1975 when there were very few cases.[5]

The three illustrious doctors in this chapter were all trained specialists appointed by the Government Medical and Health Department. These three exceptional individuals took it upon themselves to develop, expand, and advance their specialties to such an extent that their departments were equally advanced as those in Western countries. They were appointed honorary lecturers/professors at the university to teach medical students, and at the same time, they trained a cadre of doctors to carry on after them. Two of them also developed their own research program. In fact, they were not different from their university counterparts in their work. These individuals were Dr. John Ho Hung-chiu, who was the only one with dual certification in diagnostic radiology and radiotherapy; Dr. Yap Pao-meng, the first properly trained psychiatrist, and Dr. Zoltan Lett, the first anesthesia specialist in Hong Kong. Each left his footprints in the history of medicine in Hong Kong.

Ho Hung-chiu, John 何鴻超 (1916–2005)

MBBS, MD, FRCR, FACR, FRANZCR, FHKCR, CBE, Cavaliere of the Order Al Merito della Repubblica Italiana.

Professor Ho Hung-chiu, John, fondly nicknamed "Emperor Ho," was the "Father of Radiology and Oncology" in Hong Kong. His influence and contributions to his profession and to the Hong Kong community were profound.

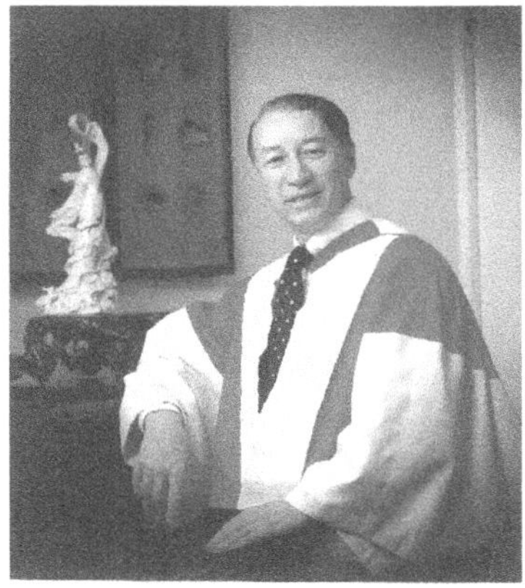

Figure 9.1 Professor Ho Hung-chiu John
Image courtesy of the Ho family

Born in 1916 into a prominent family, he was expected to have nothing short of the best performance in school. He attended St. Joseph's College and entered the Faculty of Medicine, HKU. In the HKU he enjoyed sports and excelled in swimming, diving, and long-distance running and collected a host of medals and trophies in interfaculty and university competitions.

Ho graduated in 1940, when the Japanese Army had already marched to Shenzhen border between China and Hong Kong during the Second Sino-Japanese War. Being a patriot, he responded to the call from the China Defence League for urgent relief measures and organized two ambulances packed with medical supplies to be driven into mainland China. In the mainland, he initially worked with the Medical Relief Corps of Chinese Red Cross, but later he joined the Nationalist Army.[6] He worked in field hospitals where surgeries had to be performed even without anesthesia and without disinfectants. On his return to Hong Kong in 1945, he took charge of the partially bombed-out Lai Chi Kok Infectious Diseases Hospital, which was overflowing with patients with smallpox, cholera, typhoid, diphtheria, and cerebrospinal meningitis. In 1946, he received a British Council Scholarship for further studies in England, in recognition of his wartime services in China.

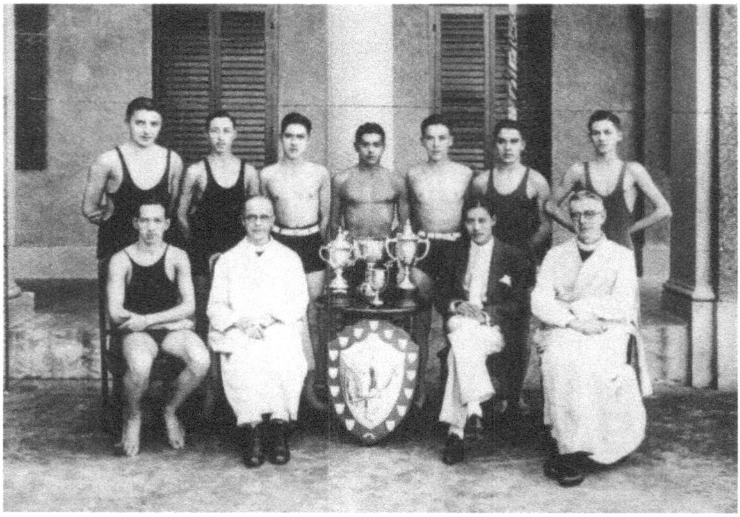

Figure 9.2 Ho Hung-chiu (standing left 2) and his swimming team of Ricci Hall, 1936
Image courtesy of the Ho Family

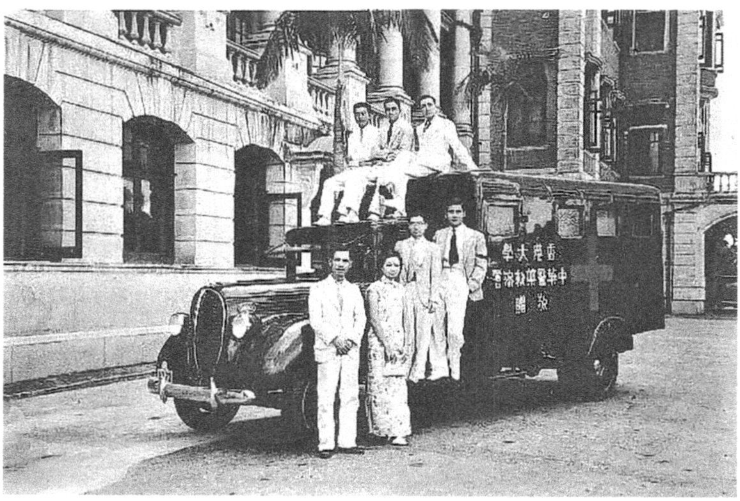

Figure 9.3 Dr. Ho Hung-chiu (sitting R1) and the ambulance packed with medical supplies for China, 1939
Image courtesy of the Ho Family

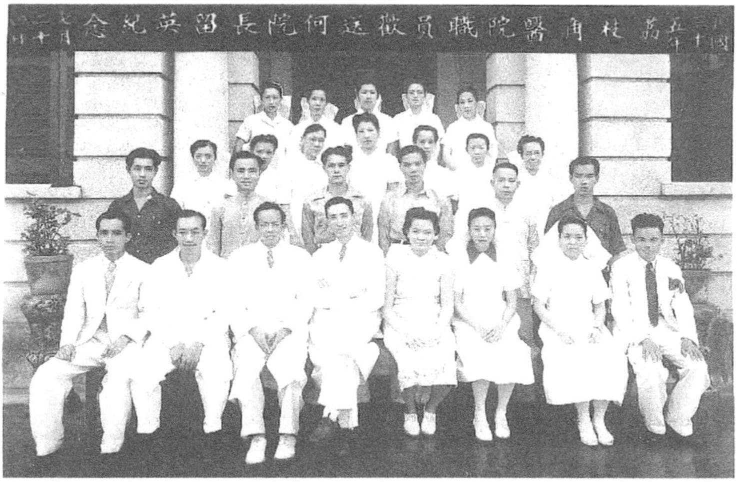

Figure 9.4 Dr. Ho Hung-chiu (front row, L4) and staff of Lai Chi Kok Hospital, 1946
Image courtesy of the Ho family

Ho's experience with surgery and tropical medicine thus far failed to arouse his enthusiasm.[7] In England, however, he found his calling. He attended the Department of Radiology of the Royal Postgraduate Medical School at Hammersmith Hospital and received a Diploma in Medical Radio-diagnosis (DMRD) of the English Conjoint Board of the Royal College of Physicians of London and the Royal College of Surgeons of England. After spending three weeks at the Radiology Department of the renowned Karolinska Institute, he returned to Hong Kong via the US, where he visited some of the best radiodiagnostic and radiotherapeutic centers in the world at Mount Sinai Hospital, the Mayo Clinic, and Moffitt Hospital.[8]

When Ho arrived in Hong Kong in 1949, he joined the Radiological Sub-Department (RSD) of the Government Medical Department headed by Dr. Frank James Farr, who retired the same year. Although the first X-ray machine was installed in Alice Memorial Hospital as early as 1910, neither the Hong Kong Government Medical Department nor the university attempted to develop radiology service to any extent before the war. The first deep-X ray machine for the treatment of cancer was installed at Queen Mary Hospital in 1939. During the war, the machine was dismantled and removed to Japan. During the immediate postwar years, prevention and control of the overwhelming prevalent infectious diseases in Hong Kong took the lion's share of the medical budget. Radiology remained a "sub-department."[9]

Due to the population increase in Hong Kong and the rising importance of X-rays as a diagnostic technique, Ho anticipated that radiology would have to expand. He began to build his empire systematically and strategically. Realizing that training of radiographers and radiotherapy technicians must be carried out locally because of the prohibitive cost of sending individuals to England, Ho successfully negotiated with the College of Radiographers in London to recognize training in Hong Kong and to have the examination locally in 1953.[10]

In 1954, Ho returned to the UK to complete his training in Middlesex Hospital. Between 1954 and 1959, he obtained Fellowships of the Faculty of Radiologists of the Conjoint Board (retitled Royal College of Radiologists in 1975) in both diagnostic and therapeutic radiology—the only person in Hong Kong with such qualifications. After he returned from the UK, he discussed with the corresponding UK college to have the local training of radiotherapy technicians recognized, and he received approval. Foundations were then laid for radiotherapy to become a specialist area in Hong Kong.[11]

Ho then turned to training of Hong Kong doctors. In October 1959, he applied to the Conjoint Board of the Faculty of Radiologists to recognize the training of qualified doctors for the DMRD and Diploma in Medical Radiotherapy (DMRT) and to have Part I of the examination to be held in Hong Kong. Successful candidates were sent to the UK for one to two years for the Part II DMRD or DMRT. In the mid-1970s, even Part II examination for the Fellowship of the Royal College of Radiologists (FRCR) was held in either Hong Kong or Singapore for Diagnosis (D) and Therapy (T) separately—an important step forward, showing the confidence of the Royal College of Radiologists in the training provided by senior colleagues in Hong Kong.[12] In the 2000s, four generations of radiographers, radiotherapy technicians, and radiologists and oncologists could trace their lineage to Ho as their original mentor; the department heads in all major oncology centers were his trainees.[13]

In 1956, the RSD of the Government Medical Department at Queen Mary Hospital was located on the first floor at the southeast corner of the main building, accommodating both diagnostic and radiotherapy facilities. Soon the RSD expanded to occupy the whole wing of the first floor. In the following decade, the pattern of diseases in Hong Kong changed, and chronic noncommunicable diseases, including cancer, constituted the main causes of death. There was a need for more sophisticated facilities for diagnosis and therapy. These included ultrasound, X-ray tomography, and radioisotope imaging equipment and at a later stage computerized scanning, magnetic resonance imaging, and positron emission tomography, and the introduction of linear accelerators for radiotherapy. A great deal more space was required for the new equipment. In 1964, Ho had the Institute of Radiotherapy and Oncology built and equipped at Queen Elizabeth Hospital, with a generous donation from the Royal Hong Kong Jockey Club. The institute accommodated all the advanced facilities for radiology, radiotherapy, and oncology, including the new high-energy radiotherapy machine for treatment of nasopharyngeal carcinoma (NPC).

Ho had the foresight to recruit Geoffrey Mauldon from Australia as early as 1956, to set up a new Physics Division and to train physicists and engineers to develop and support these services.[14] During the economic boom from the 1970s to 1990s, several major regional hospitals were built such as Princess Margaret Hospital, Prince of Wales Hospital, Tuen Mun Hospital, and Pamela Youde Nethersole Eastern Hospital. They all required radiology, radioisotope, and radiotherapy services, and the service of a physicist in the planning stage, to determine the facilities and the equipment required and to ensure the safety of the staff and patients. He was able to provide such a service.

Step by step, Ho created and developed his "empire" to provide both radiology and radiotherapy services for the people of Hong Kong. As he headed both the radiodiagnostic and radiotherapeutic services of all the hospitals in the Government Medical and Health Department in Hong Kong, he must have headed one of the largest radiology services in the world. His colleagues, Professor G. B. Ong and Professor A. J. S. McFadzean, admired and envied Ho's ability to establish such a huge service, and they fondly called him "Emperor Ho."[15]

Ho deeply cared for his patients, and they in turn trusted him. He aimed at providing them with better services and advanced therapeutic modalities. In 1956, to enable patients to receive radiotherapy at Queen Mary Hospital, which had no beds for such patients, Ho approached Oxfam for a donation to build a 32-bed hostel near Queen Mary Hospital for patients who could care for themselves.[16] In 1967, with donations from the Hong Kong Anti-Cancer Society, Ho was able to have Nam Long

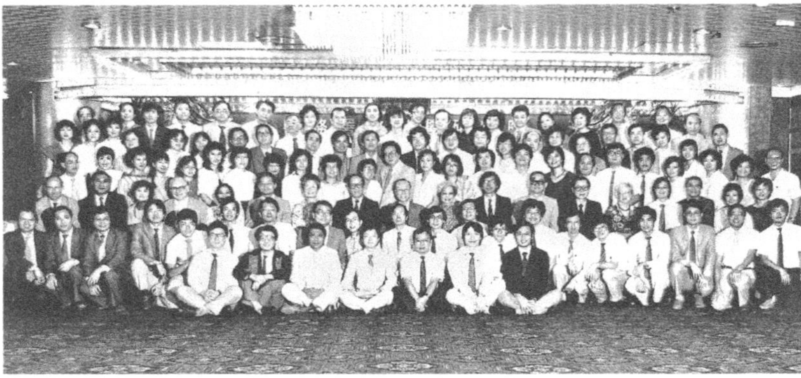

Figure 9.5 Professor Ho Hung-chiu (sitting, third row, L9) with staff of the Radiotherapy Division, 1985
Image courtesy of the Ho Family

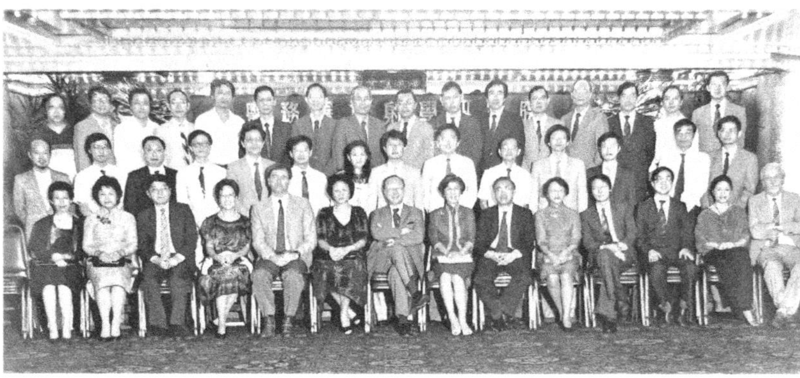

Figure 9.6 Professor Ho Hung-chiu (Front row, L7) with staff of the Radiodiagnostic Division, 1985
Image courtesy of the Ho family

Hospital built specifically for the treatment of cancer patients. Over the years the hospital increased in size, to accommodate more patients and to expand its services.[17] In 2003, Nam Long Hospital closed and was changed to a nursing home to suit the needs of Hong Kong.[18]

Although Ho treated and investigated patients with different types of cancer, it was his seminal research on NPC that he achieved international recognition. He pursued every aspect of this disease to understand its pathogenesis, treatment, methods of prevention, and early detection. NPC is common among southern Chinese. He postulated that early exposure to preserved food, especially salted fish, was a major causative factor and provided epidemiological and experimental evidence[19] to support this hypothesis. Another major finding was the strong association between Epstein-Barr virus (EBV) and NPC, leading to a method for early detection of NPC[20] and a better understanding of the pathogenesis. Ho proposed a different staging system for NPC because its behavior and therapeutic considerations are different from other head-and-neck cancers. The current staging system of the International Union Against Cancer and the American Joint Committee for Cancer Staging and End-Results Reporting for NPC was largely based on his concepts. In treating NPC patients with radiotherapy, the techniques he used achieved a 5-year disease-specific survival of 52% during 1976–1985, when the disease used to be fatal.[21]

The founding of the Hong Kong Anti-Cancer Society in 1963 was another major accomplishment of Ho. The society played a vital role in promoting prevention and early detection of cancer and providing effective treatment as well as hospice care. It offered funding for cancer research, especially studies on locally prevalent cancers, such as NPC, and lung cancer. The society contributed immensely to the development of evidence-based clinical practice for treating various cancers.[22] Ho also had the vision to establish a population-based cancer registry in Hong Kong in the 1970s. The registry was accepted by the International Association of Cancer Registries as a member, in recognition of its good-quality data. By showing changes in incidence and mortality and the patterns of cancer distribution, the registry is proved vital for planning cancer services as well as for epidemiological and clinical research.[23]

Ho was first appointed Honorary Lecturer in Radiology in 1950 and Honorary Clinical Professor of Radiation Oncology in 1983 at HKU. He and his staff were responsible for teaching medical students until the academic departments were established in CUHK in 1984 and HKU in 1991. For his students and staff, he emphasized the following: "cancer treatment must be based on scientific evidence, and if there was none available in the literature, one should try to secure the evidence through research. He placed great emphasis on accurate assessment of measurable disease, meticulous record keeping and use of correct terminology"[24]—sound advice that any researcher, in fact, any doctor should heed. He was loved by his students, trainees, and staff. He often came to the "rescue" of young trainees cornered by Professor G. B. Ong, who only revered Ho among all the doctors.

Even though Ho came from a wealthy and prominent family, he recognized the difficulties of everyday living for millions of Chinese in his time. A compassionate man, Ho was known to pick up every single grain of rice that was left on the table in front of him, saying: every grain comes with the hard work of farmers.[25] Ho donated his salary to various charities.

Professor Ho Hung-chiu, John retired in 1985. His students and colleagues set up "The Ho Hung-chiu Medical Education Foundation" as a tribute to their mentor to continue his spirit of promoting education and research. He continued to serve for another 15 years as Honorary Consultant at Baptist Hospital.

For his enormous contributions to cancer treatment and research, Professor Ho was decorated locally and in other countries as well as by international agencies. The honors that Professor Ho received are unprecedented in number and in global extensiveness. The most prestigious ones include the following: in Europe, OBE and CBE, Cavaliere of the Order Al Merito della Repubblica Italiana, and the award by the International Association for Research on EBV and Associated Diseases; in North America, Honorary Fellow of the American College of Radiology, the first Gold Medal and Inaugural Lecture of the del Regato Foundation, Gold Medal and the 5th Annual Lecture of the Gilbert H. Fletcher Society; in Australia, Honorary Fellow of the Royal Australian and New Zealand College of Radiologists; and in Hong Kong, the First Sir Patrick Manson Gold Medal, Honorary Doctor of Science, and Honorary Fellow of the Hong Kong College of Radiologists.[26]

Professor Ho was a legend in Hong Kong, an icon in the academic world, and a visionary among radiologists, oncologists, and radiotherapists, and from whom we have much to learn and emulate. He is remembered with fondness, admiration, pride, and reverence.

Yap Pow-meng 葉寶明 (1921–1971)

MA, MD, DPM, FRCPE, FRCPsych

Professor Yap Pow-meng was the founding "Father of Psychiatry and Mental Health Services" in Hong Kong[27] and a world authority on international mental health and comparative psychiatry.

Yap was born in Malacca, Malaya, in 1921. He attended the Victoria Institution, the oldest secondary school in Kuala Lumpur.[28] Being the most distinguished scholar in the family of five boys, he won several scholarships while in high school. The most prestigious, Queen's Scholarship, was offered on his graduation in 1939, thereby securing him a place in Cambridge, England, for his higher education. The Queen's Scholarship, named in honor of Britain's Queen Victoria, was inaugurated in 1885 in the Straits Settlements by Sir Cecil Clementi Smith. One of the objectives for the scholarship was to allow promising boys an opportunity to complete their studies in England. There was no university in the Straits Settlements or in the Malay States then, and most families could hardly afford to send their children to school let alone to England for a university education. As a student, Yap was very active in many extracurricular activities: a member of the debating society and the geography society, a prefect, and a member of the prefects' board, and the captain of the swimming team. He arrived in England just as World War II broke out in Europe.

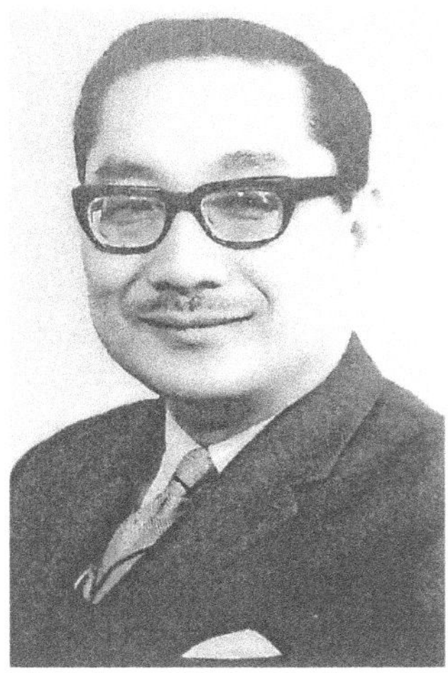

Figure 9.7 Professor Yap Pow-meng

Source: "Professor P. M. Yap Memorial Lectures," *Hong Kong Journal of Mental Health*, 28 (1&2) (1999), 2.

Yap entered Sidney Sussex College of Cambridge University and obtained his BA in moral sciences (psychology) in 1943 and MB in 1946. He went on to receive postgraduate training at Maudsley Hospital and received a Diploma of Psychological Medicine (DPM) in 1948. The same year he began his career in Hong Kong, when he took up the position of Medical Superintendent of Victoria Mental Hospital at High Street.[29]

In the early twentieth century, mental patients in Hong Kong were kept in asylums, one for males and one for females; Europeans were also separated from Chinese. In 1925, the asylums for Europeans and Chinese were merged to form Victoria Mental Hospital, which had only 23 beds in the beginning. Later it was enlarged to hold 84 patients. Despite the progressive increase in population in Hong Kong, the number of beds remained the same. The government sent Chinese patients, who could not be accommodated, to John G. Kerr Refuge for the Insane in Fangcun in the southwestern part of Guangzhou and remitted funds to the refuge each year to cover the patients' expenses.[30] After the founding of People's Republic of China (PRC) in 1949 and closure of the border in 1951, patients could no longer be repatriated to Guangzhou. The Hong Kong government had to care for its own mental patients and it planned building a psychiatric hospital in Castle Peak.

Yap was at the right time to introduce contemporary concepts and Western psychiatry to Hong Kong when psychiatric facilities were beginning to be developed. Under his leadership, mental health services developed systematically. There was a great deal of societal prejudice against patients with mental illness in Hong Kong. He spent the first few years educating the public on mental illness[31] and on mental abnormality.[32] He lectured on mental hygiene and how to prevent mental illness, and urged the establishment of guidance clinics for school children.[33] He told the people of Hong Kong, "It has been said that in the manner in which a country treats its mentally diseased people, you can estimate its level of civilization." In 1954, he organized a mental health study group, which developed into the Mental Health Association of Hong Kong—a NGO to promote mental health education and mental healthcare for psychiatric patients.[34] This organization provided facilities for rehabilitation for mental patients. In 1960, Mental Health Ordinance (Cap. 136) was enacted to provide for the care of patients with mental illness, and the old Mental Hospital Ordinance was repealed.[35]

In 1957, the first phase of Castle Peak Hospital was opened. Yap organized a voluntary treatment center for narcotic dependence, to occupy the first 120 beds in Castle Peak Hospital. When the narcotic treatment center moved out of Castle Peak Hospital in 1965,[36] Yap remained as an honorary advisor to the Society for the Aid and Rehabilitation of Drug Abusers (SARDA). When completed in 1961, Castle Peak Hospital had 1,000 beds. It replaced Victoria Mental Hospital, and Yap, who was appointed the superintendent, was very proud of this hospital.[37] He introduced modern psychiatric treatment to the hospital and equipped it with a multidisciplinary team of doctors, nurses, medical social workers, occupational therapists, two psychologists, and a pharmacist. The advent of psychotropic drugs for the treatment of mental illness permitted some patients to leave the hospital and enabled them to have a productive life outside while taking medications. However, they needed to be rehabilitated and closely monitored in outpatient clinics.[38]

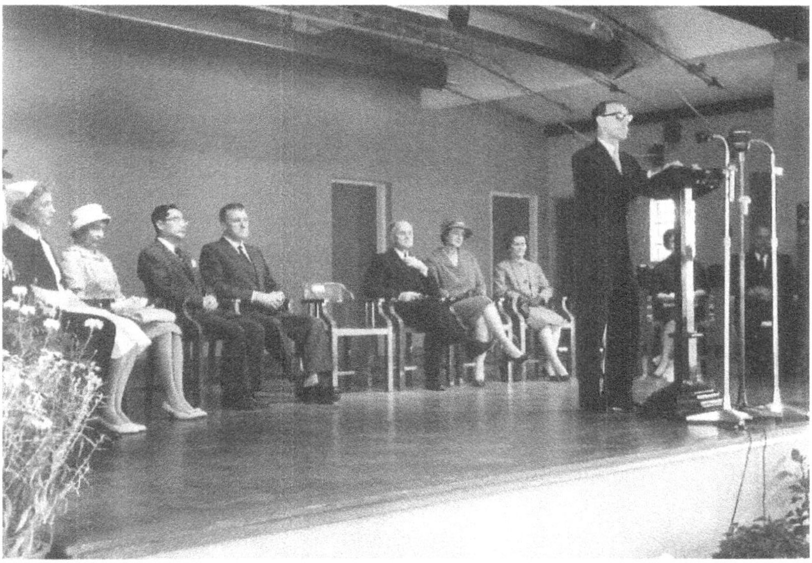

Figure 9.8 Opening of the Castle Peak Hospital, Dr. P. M. Yap (sitting, L3) in 1961. The hospital was opened officially by the Governor Sir Robert Black.

Source: "Brief History of Psychiatric Service in Hong Kong" published by the Institute of Mental Health, Castle Peak Hospital.

Dr. Yap was a pioneer of rehabilitation and community care of psychiatric patients. He aimed at returning psychiatric patients to society with gainful employment. For this to happen, there had to be psychiatric outpatient clinics and halfway houses, as most of the patients had been in hospital for a long time, and they needed readjustment to return to the community. The first halfway house was opened in 1964 by the New Life Mutual Aid Club, a non-profit NGO, for discharged patients from Castle Peak Hospital.[39] It set up the first male halfway house at To Kwa Wan.

In the following year, the New Life Mutual Aid Club was renamed the New Life Psychiatric Rehabilitation Association, which set up agricultural and industrial sheltered workshops for men, and in 1972, the first female halfway house at Kwun Tong.[40] For a long time, the responsibility of rehabilitation was provided mainly by NGOs such as the Mental Health Association of Hong Kong and the New Life Psychiatric Rehabilitation Association.

Yap believed in moving psychiatric services to the community by establishing several psychiatric or mental health centers and units. This took the form of day hospitals and outpatient services for follow-up of discharged patients from psychiatric hospitals. The new Yau Ma Tei Psychiatric Center with various types of psychiatric services, including outpatient clinics for adults and children, was opened in 1966 to replace Tsim Sha Tsui Psychiatric Center.[41] The Hong Kong Psychiatric Center, created in 1968/1969, was and still is the reference center on Hong Kong Island.[42] More halfway houses and outpatient services were developed after Yap left Hong Kong in 1969. The change from institutional care to rehabilitation and returning the patient to society under community care was painfully slow in Hong Kong because of the strong societal prejudice against those with mental illness. It was only after the turn of the millennium that the number of psychiatric hospital beds was reduced by one-third from 5,395 in 2000 to 3,607 in 2012 and more patients attending outpatient clinics.[43]

Throughout the period that he was in government service, Yap was a lecturer in the Department of Medicine at HKU. At that time, psychiatry was taught as a subject within the medicine curriculum. He was an inspiring teacher and interested in his students. He spoke English almost as his first language but did not master Cantonese well enough to communicate satisfactorily with his patients. Students found it hilarious when Yap conducted a psychiatric interview, using very awkward phrases to elicit sexual history from his patients.

While busily organizing the mental health service in Hong Kong, Yap still carried out his research. He conducted an epidemiological study on suicide in Hong Kong, investigated into its incidence and trend, and analyzed the factors predisposing to suicide.[44] He found an increasing tendency for suicide between 1946 and 1955, and the prevalence greater in men than in women, except in the older age group, when the reverse was found. Poverty, illness, and unemployment were the most important causes for suicide.[45] The result of this study formed the basis of his MD thesis in 1957. He was best known for his work on transcultural psychiatry and coined the term "culture-bound syndrome." He published his classic paper describing koro as a culture-bound depersonalization syndrome in the *British Journal of Psychiatry*.[46] He examined the condition latah syndrome, and dissected the nosology of the condition and argued that "latah is a specialized form of fright neurosis, with minimal hysterical features, culturally maintained and found only in persons whose powers of mastery and of defense are limited by the level of their own cultural development."[47] He utilized his excellent command of the English language fully and became a prolific contributor at international seminars as well as various journals covering not only his legendary culture-bound syndrome and comparative psychiatry but also other topics such as drug dependence, suicide, aging, and nosology.[48] His findings were widely quoted in literature.

As he became increasingly recognized in the field of international mental health and comparative psychiatry, Yap received invitations to deliver lectures in psychiatric centers around the world and to address conferences. In 1963, he was a member of the Expert Advisory Panel on Mental Health of the WHO. In 1966, he spent six-months in Honolulu doing research at the East-West Centre preceding the Conference of Mental Health Research in Asia and the Pacific. In 1969, he left the Hong Kong Government Medical Services to become Associate Professor at Clarke Institute of University of Toronto.[49] However, in 1971, he returned to Hong Kong as the first Professor of Psychiatry at HKU.[50] Unfortunately, his career was cut short by his sudden death in November of that year while attending the Fifth World Psychiatric Congress at Mexico City. He was survived by his wife and two children.[51]

Professor Yap Pow-meng is remembered as a scholar, an intellectual, and a profound philosopher with a keen interest in people. According to his students, he was always kind, considerate, courteous, and helpful. He dedicated his life to the understanding of the minds of people.

Zoltan Lett (1916–2014)

MD, DA, FRCA, FFARCS, FANZCA, FHKCA, FHKAM (Anaes)

Dr. Zoltan Lett, known as Lefty to his friends, was the "Father of Anesthesia" in Hong Kong. He was responsible for the development of anesthesia and for the training of anesthetists until the establishment of the Department of Anesthesia in the two universities in Hong Kong. He founded the two professional organizations of anesthesia—The Society of Anesthetists of Hong Kong and The Hong Kong College of Anesthesiologists. He was also instrumental in the establishment of the Society of Critical Care Medicine.

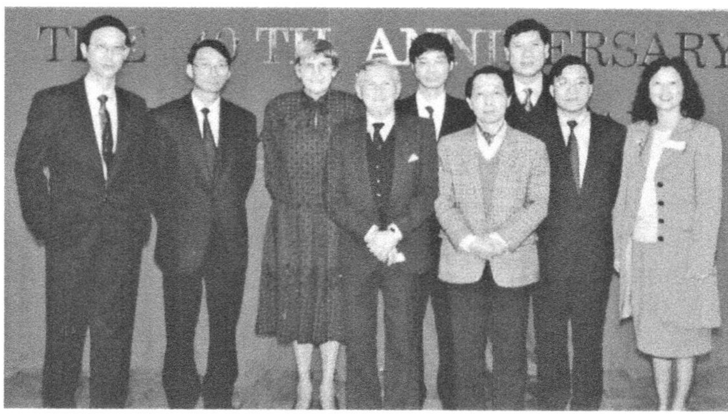

Figure 9.9 Dr. Zoltan Lett (L4) and past presidents and vice presidents of SAHK during its 40th anniversary, 1995
Image courtesy of Dr. C. T. Hung

Born in 1916 in Czechoslovakia, Lett was a fifth-year medical student when Nazi Germany took over his country. Lett left for England and joined the Czech Free Force in 1939. When the Czech government in exile decided to send students to continue their education in England to rebuild the country after the war, Lett completed his medical training at University College Hospital in London. He was one of 23 Czech graduates to receive their medical degrees from Oxford in 1942. After graduation, he joined the Royal Army Medical Corps and was deployed to Burma, where he worked as an anesthetist. After the war, he received further training in anesthesia and obtained a Diploma in Anesthetics and later Fellowship of the Faculty of Anesthetists of the Royal College of Surgeons (FFARCS).[52] He then worked as a registrar in anesthesia in the National Health Service. In Nottingham where he was posted, he met Dr. K. C. Yeo, then Director of Medical and Health Services of Hong Kong.[53] Yeo recruited Lett to take up the first ever specialist anesthetist position in Hong Kong.[54]

Lett arrived in Hong Kong in 1954. He was to provide and develop anesthetic services to government hospitals in Hong Kong and to teach medical students at HKU on a part-time basis. There were only three government hospitals: Queen Mary Hospital, Tsan Yuk Hospital, and Kowloon Hospital. There were few anesthetists in Hong Kong, and none had received proper postgraduate training in anesthesia, with the exception of Dr. Horatio Percy Loui Ozorio, who was of Portuguese descent and a graduate of the Faculty of Medicine, HKU. Ozorio practiced obstetrics and gynecology and anesthesia, and he gained vast experience working with Professor Kenelm Digby at HKU before the war.[55] Lett and Ozorio collaborated to develop anesthesia in Hong Kong until 1960, when Ozorio left for the UK. The two founded the Society of Anesthetists (now anesthesiologists) of Hong Kong (SAHK) in 1954,[56] which had only a handful of anesthetists and a few interested surgeons. The objectives of SAHK were to raise the awareness of anesthesia as a component of medicine, to provide an optimal training environment for anesthesiologists, to create opportunities for continuing clinical education, and to improve public perception of anesthesiology as a medical discipline. The scientific meetings organized by SAHK with overseas speakers were popular among local anesthetists, as it was rare for them to attend conferences overseas in those days. Three years after its founding, SAHK was admitted to the World Federation for Societies of Anesthesiologists as a full member. Lett served as president for 17 years.

Due to the increasing number of hospital beds in the public sector, there was increased demand for doctors, including anesthesiologists. Anesthesiologists in the Government Medical and Health Department could not assume senior position unless they were accredited through examinations of Faculty of Anesthetists of the Royal College of Surgeons in England (FFARCS) or the Royal Australasian College of Surgeon (FFARACS).[57] In the 1960s, the government's policy was to send an individual for one to two years to England to receive training and to take the fellowship examination. The government paid the expenses. The whole process of postgraduate training was far too slow to fulfill the demand for anesthesiologists. The solution was to train them locally.

Because of his dedication and his friendly and gregarious nature, Lett had built up an international network of friends in anesthesiology, and they helped him to advance his vision of a high standard of anesthesia in Hong Kong. Lett negotiated for the training in Hong Kong to be recognized by the Faculty of Anesthetists within the Royal Australasian College of Surgeons. In the 1960s, the Australian Faculty of Anesthetists sent examiners to conduct training and mock examinations of candidates in Hong Kong. Lett, through SAHK, organized refresher courses during which they and other senior colleagues lectured on anesthesia, and basic scientists from HKU lectured on physiology and pharmacology. He also established an educational foundation to sponsor tutors from Australia to conduct courses in Hong Kong.[58] In 1969, the first primary examination of FFARACS was carried out by Australian examiners in Hong Kong. In later years, the examination was carried out by Hong Kong anesthesiologists.[59]

During the golden era of hospital building in the 1970s and 1980s, more anesthesiologists were needed, and a proper training program was necessary. Up to that time, there had been no formal postgraduate training program in Hong Kong not only for anesthesia but also for other specialties. Lett held a part-time appointment as honorary clinical lecturer in the Department of Surgery in HKU. On his retirement from government service in 1976, he was renamed full-time Lecturer and later Reader of Anesthesia at the Department of Surgery, devoting more time on the training program until his second retirement in 1983. A review of the situation of anesthesia in Hong Kong was carried out by Dr. Michael D. Vicker, a British anesthesiologist, at the request of the British Council Committee for International Cooperation in Higher Education. Dr. Vicker recommended that an independent department of anesthesia be established in the university. In 1987, the Department of Anesthesia was founded within the Faculty of Medicine in HKU, four years after CUHK had established a Department of Anesthesia in the Faculty of Medicine.[60]

Intensive care medicine as a specialty developed relatively late compared to other specialties. It was first established in 1953, when a number of patients required controlled ventilation during an epidemic of poliomyelitis. These patients were put together in a unit and headed by an anesthetist.[61] The first Society for Critical Care Medicine was formed in the US in 1970.[62] Lett founded the Hong Kong Society of Critical

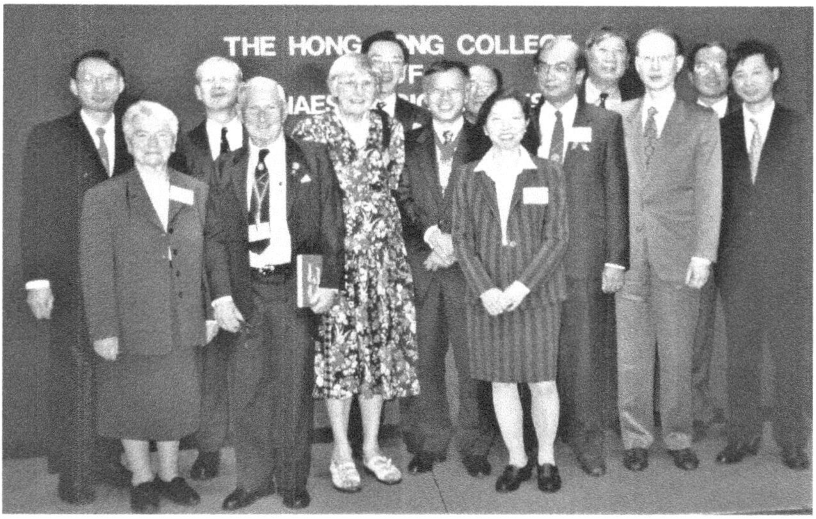

Figure 9.10 Dr. Zoltan Lett (Front, L2) at Hong Kong College of Anesthesiologists annual meeting 1999
Image courtesy of Dr. C. T. Hung

Care Medicine (HKSCCM) in 1984 and was its inaugural chair. He was also the promoter and one of the founders of the Hong Kong College of Anesthesiologists (HKCA) in 1989. The objective of HKCA was to assume professional authority for accreditation and setting standards in anticipation of the establishment of Hong Kong Academy of Medicine which was launched by government legislation in 1993. The College of Anesthesiologists was one of the founding colleges of the academy.

Lett encouraged clinical research and had published in peer-reviewed journals. He was the author of several books: a textbook on anesthesia and two books on the history of anesthesia and intensive care in Hong Kong.[63] He stressed the importance of a sympathetic approach to patients. He said in an interview, "pre-operative sedation with modern drugs is undoubtedly efficacious, but one should not forget the tranquilizing effect of a visit by a wise, experienced, and sympathetic anesthetist who can gain the patient's confidence and respect. The beneficial effects of a good anesthetist's personality ... are non-toxic, not depressant on the vital centers ... do not depress respiration and are neither addictive or habit-forming. All these are in marked contrast to many of the chemical substances at our disposal for sedation."[64]

When Lett retired the second time from HKU in 1983, he was immediately recruited by Caritas Medical Centre to head their Anesthesia Department. He served until 1993, when he began to travel extensively for several years before settling in the UK. He remained closely associated with SAHK and HKCA, until he finally retired from clinical practice. Lett passed away in 2014, at the ripe old age of 98.

According to Dr. Ronald Lo, past president of HKCA, Dr. Zoltan Lett was not only an effective administrator, clinician, and teacher but also a mentor and friend to many anesthesiologists who were trained in Hong Kong. His contributions to anesthesia are recognized both locally and internationally. He was awarded Honorary Life Membership of the Society of Anesthetists of Hong Kong as well as the Philippine Society of Anesthesiology, and emeritus professorship from the University of Philippines. He received fellowships from many anesthesia colleges around the world. Dr. Lett was the lynchpin in bringing Hong Kong anesthesia from a primitive state after World War II to the sophisticated system with a high standard of clinical care that Hong Kong has today. He dedicated himself to the specialty of anesthesia and served Hong Kong well for 40 years.[65]

10. Postwar University Educators
Producing Doctors and Training Specialists

In the Western world, the division of medicine into various specialties, such as medicine, surgery, gynecology and obstetrics, can be dated to hundreds of years ago, and medical practitioners have long been specialized to practice in an area of their interest. By the beginning of the twentieth century, the number of specialists had steadily increased in urban areas in the Western world.[1] In the US, there were more specialists than general practitioners by the 1940s, and this phenomenon persists today.

In Hong Kong, Western medicine was also divided into special branches early. Surgery was performed early at Government Civil Hospital when it was first established in 1850, but a proper operating theatre was only established around 1890. Beds for confinement were introduced by Dr. P. B. C. Ayres in 1890 to Government Civil Hospital, but only women in moribund conditions from difficult labor were admitted. When Alice Memorial Hospital and Nethersole Hospital were founded, there were beds for women, but again, few used them for confinement until the opening of Alice Memorial Maternity Hospital and the arrival of Dr. Alice Hickling (née Sibree) in 1904. Nevertheless, by the late nineteenth century, there were three basic branches of medicine: medicine, surgery, and gynecology and obstetrics in Government Civil Hospital and Alice Memorial and Affiliated Hospitals.

When HKCM for Chinese was established in 1887, the curriculum included various areas of Western clinical medicine: medicine, surgery, obstetrics and gynecology. The teaching of these subjects was carried out by doctors who were working in these areas. These teachers were not usually trained as specialists but developed their skills through years of practice.

Despite the founding of HKU and the Faculty of Medicine in 1911, clinical departments were developed much later only with the endowment of the Rockefeller professors in medicine and surgery in 1923, and in obstetrics and gynecology in 1924. Medical students had clinical training in these three areas during the last three years of the curriculum and had to be examined in each one during the final examination. Up to the beginning of World War II, when medical students graduated, they were allowed to practice in one branch or all three basic branches of medicine as they wished without further training. They did not require one year of internship before registration. There was no postgraduate training in HKU.

Although World War II ended in August 1945, the university did not reopen officially until mid-1948, and there was a great deal of controversy as to whether it should even be reopened. Although Admiral Harcourt took over Hong Kong from the Japanese, it was unclear whether Hong Kong would remain a British colony. The university campus had been badly damaged both by bombing and by looting, and the library had been partly destroyed. The colonial government, its infrastructure also greatly damaged, had little cash to spare. Many felt that Hong Kong did not need a university, because only 25% of the students were local, and its higher educational needs could be met in other ways.[2] After two years, it became obvious that there was a great demand for university graduates in all fields of work in Hong Kong, as few expatriates were willing to return from England. The few who were available demanded much higher salaries than the locals earned. Governor Alexander Grantham brought the uncertain fate of the university to an end by offering a special fund of HK$4 million from the Hong Kong government for the reestablishment program and increasing the annual grant to HK$1.5 million.[3] The university was formally reestablished on 7 April 1948.

The faculty members of HKU were also badly affected. Of the 25 positions filled by Europeans, only seven were still occupied; some had died, and others did not return. In the Faculty of Medicine, only Lindsay Ride, Professor of Physiology, and Gordon King, Professor of Obstetrics and Gynecology, remained. Ride and King, together with dedicated new recruits in 1948, which included Hou Pao-chang, Professor of Pathology, Alexander James Smith McFadzean, Professor of Medicine, will be discussed in this chapter. They played invaluable roles in the rebuilding of HKU.

As the population of Hong Kong increased rapidly after World War II, there was a shortage of doctors. In 1960, the government made an urgent request to the university to increase medical student enrollment by one-third, granting the university a subsidy, with guaranteed increases for the next seven years. For the first time in its history, the university could embark on a program of expansion—a great cause for celebration in its Golden Jubilee (1961).[4] Until 1980, there was only one medical school in Hong Kong. As noted, although the total number of medical student enrollments in HKU Faculty of Medicine had increased by almost three times from the 1950s to 1972, because of the dramatic increase in the population, the number of doctors per 1,000 population only increased marginally.[5] The government decided in 1974 to establish a second medical school at CUHK.[6]

Medicine developed very rapidly after the World War II. Advances in technology led to the discovery of many new diagnostic and treatment modalities. Although medical students were taught the basic branches of medicine—medicine, surgery, obstetrics, and gynecology—it was no longer possible for a doctor to be able to know all the recent advances in each branch of medicine. It became necessary for some doctors to acquire expertise in different specific areas—to become specialists. It is the task of universities to develop different specialties to provide clinical service equipped with latest technology required for patient care, teaching, and research in these specific areas.

To become a specialist requires several years of postgraduate education. Before World War II, medical specialists were all trained overseas. In the 1950s, medical graduates, fresh out of a one-year internship, would spend the next three or four years gaining local clinical and research experience under the guidance of their seniors. There was no formal, coordinated local postgraduate training, and the opportunities were usually only available to the cream of the student body.[7] After the local apprenticeship, trainees usually went to the UK for further postgraduate training and, if needed, to acquire more research experience in their field of interest. To be eligible to practice as specialists in the British Commonwealth, candidates had to pass Royal College examinations in their respective specialties. However, as Hong Kong would be returned to China after 1997, it could no longer depend on the Royal Colleges in the UK to certify its medical specialists. In the late 1980s and early 1990s, colleges of different branches of medicine were formed in Hong Kong to set their own training guidelines, assessment criteria and procedures for selection of trainers, and evaluation of training programs. As a result, postgraduate training became formalized. The final step was to establish the Academy of Medicine by statute, to coordinate the activities of all the colleges of different branches of medicine to foster development of postgraduate training and continuing medical education.[8] This difficult task was carried out by a committee chaired by Professor David Todd.

This chapter presents the stories of six postwar professors in the Faculty of Medicine of HKU, who were responsible for rehabilitating, rebuilding, and developing their departments. They were Professors Hou Pao-chang, James Gibson, A. J. S. McFadzean, David Todd, Arthur Ralph Hodgson, and Ong Guan Bee. These extraordinary individuals recognized the importance of their tasks and dedicated themselves to bring about state-of-the-art clinical service for patient care and research and above all, to teaching to produce doctors and specialists. During the course of their career, they became well recognized researchers and leaders and placed Hong Kong on the world map in their areas of interest. As a result of their endeavor, Hong Kong's healthcare system was staffed by their students and trainees, and soon their students became trainers, professors, or chief of service in most branches of medicine in HKU and CUHK. It is due to their devotion and hard work that we have our current healthcare system comparable to those of Western countries today.

Pathologists

Hou Pao-chang 侯寶璋 (1893–1967)

MD, DSc

Professor Hou Pao-chang was a pioneer in pathology in China and had a long and distinguished career nationally and internationally. He became the first postwar Professor of Pathology in Hong Kong (1948–1960) and rebuilt the department from scratch.

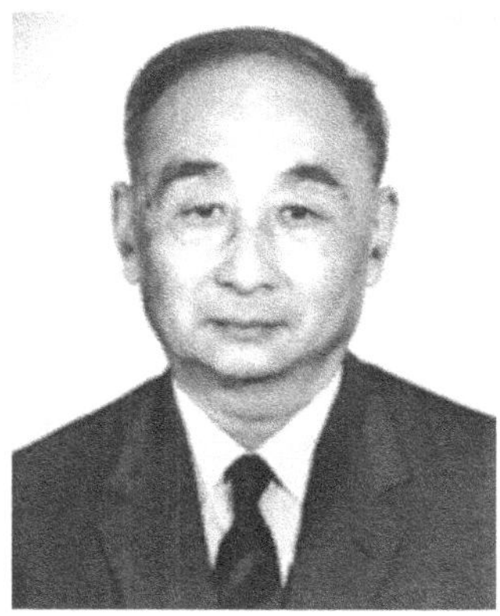

Figure 10.1 Professor Hou Pao-chang
Image courtesy of HKMMS

Hou was born in 1893 in Anhui province in China. He claimed that he owed his career to his liberal grandfather, who had a profound influence on his thinking and his life. He left home at a young age because he was unable to get along with his conservative father, a Chinese medicine practitioner. From then on, he supported himself through high school working as a laboratory assistant in a local hospital. His careful work and diligence won the attention of the authority in the hospital, which supported him through high school and university in Union Medical College in Peking. It was under very difficult circumstances that required courage and indomitable will that Hou graduated with distinction from medical school in 1920.

In his undergraduate days, Hou joined other students to demonstrate against the Chinese government's weak response to the decision of the Treaty of Versailles in allowing Japan to take over the territories in Shandong that China had surrendered to Germany after the Siege of Tsingtao in 1914. The demonstrations sparked nationwide protests and spurred an upsurge in Chinese nationalism. Hou actively participated in the May Fourth Movement, an intellectual revolution and sociopolitical reform movement that occurred in China between 1917 and 1921.[9]

After graduation, Hou returned to serve the hospital that had supported him through school and university for a period of three years. He then accepted a position in the Department of Pathology at Cheeloo University, where he also took part in translation of foreign books into Chinese, an important project to bring Western sciences into China. The opportunity for overseas training came in 1926, when he was offered a Rockefeller Foundation Scholarship that enabled him to study histology under Maximow in the US and pathology under Ludwig Pick in Berlin. From these two distinguished men he learned the thorough methods of investigation. In a subsequent visit to England, he was impressed with the work of the British schools in pathology and eventually accepted the British model.[10]

When the Japanese invaded Manchuria in 1931 and gradually occupied more territories in northern China, Hou joined the medical relief team to give medical assistance to the Chinese national army. In 1936, he was appointed Professor and Head of the Department of Pathology at Cheeloo University, a post he held for the next 10 years. When the Second Sino-Japanese War broke out in 1937, many universities, such as Peking University, Tsinghua University, and Nankai University merged to form Changsha Temporary University in Changsha and later renamed National Southwestern Associated University (Lianda) when they had moved to Kunming and Mengzi, Yunnan province. Hou decided to move with Cheeloo University to Chengdu, where he became Dean of the Medical Faculty of Cheeloo University and the Head of the Pathology Department of West China Union University. Despite the poor pay and hardship, Hou often donated part of his salary to support students who would otherwise have to leave the university.[11]

After the war, he was invited to lecture in the US and the UK. During his tour to the UK in 1947, he accepted an invitation to be Professor of Pathology at HKU,[12] at the time when civil war was intense in China. Hou arrived in Hong Kong to find the university dilapidated, as many buildings were either looted or bombed during the war. The Department of Pathology, located in the Pathology Building in the main campus, was left empty. All the benches and counters were gone, and the museum specimens disappeared. He used his ingenuity to improvise everything to get the laboratory work started and the clinical work going and at the same time began teaching and conducting research with the help of two laboratory assistants. He applied to the China Medical Board (CMB) of Rockefeller Foundation for funds to rehabilitate the department. With these funds he began to develop and establish different special divisions in the department: bacteriology, parasitology, and chemical pathology. In addition, he initiated a museum collection to keep the specimens and an archive of the wealth of materials.[13] As the economy of Hong Kong expanded in the late 1950s, the government invested more resources in the university. In 1958, a new pathology building was completed near Queen

Mary Hospital, under the close supervision of Hou. At long last, Hou was able to bring teaching and research in a clinical setting. The Pathology Building served Hong Kong for the next 60 years.[14]

Han Suyin, the celebrated author of *A Many Splendored Thing*, worked as an assistant to Hou for a brief period when she was in Hong Kong after the war. She wrote in her autobiography *My House Has Two Doors* about how Hou must have felt as she did, working and living in Hong Kong under the colonial administration:

> As for Hou Paochang, there was ecstasy upon his face as he plunged his hands into a corpse and palpated an unsuspected cancer....
>
> Prof. Hou had come from China which made understanding of our similar hesitancies, dilemmas, and self-questioning immediate and our relations excellent. He too was waiting for the dust to settle. We both hated colonial subjugation, but we were also products of this subjugation, and in this duality became supple, flexible, knowing our quandary not havoc ... neither he nor I were guilt-complex ridden, despite our respective Christian upbringings. We accepted ourselves, tolerating well the perpetual discomfort of being never entirely right, never entirely true, but in our imperfect way entire and flawless in our faith to our only religion, China.[15]

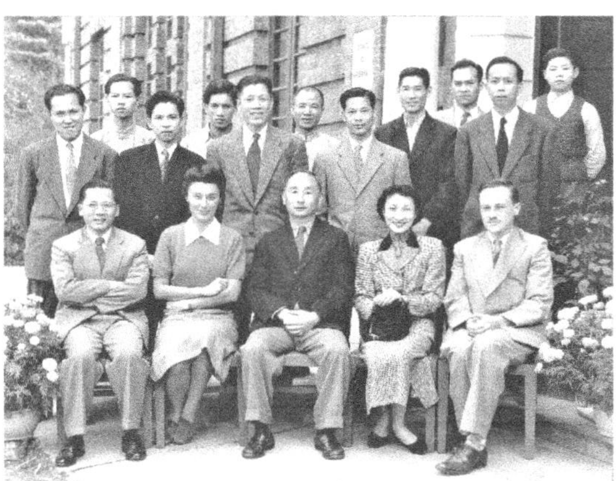

Figure 10.2 Professor Hou Pao-chang (sitting, center), Dr. C. T. Huang (sitting, L1), Han Suyin (sitting, L2) and other staff of the department, 1950

Source: HKMMS, reproduced with permission

It was expected that Hou would return to China to serve his beloved country after his retirement from Hong Kong in 1960.[16] His enormous contributions to HKU in reestablishing and expanding the department out of an empty building after the war were recognized by the title of Emeritus Professor on his retirement and in the following year, honorary Doctor of Science.[17]

While working in Hong Kong, he attended conferences abroad and lectured in different parts of the world, gaining international reputation for his research. He also visited China several times to lecture and to share information and knowledge with his colleagues in various universities. His reputation caught the attention of the medical and political circle in Beijing, and he was received by Premier Zhou Enlai. After his retirement, he was offered positions in a number of Western universities but chose to return to China. He became Professor of Morbid Anatomy and Vice-President of Peking Union Medical College, his alma mater. There he continued to train pathologists and to conduct research.[18] Unfortunately during the Cultural Revolution, which began in 1966, Hou and his family suffered under the Red Guards. He passed away in 1967 at the age of 74.[19]

During his life time, Hou had many students in China and in Hong Kong, and some became well-known pathologists. He was one of the most admired and respected teachers while at HKU. Some rated him as their best. One wrote: "Prof Hou's lectures were concise and succinct. He used words that were carefully chosen.... He possessed the true humility and dignity of a true Chinese scholar, greeting his students with a warm smile and almost a bow!" Many were impressed by his selfless patriotism. They were all proud to be a student of Hou. Professor Sir David Todd thought that Professor Hou was a blessing from God to HKU. He enjoyed the delightful time listening to the discussion on Chinese art and culture between Professors Hou and McFadzean and the gracious hospitality of Mrs. Hou. Professor Rosie Young was a student and later a colleague of Professor Hou. They collaborated on research projects on biliary cirrhosis and liver cancer. She said that Professor Hou focused on teaching principles and not details, and she learned a great deal from him.[20]

Hou's research interests were broad, including cirrhosis of the liver, primary liver cancer, nasopharyngeal carcinoma, "black fever," and others. It was the discovery of the relationship between the infestation of *Clonorchis sinensis* and biliary cirrhosis and primary carcinoma of the liver that pushed him to the forefront of cancer research. He demonstrated that infestation of parasites could lead to cirrhosis and then cancer—a novel hypothesis at the time.[21] Many researchers took shortcuts in their research. They did not form a hypothesis before the research but rather formed an opinion on the results and set about to prove it. Hou believed that a study with negative results is just as valuable, as it helped later researchers not to repeat the same path.[22]

Hou was also an expert in the history of Chinese medicine, applying his deep understanding of Western medicine to the historical investigation of Chinese medicine.[23] In his book *A History of Anatomy in China*, he traced the history of Chinese anatomy through the medical classics written in ancient China. He compared descriptions from ancient medical classics with modern medical knowledge on the physical dimensions of human organs and found a rough match. He believed that Chinese investigators had practiced human dissection before the Tang Dynasty (618–907 CE). He also studied the history of malaria from Tang poetry and of diabetes in the Western Han dynasty.[24] In his book *Science and Civilization in China*, Professor Joseph Needham referred to Professor Hou as "a pathologist and historian of anatomy and medicine."[25]

During his Chengdu days, Professor Hou was frequently found in the company of illustrious Chinese writers and historians. Of these, Lao She remained in contact with him after the war. Hou was a connoisseur of arts, calligraphy, and painting. In Chengdu, he visited old curio shops and stores of old books and collected many valuable items. He did the same in Hong Kong and bought the artifacts with any spare money he had, to prevent losing these precious items overseas. On his return to China, he donated his entire collection to the Palace Museum, consisting of 804 paintings, 506 ceramic works, and 2,067 books, all precious objects.[26]

Professor Hou left behind a fine tradition of research of high quality. His culture and scholarship, his great humility, dignity, kindness, and his love and devotion to his profession and his country were appreciated by all his friends and students.

James Blackburn Gibson (1921–1994)

MD (Western Reserve), MB, ChB (Edin), PhD (Edin), OBE, Hon DSc (HK).

Professor James Blackburn Gibson held the Chair of Pathology at HKU from 1963 to 1983. He extensively advanced pathology practice and service, thereby improving medical care in Hong Kong. He defined and shaped the standard of pathology practice of the Pathology Department.

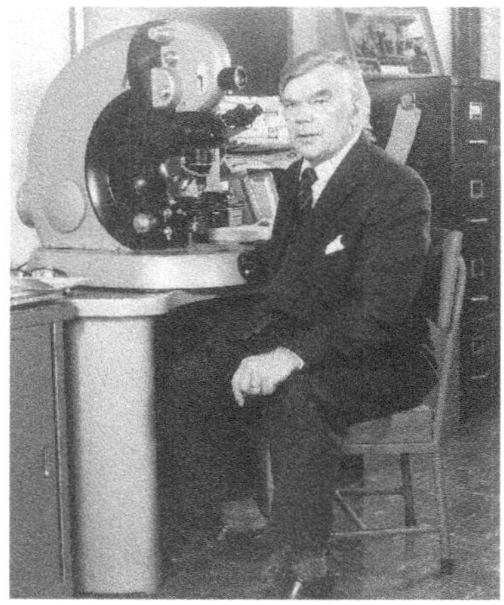

Figure 10.3 Professor James Blackburn Gibson
Image courtesy of Department of Pathology, School of Clinical Medicine, HKU

After graduating from Dundee High School, Gibson entered University of Edinburgh in 1938.[27] In 1941, he left Edinburgh University to complete his study of medicine at Western Reserve University, Cleveland, as a Rockefeller student. He graduated from Western Reserve with an MD degree and an MBChB from the University of Edinburgh in 1943. He then enlisted with the Royal Navy and served as a surgeon for two and a half years.[28] After the war, Gibson joined the Department of Pathology at the University of Glasgow. After seven years at the University of Glasgow, he was appointed Lecturer in Pathology at Queen's University, Belfast. In 1958, he obtained his MD "with high commendation" from the University of Edinburgh. His thesis was entitled "The Hepatic Veins in Health and Disease."[29]

In 1963, he was appointed Professor and Head of Department of Pathology at HKU. In his inaugural address, Gibson said, "Medicine without the audit of pathology is medicine neglectful of standards." During the next 20 years, he put these principles into practice and improved every area of pathology service as well as the training of professional and technical staff to deliver excellent service. The number of professional staff members in the Department of Pathology grew from about 6 in 1963 to 30 in 1983, at the time of his retirement.[30]

Pathology had rapidly advanced in many special areas after the Second World War. At the time, infectious diseases were still one of the major killers in Hong Kong, and microbiology was a branch within the Pathology Department. Gibson wisely established microbiology as a separate department in 1968, to allow it to grow under the expert hands of Dr. Huang Chi-to, who became the founding Professor of the Department of Microbiology. In the 1970s, Gibson set up a cytology service and an immunology service and in 1980s, a tissue typing service and the clinical biochemistry unit. He also founded a central electron microscopy unit in HKU.[31]

By the late 1960s, the Pathology Building at Queen Mary Hospital built in the 1950s was no longer capable of accommodating the growing number of services. The Clinical Pathology Building, which was built with Gibson's careful planning, was opened in 1972, to provide laboratory services for the hospital. Gibson formed the HKU Hospital Pathology Service in Queen Mary Hospital to provide high-quality pathology service to the hospital until the 1990s, when the Hospital Authority took over the service.[32] Such an arrangement at the time allowed the Pathology Department to expand and facilitate the training of personnel.

Shortly after his appointment, Gibson took on the chairmanship of the Management Committee of Extramural Studies and pioneered the in-service training of medical laboratory technicians, which led to the establishment of technician certification at two levels (ordinary and higher), equivalent to that of the UK. This expedited the enactment of Supplementary Medical Professions Bill 1980 to regulate the practice of medical laboratory technology in Hong Kong and resulted in an improvement in laboratory services in government, subvented, and private hospitals in Hong Kong. His trainees in pathology were the first to pass the Royal College of Pathologist membership examination.[33]

In Hong Kong, Gibson's contribution was not limited to pathology. He was a pioneer in postgraduate medical studies, encouraging students to further their studies and to spend time in medical research. He was the prime mover in helping establish the HKU/CMB Fellowship Scheme. As readers recall, the CMB was established in 1920 from the Rockefeller Foundation, focusing on development of Western medical education in China. The Board established PUMC. Hong Kong also benefited in receiving an endowment to establish three Rockefeller professorships which enabled HKU Faculty of Medicine to establish the clinical departments. After the founding of the People's Republic of China, PUMC became nationalized and the CMB had to withdraw from China. Between 1951 and 1973, the CMB brought more than 700 fellows from 30 leading institutions in Asia for advanced training in the US. Hong Kong also benefited from its fellowship program. However, instead of returning to serve their own countries, many fellows ended up staying in the US. This program was discontinued in the mid-1970s.[34] Another program was instituted for the East Asian and Southeast Asian doctors to receive further training in Hong Kong or Singapore where medical development was considered advanced in the Far East instead of going to the US. Through this scheme—the HKU/CMB Fellowship Program, individuals who received the fellowship award from Southeast Asia had the opportunity to receive postgraduate studies in Hong Kong. When China opened up in the 1980s, academic exchanges between mainland China and Hong Kong were feasible, and a number of medical teachers from China were able to come to Hong Kong.[35] Over the years, hundreds of doctors from the mainland benefited from this program. In 1997 CMB discontinued its funding to Hong Kong but the program continued through the generous donation from Dr. Cheng Yu-tung. [36] Gibson was chiefly responsible for this program until his retirement in 1983.

Gibson also played a role with the Hong Kong Medical Council in establishing the Licentiate Committee, which is responsible for administering and conducting licensing examinations for non-local medical graduates in Hong Kong. Gibson was appointed medical consultant to different organizations and external examiner for local and overseas universities. He was elected Dean of the Faculty of Medicine for two consecutive terms, was twice Pro-Vice-Chancellor, and Acting Vice-Chancellor on a number of occasions.[37] Despite the numerous administrative duties, he did not neglect his own research and had 60 publications to his credit. He was a world authority on the pathology of the liver and biliary tract, and his department was the organizational center for a multicenter collaborative study of the WHO on the classification of liver tumors. This resulted in the publication of a WHO book in 1978 entitled *Histological Typing and Tumors of the Liver, Biliary Tract and Pancreas*.[38]

Gibson retired in 1983 and was awarded an honorary Doctor of Science by HKU and became an Emeritus Professor of the University. He returned to Scotland, where he enjoyed the pastime of hiking, but he continued to keep an interest in the pathology profession in Hong Kong.[39] He passed away in 1994.

Dr. Rayson Huang, who was Vice-Chancellor of HKU (1972–1986) and a personal friend of Professor Gibson, wrote in the eulogy, "Strong in resolve and resolute in purpose, he held well-reasoned, clear cut and well-articulated views, but he always respected others' opinions and as always ready to give them the benefit of his consideration. He was a man of his word ... I have always thought that of the things on which the quality of a university depends, none is more vital than the caliber of its staff, apart from the academic ability, their loyalty to the institution and their devotion to their calling. Hong Kong University has been fortunate to have a good many of its staff who fit this description, and among their leaders a man of James' caliber."[40] It was another blessing from God to HKU that Professor Gibson survived the carnage at the Normandy Landings, as his ship was stationed off Omaha Beach during World War II.[41]

Professor James Blackburn Gibson lived a highly rewarding life, fulfilling his pursuit of knowledge and his principle that "medicine without the audit of pathology is medicine neglectful of standards." His outstanding service to his profession, to HKU, to teaching, and to healthcare for the community will be long remembered with gratitude by his students, friends, and colleagues. He was awarded the OBE in 1976, for his enormous contributions to Hong Kong.

Physicians

Alexander James Smith McFadzean (1914–1974)

MD, FRCP, FRCP Edin, FACP, DSc, OBE

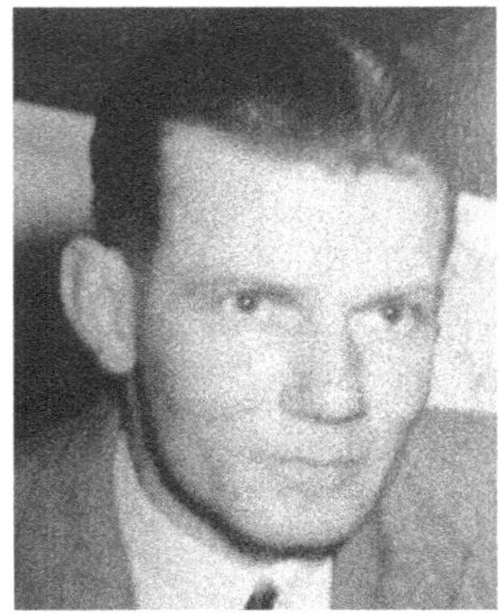

Figure 10.4 Professor A. J. S. McFadzean

Image courtesy of the Department of Medicine, HKU

The appointment of Professor Alexander James Smith McFadzean as Chair in 1948 marked the beginning of the modern Department of Medicine at HKU. He was the longest-serving head in the history of the Department of Medicine. He also served as Vice-Chancellor in 1965 and Dean of the Faculty of Medicine from 1967 to 1972. He expanded the Department of Medicine and brought about specialization and helped the great expansion of the Faculty of Medicine as a whole.

Born in Troon, Scotland, on 28 January 1914, McFadzean graduated with honors in 1936 from Glasgow University and was the most outstanding student of the year. After graduation he worked in Glasgow Infirmary, Hawkhead Mental Hospital, and Anlaby Road Hospital, Hull. During World War II, he volunteered for service with the Royal Army Medical Corps and became a medical specialist with the Middle East Command in 1943. After the war, he was elected a member of the Royal College of Physicians, London, and became Senior Lecturer in the Muirhead Department of Medicine, Glasgow University. In 1948, he was appointed Professor of Medicine at HKU.[42]

McFadzean's 26-year term covered the period of rapid expansion of the Faculty of Medicine and the Department of Medicine, enrollment of medical students surging from under 60 in the late 1950s, to 150 by 1972. He seized the opportunity to fully increase the number of staff in the department, as well as the number of hospital teaching beds. In addition, he ensured that the department would provide modern, state-of-the-art clinical service for patient care and clinical teaching, commensurate with advances in medicine and medical technology. He and his staff also conducted research on different diseases that were prevalent in Hong Kong. Apart from scientific curiosity, he was hoping to improve the treatment and prevention of these diseases.[43]

In the 1940s and 1950s, pediatrics and psychiatry were taught within the Department of Medicine. McFadzean persuaded the university to provide adequate resources to establish separate departments for these two branches of medicine. In 1962, Elaine Field joined the department as Professor of Pediatrics, and the Department of Pediatrics was established in 1964.[44] A separate Department of Psychiatry was founded in 1972, when Dr. P. M. Yap was appointed the Chair.[45] These two departments were able to grow independently, more adequately to address the needs of Hong Kong.

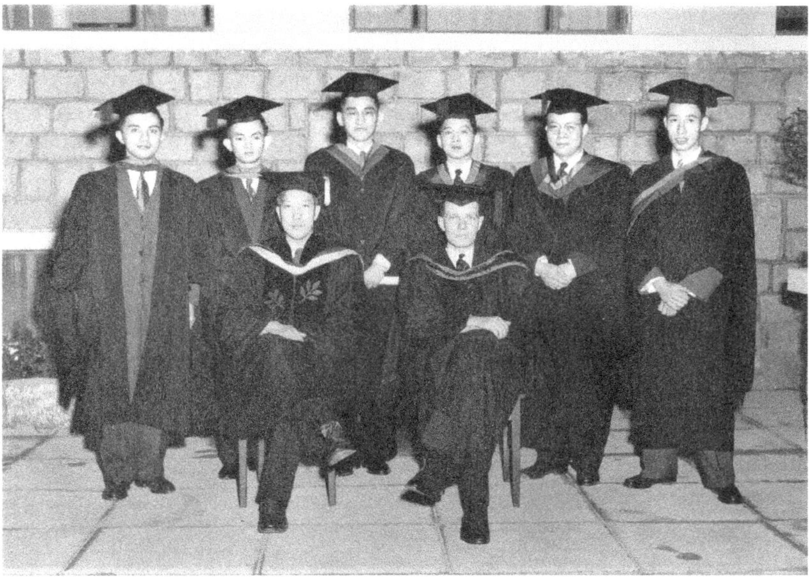

Figure 10.5 Professor A. J. S. McFadzean (sitting, right), Dr. Stephen Chang (sitting, left) and graduates of 1951

Source: HKMMS, reproduced with permission, photograph donated by Dr. Joseph Pan

In 1948, the Department of Medicine had only five full time staff: a professor, one senior lecturer, one lecturer, and two clinical assistants. At the time of his retirement in 1974, the department had a staff of about 50. The physicians who worked in the Department of Medicine in McFadzean's era were impressive, including some of the most accomplished physicians of the day, such as Drs. Stephen Chang, Gerald Choa, Joseph Pan, Wong Cheung-chih, Kwaan Hau-cheong, and Fong Chun-piu.[46]

Although the leading causes of death in the 1950s were infectious diseases, in the 1960s, these diseases gradually faded into the background due to the availability of antibiotics and improved sanitation and nutrition. By the 1970s, malignancy and other chronic noncommunicable diseases, such as heart diseases, cerebrovascular diseases, and cancer, became the leading causes of death.[47] With changes in disease pattern and the complexities of chronic diseases, McFadzean recognized the need for doctors to acquire expertise in these newer specific areas of medicine. This would not only provide appropriate clinical service but also future leaders in the profession. He sent members of his junior staff overseas for training, and they returned as specialists to develop their area of interest. As a result, he trained important and influential physicians including David Todd and Rosie Tse-tse Young, and many others in the department. Each one of them became founders and pillars of their respective specialties.[48]

Despite his eagerness for young doctors to acquire knowledge, skill, and experience in various specialties, McFadzean always preached holistic care, insisting that a sound knowledge of general medicine acquired during the basic physician training period was the foundation of all professional training. He was adamant that a physician should not lose sight of his/her role as a generalist even after special training in a certain branch of medicine. He would certainly be unhappy with the present-day tendency of specialists confining themselves to the narrow paths of their chosen specialties, shuffling patients from one specialist clinic to another.[49]

McFadzean was a remarkable clinician. His clinical acumen and knowledge were legendary. He emphasized the value of a detailed history and a good physical examination, rather than the current emphasis on laboratory investigations and imaging. He was selected to be the Gordon Wilson Lecturer by the prestigious American Clinical and Climatological Association.[50]

Being the first Professor of Medicine after World War II, McFadzean devised a curriculum that would produce competent doctors to treat primarily Chinese patients and satisfy the General Medical Council of the UK to gain recognition of the MBBS degree. The curriculum included genetics and molecular biology—advances in medicine then.[51] He stressed the importance of principles, and encouraged clear and logical thinking rather than rote recall. As a teacher, McFadzean was dreaded and respected. He was a disciplinarian. All students had to be neatly dressed;

men had to wear ties and women skirts and short hair. Students were not allowed to take notes. They had to listen and remember what he said. There was no lack of anecdotes about the professorial Thursday Clinic, which were excellent training sessions and provided invaluable experience for the senior students and the attending staff.[52] All students arrived early to take a back seat, to escape being called upon to answer his questions, leaving the first few rows relatively empty. However, no place was safe. Dr. Arthur Van Langenberg, a student then, wrote a poem to memorialize the celebrated professorial Thursday Clinic, and it was published in the journal *Elixir*,[53] causing quite a stir:

The Thursday Clinic

The Thursday Clinic is a sheer delight!
It always is so merry and bright!
Nothing Else has what it's got
When it's run by that cheery old Scot!
As the clinic begins the dear man smiles…
You can see his fangs from miles and miles!
His cold clear voice, like the waters of Loch Fyne
Can curdle your blood and chill your spine!

Professor Donald Yu, one of his protégés, wrote in the centenary tribute of McFadzean, "Behind a stern, fierce façade, one found a compassionate fine actor with a sense of humor. Many times, after admonishing a student he would turn round to chuckle to himself. Not infrequently one could catch a mischievous gleam in his eye amidst a barrage of angry fiery words."[54]Another story was told by Professor David Todd: "The Professor was in great form waxing eloquent on the subject of subacute bacterial endocarditis. Suddenly he excused himself and reappeared about ten minutes later, looking somewhat pale and shaken but the Clinic continued. It was learnt afterwards that he had suffered a hematemesis and we marveled at this man who placed finishing a teaching session before his own comfort."[55]

McFadzean was interested in hematology at the Glasgow University. In Hong Kong he extended his interest on prevalent local diseases, often to answer questions related to a clinical problem. His research on diseases of blood, liver, thyroid, and spleen was renowned.[56] According to Professor Rosie Young, McFadzean's intellectual curiosity was contagious. Before long, all members in the department were engaged in research, and some registered for an MD degree at HKU. McFadzean strongly believed that teaching, research, and clinical service must go hand in hand, and stressed the application of research to clinical practice. He also emphasized laboratory research. In the 1950s, despite the lack of facilities and proper laboratories, his staff conducted laboratory research under difficult circumstances. However, in the early 1960s, Wellcome Laboratory was built for animal studies and isotope work. In 1967, when the Professorial Block was constructed next to the hospital, the Department of Medicine was assigned two floors, one for offices and the other for laboratories, vastly improving the infrastructure for research. He also had the foresight to recruit the first scientist, Vivian Chan (PhD), to join the department and provide new research techniques including molecular biology.[57]

McFadzean was devoted to his students and staff. As Dean of the Faculty of Medicine, he discovered that many students came from poor families and could not afford to buy expensive equipment such as microscopes or ophthalmoscopes. His "Dean's Loan Fund" for students in need required no IOU, as McFadzean truly believed that "a man is as good as his word." All students returned the borrowed money after graduation, most donating to the fund as well. McFadzean also redressed a long-standing problem of unequal salaries of individuals doing the same job. In those days, remuneration for doctors in the government service was higher than that for university employees, making it difficult for the university to recruit bright young doctors. Female doctors of the same rank received only 75% of the pay of male doctors. McFadzean negotiated directly with the Financial Secretary to put the salaries of university medical staff on par with those of government medical staff. This won him the hearts and respect of all university staff.[58] Gender parity, however, was only achieved in the 1970s.

McFadzean tended to be autocratic, making all important decisions himself. Professor Lee Sum-ping, Dean of Medicine (2008–2013), remarked on McFadzean's style of leadership as "more like a dictator—a benevolent, efficient, and effective dictatorship, but always without fail, with the common good in mind."[59] His other interests were golf, history, poetry, and Chinese antiques. He spent many hours with Professor Hou Pao-chang discussing and learning about Chinese Art.[60]

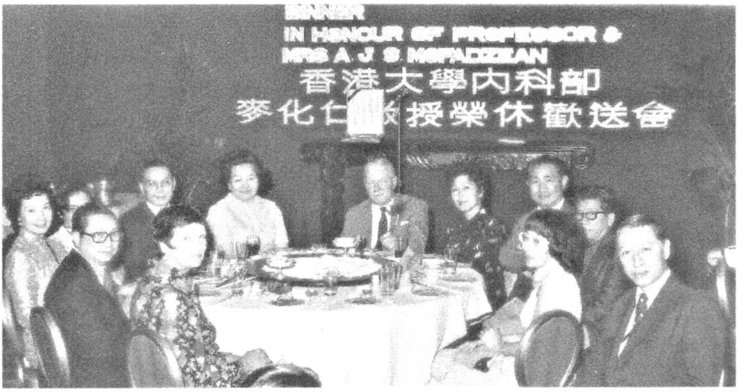

Figure 10.6 Farewell dinner to Professor A. J. S. McFadzean (center), Dr. Harry Fang (R4), Dr. C. C. Wong (R3), Dr. John Ho Hung-chiu (R1), 1974

Image courtesy of the Department of Medicine, HKU

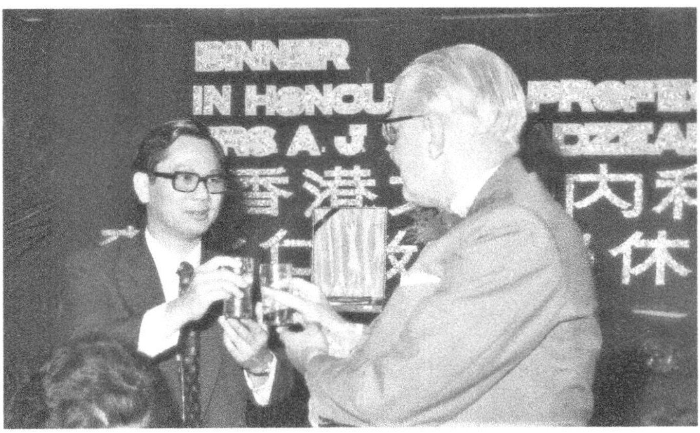

Figure 10.7 Professor David Todd toasting to Professor A. J. S. McFadzean during the farewell dinner

Image courtesy of the Department of Medicine, HKU

When he retired in 1974, Professor A. J. S. McFadzean had fully accomplished the two missions he had for Hong Kong: 1) to educate and train local doctors to staff the healthcare system in Hong Kong; and 2) to pass on the chair to a local graduate. Professor David Todd succeeded him.[61] On his retirement, to honor him for the perfect example he had set, both past and present members of the Department of Medicine presented him with a bronze plaque on which was inscribed a passage from Kahlil

Gibran's *The Prophet*: "And all knowledge is vain save when there is work, and all work is empty save when there is love.[62] He left Hong Kong with his family in June 1974 for Scotland. Sadly, he died on 29 November the same year.

His passing was a great loss to the medical community in Hong Kong, especially to those who had been closely associated with him, and marked the end of an era of medicine in Hong Kong.

David Todd 達安輝 (1928–2017)

CBE, OBE, MBBS Hong Kong, MD, FRCP Edin, FRACP, FRCP Lond, FRCP Glasg, Hon FAMS, Hon DSc CUHK, FRCPath, Hon DSc HKU, Hon FHKCFP, Hon LLD Lingnan, Hon FHKAM, Hon FHKCP, Hon FRCPS, JP

Professor Sir David Todd was the doyen of medicine in Hong Kong and respected and admired by his colleagues, students, and patients. He taught generations of physicians locally. He greatly expanded the Department of Medicine at HKU, firmly established many specialties, and promoted research within the department. He founded the Hong Kong College of Physicians and the Hong Kong Academy of Medicine to achieve and maintain the high standard of practice in Hong Kong. A man of letters, he was one of the most decorated physicians in Hong Kong.

Todd's life in medicine began early—his adoptive parents were missionaries from the US. His father, Dr. Paul Todd, had played a leading educational role both as an administrator and teacher in medical schools in Guangzhou, having started Kung Yee Hospital in 1909 and a medical school, Kung Yee Medical College—one of the first medical schools in Guangzhou. The medical school later merged with Sun Yat-sen University to become Zhongshan School of Medicine. Dr. Paul Todd also established the Paul Todd Clinic and Hospital to serve the poor and needy; this was renamed Second People's Children Hospital in 1949.

When Guangzhou fell to the Japanese in 1938, Todd left Guangzhou for Hong Kong and entered Diocesan Boys' School.[63] It was likely that at DBS he acquired a love of classical music from the two successive headmasters, Mr. Sargent Christopher and Mr. Gerald Goodban. After the fall of Hong Kong to the Japanese on Christmas Day 1941, Todd, at the tender age of 13, made his own way from Hong Kong to northern Guangdong, Kukong, now Shaoguan, to study at Lingnan Middle School. After the war, he was admitted to Lingnan University Medical School, but civil war in China brought him to HKU to complete his medical degree in 1952.[64] He won many prizes and gold medals during his undergraduate days.

Professor A. J. S. McFadzean recognized Todd's talents early. In 1953, as soon as Todd completed his internship, he was invited to join the Department of Medicine. He then went on a Sino-British Fellowship for postgraduate study in the UK as a registrar at Muirhead Department of

Medicine, Royal Infirmary Glasgow, where his mentor was trained. He became a Lecturer in the department on returning to Hong Kong,[65] and remained in the department until his retirement. According to Professor Rosie Young, over the next two decades, the "McFadzean and Todd dream team" launched training programs in different medical specialties and initiated a number of ground-breaking research projects. Not surprisingly, Todd rose rapidly in rank to a personal professorship in 1972 and succeeded McFadzean when the latter retired in 1974.[66] Todd was also Sub-dean from 1976 to 1978 and Pro-Vice-Chancellor from 1978 to 1980, contributing greatly to the development of the Department of Medicine, Faculty of Medicine and the University.

When Todd took over the department, there were eight specialties which he helped McFadzean establish: cardiology, endocrinology and metabolism, gastroenterology and hepatology, hematology and medical oncology, nephrology, neurology, respiratory medicine, and rheumatology and immunology. During his own tenure, he added two more specialties, clinical pharmacology and general practice. Each staff member belonged to one of the above specialties. Under his leadership all specialties were given the freedom to develop; if he was not paving the way, he would be assisting in the background.[67]

Because medicine advanced very rapidly in the 1980s and 1990s, Todd encouraged each specialty to bring in new diagnostic and treatment modalities for patient care. The department greatly expanded as a result. A combined gastrointestinal unit had been set up between the University Departments of Medicine and Surgery, providing a strong basis for clinical services as well as postgraduate training and research.[68] A new cardiothoracic unit, the first in Hong Kong, was started at Grantham Hospital in 1968.[69] A unit specializing in the care of patients with end-stage renal failure was first established by the renal team at Tung Wah Hospital in January 1980. A diabetes center was set up at Queen Mary Hospital to promote patient education.[70] Hematology was divided into a clinical division in the Department of Medicine, and laboratory hematology in the Pathology Department. The medical hematology subspecialty was able to concentrate on developing bone marrow transplantation, treatment of hemic malignancies, and research.[71] Many specialists were desperately needed in Hong Kong at the time,[72] and the Department of Medicine trained quite a few in different specialties. Recognizing the importance of primary care beside specialized care, Todd

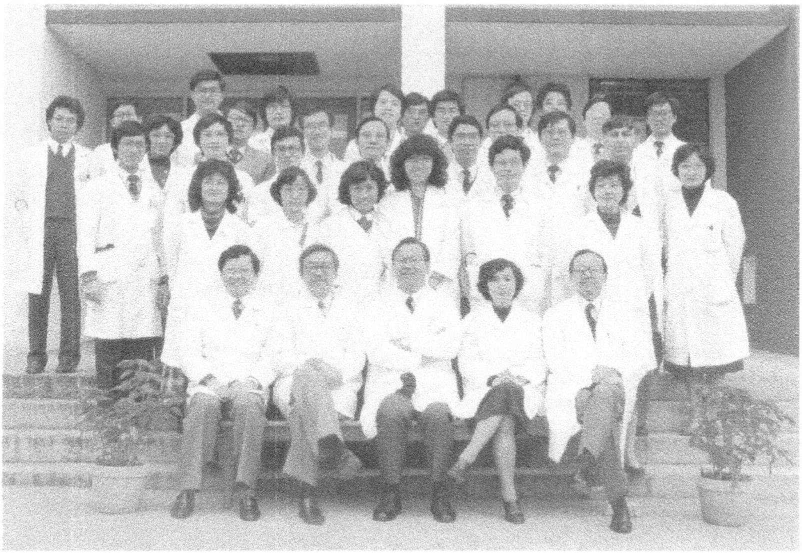

Figure 10.8 Department of Medicine in 1985 showing the large number of staff. Professor Todd was in the front center with Professor Rosie Young next to him on the right.

Image courtesy of Department of Medicine HKU

strongly encouraged the development of family medicine and supported training of academic family physicians.[73]

Research for universities had been poorly funded. However, in 1979, the Croucher Foundation and in the early 1990s, the Research Grants Council of the University and Polytechnic Grants Committee were established. Together with generous donations from patients and their families, the chances of obtaining funds for research improved. Todd encouraged collaborative research with other departments inside and outside the Medical Faculty and took leadership to establish the Institute of Molecular Biology, a university-wide centre for molecular biology research.[74] He frequently lamented on the meager government funding for research. In 2014, the budget for R & D for all fields in Hong Kong was the highest ever, but at just 0.74% of the GDP[75] still very small compared to 2.05% in China, 2.74% in the US, and 3.58% in Japan.[76] Despite busy administration, he did not forget his own research projects. His research team studied two inherited blood diseases, thalassemia and G-6-PD deficiency, and was able to isolate the gene responsible for the disease in thalassemia. In addition, the team researched the treatment of leukemias and lymphomas and was the first to use arsenic in the treatment of chronic myeloid leukemia with good results. For his seminal research in thalassemia and lymphomas, he was awarded the Carl de Cruchy Medal of the Hematological Society of Australia in 1979.[77]

A great proponent of postgraduate and continuing education, Todd established the A. J. S McFadzean Library, ensuring that his staff and trainees always had access to up-to-date books, monographs, and journals to facilitate continuous self-education.[78] At that time, to be eligible to practice as a specialist in the British Commonwealth, candidates had to pass the Royal College examinations of their specialty. Todd had been an Overseas Examiner for Membership of the Royal Colleges of Physicians for the United Kingdom (MRCP [UK]) since 1980. As a result of his efforts and the trust of the Royal College, both parts 1 and 2 of the MRCP (UK) examination were held in Hong Kong in 1985—the first time in the history of the college that the entire examination was held outside Britain.[79]

In those days, local postgraduate medical training was not coordinated but available only to a few, on competitive merit. An enquiry was carried out on postgraduate medical training in Hong Kong. The Halnan Report, which was published in 1988, found that the training was

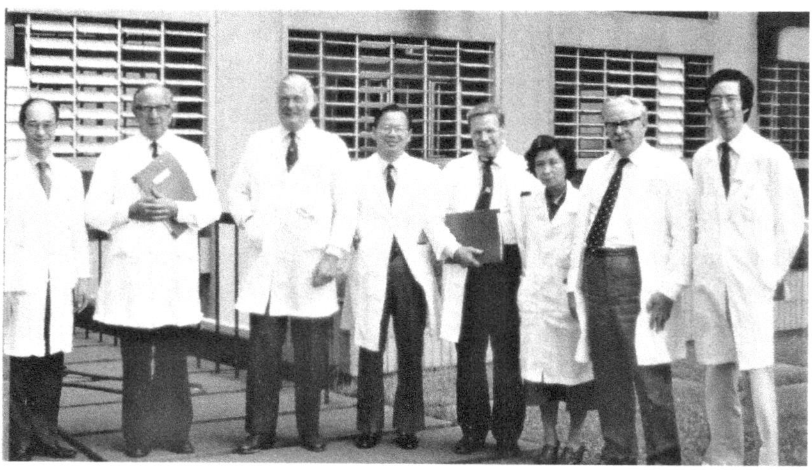

Figure 10.9 Profssor David Todd (L4) and Professor Rosie Young (R3) with examiners from the Royal College of Physicians, to conduct Part 2 membership examination in Hong Kong the first time in 1985
Image courtesy of Department of Medicine, HKU

poorly organized and inadequate, and recommended the establishment of a formalized, locally based postgraduate and continuing medical education (CME) program to ensure a suitably high level of clinical competence.[80]

Todd took the initiative to establish the Hong Kong College of Physicians (HKCP) in 1986 and became its first president. He chaired the Education and Accreditation Committee, to develop training guidelines, assessment criteria, and procedures for selection of trainers, and evaluation of training programs for Specialty Boards. In the beginning, the College had established 12 such Specialty Boards; four new specialties were later added. Todd also helped establish colleges of other branches of medicine. In addition, as Hong Kong would no longer be part of the Commonwealth in 1997, after the handover of Hong Kong to China, there was an urgent need for Hong Kong to have an institution, preferably constituted by statute, to provide the legal basis for the administration of medical standards in the territory. The institution should have the ability to award internationally recognized medical specialist qualifications. Todd was the chairman of the preparatory committee.[81] In December 1993, Todd became its first president when the Hong Kong Academy of Medicine was established by statute. The academy's main functions include coordinating the activities of all the colleges of different branches of medicine, fostering the development of postgraduate training and continuing medical education, promoting the integrity and ethical behavior of the medical profession, and safeguarding and improving healthcare in Hong Kong. At the time of its founding in 1993, there were 11 colleges: anesthesiology, community medicine, general practice, medicine, obstetrics and gynecology, orthopedics, pathology, pediatrics, psychiatry, radiology, and surgery. Later additions would include dental surgery, ophthalmology, otorhinolaryngology and emergency medicine.[82] The academy developed general guidelines for recognition of academy colleges, training of specialists, recognition and visitation of local training units, and training units outside Hong Kong. In addition, it produced a document on Continuing Medical Education (CME) Principles and Guidelines.[83] As of January 2005, all practicing specialists are required to participate in the three-year CME cycle and fulfill its requirements in order to remain in the Specialist Register—a major milestone in the development of medicine in Hong Kong. For non-specialists, the CME program is strongly recommended although not mandatory.

It was not an easy job to have the cooperation from so many colleges and different personalities to form the Academy of Medicine. Many believed that only Todd could master such a difficult job. He was not only an accomplished academician, a practicing physician of the highest caliber, an experienced administrator, but also a skillful politician who commanded tremendous respect from the medical community. The founding of the Hong Kong College of Physicians and the Hong Kong Academy of Medicine constituted one of the most important contributions of Todd to the medical community of Hong Kong.

In addition to serving the Hong Kong College of Physicians and the Academy of Medicine, Todd served many public institutions in various capacities, including: AIDS Trust Fund (Chairman),[84] Health Services Research Committee, the Croucher Foundation, University and Polytechnic Grants Committee (1986 to 1993, Chairman), the S. K. Yee Medical Foundation (Vice-chairman), and a trustee of the Sino-British Fellowship Trust. In an interview by the *South China Morning Post*, Todd admitted that although he felt his work on these committees had been most satisfying, nothing in his experience prepared him for the task of conducting the inquiry into the government controversial raid at Whitehead Vietnamese Detention Centre for Vietnamese refugees in 1994. He had to visit the detention centre and interview the Correctional Services Department officers and the refugees themselves.[85] Eventually, the Whitehead Detention Centre was closed.

In recognition of his outstanding academic achievements and influence on the medical profession, CUHK and HKU conferred on him an honorary degree of Doctor of Science in 1990 and 1992 respectively. For his distinguished public service, he was made an OBE in 1982, a CBE in 1990,[86] and a Knight Bachelor in 1995.[87]

Todd's network was not limited to local physicians, which enabled him to found the Academy of Medicine. His international network included links with North America that enabled prominent US physicians to visit Hong Kong and participate in teaching, discussions, and research, with great benefits to students and staff. He was also appointed Councillor of Royal Australian College of Physicians (RACP), 1980–1986, a singular honor for a person outside Australia. He was, indeed, a "man of many continents" and won the admiration and respect of many with his sincerity, and unassuming and unpretentious manner. He was awarded an honorary member of the Singapore Academy of Medicine for his influence on postgraduate teaching at National University of Singapore. Dr. P. H. Feng, in presenting him for admission to the Singapore Academy of Medicine, aptly described him as follows: "His analytic mind, incisive intellect, quiet manner and compassion for his fellow man epitomizes the best from both East and West and make him what he is—a gentleman extraordinaire."[88]

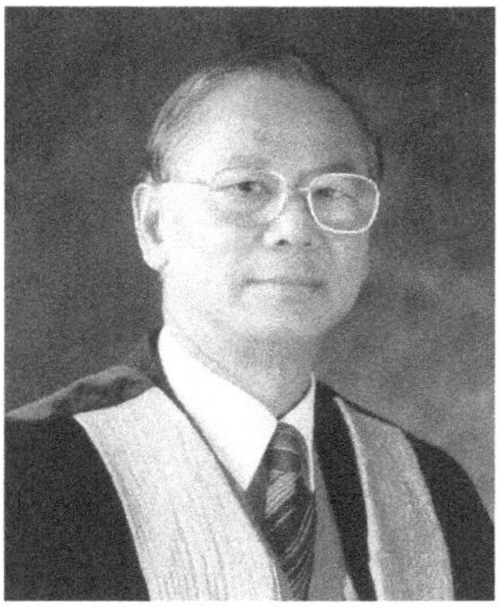

Figure 10.10 Professor Sir David Todd, Founding President of the Academy of Medicine

Image courtesy of Department of Medicine, HKU

Sir David was a great lover of classical music. He contributed as a classical music critic to the *South China Morning Post*. He had a great breadth of knowledge and insight to works across the board from Bach to Wagner, and beyond. For personal pleasure, he made many trips to music festivals in Britain and Germany, especially after his retirement.

Regarded as a formidable teacher and mentor by his students and colleagues, his popularity among them was legendary. His graciousness, consideration, and kindness underscore the secrets of his popularity. After his retirement, he was busy receiving visits from former colleagues and students, irrespective of whether he was living in Hong Kong or in Cambridge, amply witnessing the love and respect his students had for him.

Professor Sir David Todd passed away on 16 August 2017, after a courageous battle against cancer. His passing put the whole medical profession in Hong Kong into mourning, losing their beloved leader who was an irreplaceable model as a teacher, clinician, scientist, and mentor. Hundreds of messages of condolences poured in from all over the world to his family. Many told their experience working with or contact with Sir David and how these unique experiences had influenced their lives.[89] Sir David will long live in our memory for his kindness, generosity, consideration, integrity, humanitarian spirit, leadership, and unwavering professionalism.

Surgeons

Arthur Ralph Hodgson (1915–1993)

MBBS, FRCS, OBE

Professor Arthur Ralph Hodgson, the founding Professor of Orthopedic Surgery Department at the University of Hong Kong, placed Hong Kong on the world orthopedic map with a new procedure of anterior approach to the spine called "Hong Kong Operation" in the 1960s and the 1970s.

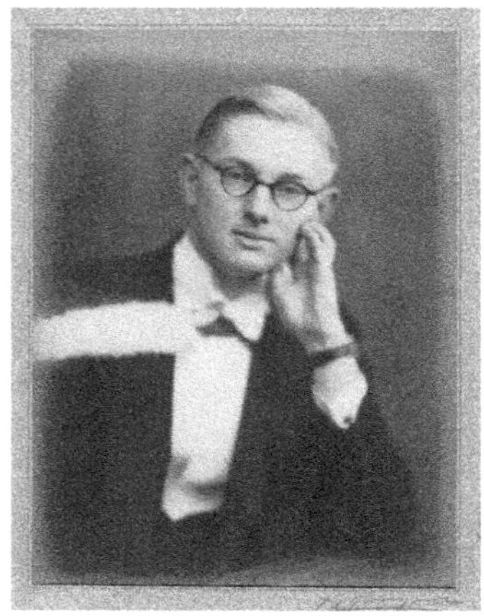

Figure 10.11 Professor Arthur Ralph Hodgson
Image courtesy of Department of Orthopedics and Traumatology, HKU

Hodgson was born in 1915 in Uruguay of British parents and was educated mostly in the UK. After graduating from the University of Edinburgh with an MBBS degree in 1939, he went for postgraduate training in an orthopedics unit in Norfolk, under Dr. George Kenneth McKee and Dr. H. A. Brittain, who greatly influenced his choice of career. In 1944, he joined the Royal Army Medical Corps as a trainee specialist and served in different parts of the world, including India, Burma, and Singapore. On discharge, he was promoted to specialist. On returning to England, he took the professional examination and was made FRCS in 1948. He then joined St. Bartholomew's Hospital as a senior registrar.[90]

In 1951, HKU decided to expand the Department of Surgery by creating an Orthopedics Unit, which would consist of a Senior Lecturer in Orthopedics who would be paid by the university, and four junior supporting staff paid by the Medical Department. Hodgson applied for the senior lecturer position and was accepted. As there was no Department of Orthopedic Surgery at the time, Hodgson was a member of the Department of Surgery with Professor Francis E. Stock as the head. Within six months, the government changed its mind and would no longer pay for some of the staff of the unit. Not only was there a lack of staff, but Hodgson also found that he had to be Acting Head of the

Anatomy Department when the head went on leave, followed by another acting headship, this time for the Head of the Department of Surgery.[91] In the 1950s, the university's budget was very tight; when a staff member went on leave, someone in the department or the university just filled in. By the time he completed the acting headships, Hodgson found that it was time for him to go on his own leave. Hodgson was a disciplined and hard-working man and performed the work of his own unit and that of the Department of Surgery very well when he was Acting Head.

Although the university had decided in principle to have a separate Department of Orthopedic Surgery in 1955, there were no funds to do so. In 1961, the Department of Orthopedic Surgery was finally created, Hodgson as the Chair and Head of the Department. It was thought that the order came directly from Sir Robert Black, who was the Chancellor of HKU then and who had successful surgery for slipped disc carried out by Hodgson.[92]

Hodgson became internationally renowned to orthopedic surgeons around the world for the operation known as the "Hong Kong Operation."[93] It was a new procedure which he and Stock pioneered—anterior approach to the spine—for treating patients with TB of the spine, which caused destruction of vertebrae and abscess formation and may result in compression of the spinal cord causing paraplegia and marked deformity. In the early 1950s, the incidence of TB was very high in Hong Kong, close to 700/100,000. Although the lung was the most common affected site, other sites were involved too, and TB of the spine was common. Although anti-TB drugs were available in Hong Kong by the late 1950s, the diagnosis might not have been made soon enough, and patients might not take medications prescribed because of frequent side effects and prolonged duration of treatment. There were also some doubts about how well the drugs would penetrate to the diseased area. Because of all these considerations, Hodgson felt that early drainage of the abscess and bone grafts to replace the destroyed vertebrae might lead to early fusion and thus stabilize the spine. This would prevent paraplegia and allow early mobilization. In those days, during surgery, the spine was usually approached from the back where it is most accessible, but the disease usually affects the vertebrae anteriorly.

The first operation for TB spine using the anterior approach was performed in late 1955 by Hodgson and Stock and was a great success. The case was reported in the *British Journal of Surgery* in 1956 by Hodgson and Stock, and it remains a classic today.[94] Since then, Hodgson and his team carried out a number of clinical studies on the "Hong Kong Operation" with favorable results. The Medical Research Council of Great Britain subsequently conducted a randomized study comparing the "Hong Kong Operation" with more conservative treatment of limited surgical debridement when both groups also received anti-TB drugs. The study showed favorable outcomes in both groups after three years of follow-up. However, bone fusion occurred in 93% of those who received the "Hong Kong Operation," and in 67% of those who only had limited debridement.[95]

Hodgson's concern for people with disabilities led him to initiate the Hong Kong Society for the Relief of Disabled Children in 1955. He persuaded the Rotary Club to build the Sandy Bay Convalescent Home for children, and it was opened in 1956 with 50 beds.[96] In 1971, the Convalescent Home was expanded to become a proper hospital with operation and laboratory facilities and was renamed the Duchess of Kent Children's Hospital.[97] Hodgson was also instrumental in forming the Hong Kong Society for Rehabilitation in 1959. He and Dr. Harry Fang raised funds to build two rehabilitation centers for adults.

The increase in demand for spinal surgery resulted in increase in the number of beds in the Orthopedics Unit. By 1958, the unit was responsible for 40 beds at the Queen Mary hospital, 60 at Lai Chi Kok Hospital, 50 at Sandy Bay Convalescent Home, 40 at Grantham Hospital, and all patients with TB spine at Ruttonjee Hospital.

Hodgson presented the results of the "Hong Kong Operation" at international conferences and generated a great deal of interest. At times when he was asked to give a presentation and the host organization was unable to pay for his travel, the problem was often solved by the host organization finding wealthy patients who needed the procedure. The generous fees would pay more than the travel cost. In 1966, Hodgson went on a world lecture tour during his regular leave. As a result, visiting orthopedic surgeons from all over the world came to Hong Kong to learn about the "Hong Kong Operation." Hodgson earned the department a worldwide reputation and placed Hong Kong on the world map of orthopedic surgery.[98]

Between his international travels, Hodgson continued to work hard on his research at home. He carried out original clinical research and produced a series of important publications. He experimented using the anterior approach to other spinal problems. Dr. Anthony Dwyer used the anterior approach for treatment of scoliosis and shared the idea with Hodgson. During Dr. Dwyer's visit to Hong Kong, they worked on the design and application of a screw-cable system.[99] Research of the spine remains one of the major foci of research of the department today although it has also branched out in other areas.

Hodgson was twice elected Dean of the Faculty of Medicine, showing his popularity among his colleagues. However, Professor McFadzean, Head of the Department of Medicine, and Hodgson did not see eye to eye. When McFadzean was Dean, he complained to the Vice-Chancellor that Hodgson often refused to advertise openings in his department but insisted on seeking out someone on his own.[100] Nevertheless, Hodgson trained and chose his own successor well. Dr. Arthur Yau was promoted to personal chair in 1972, and when Hodgson retired in 1975, Yau succeeded him. After a highly successful career in Hong Kong, Hodgson did not return to the UK on retirement. Instead, he started private practice at Canossa Hospital. He continued to serve as Chairman of the Society for the Relief of Disabled Children.

Professor Arthur Ralph Hodgson died in 1993. He was the first Professor of Orthopedic Surgery in HKU and is remembered for his "Hong Kong Operation." He left a strong department which has been over the years one of the leading international centers for spinal surgery.

Ong Guan Bee 王源美 (1921–2004)

MD (Shanghai), MBBS (Hong Kong), LRCP, FRCS (Edin.), MRCS, FRCS, FACS, FRACS, FRS (Edin.), DSc, OBE, PSM, Hon DSc (Hong Kong)

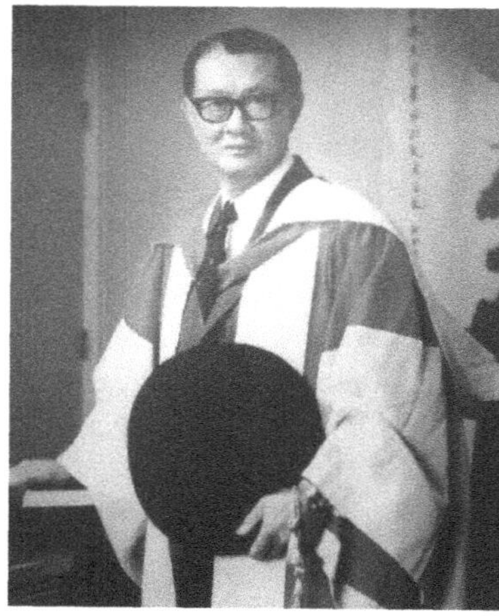

Figure 10.12 Professor G. B. Ong
Source: Department of Surgery, HKU

Professor Ong Guan Bee, or G. B. as known to his many friends and colleagues around the world, was a distinguished Professor of Surgery at HKU (1964–1982), a pioneering surgeon, an innovator, and a skillful crafts person. He was an inspirational and dynamic leader and known for his bold approach to surgery.

Ong was born in Kuching, Raj of Sarawak, and went to boarding school in Singapore, where he discovered his manual dexterity. Appointed as school barber without any prior experience, he trained himself in the art of cutting his classmates' hair to perfection.[101] He could have been elected a fellow of the Company of Barber-Surgeons in the fourteenth century, the forerunner of the Royal College of Surgeons. Although he wanted to be an electrical engineer, his father told him that it is "no good working for someone else. Better do medicine." An obedient son, he followed his father's advice and applied to Singapore Medical College. However, he was not accepted, and he left for HKU instead. Like many students in HKU, his education was abruptly interrupted in 1941 with the Japanese invasion. Ong and several other students escaped into China, making a hazardous journey on foot to Chongqing, where Professor Gordon King arranged for students to continue their studies in different universities in China. Ong continued his studies at Shanghai Medical School, which had moved from Shanghai during the war. He graduated with an MD from Shanghai Medical School and, on returning to Hong Kong, he obtained an MBBS degree in 1947. He had no difficulty in deciding which special field to go into. For the next 10 years, he received postgraduate training in surgery in Hong Kong and in the UK, where he obtained an FRCS from both Royal College of Surgeons of England and Edinburgh.

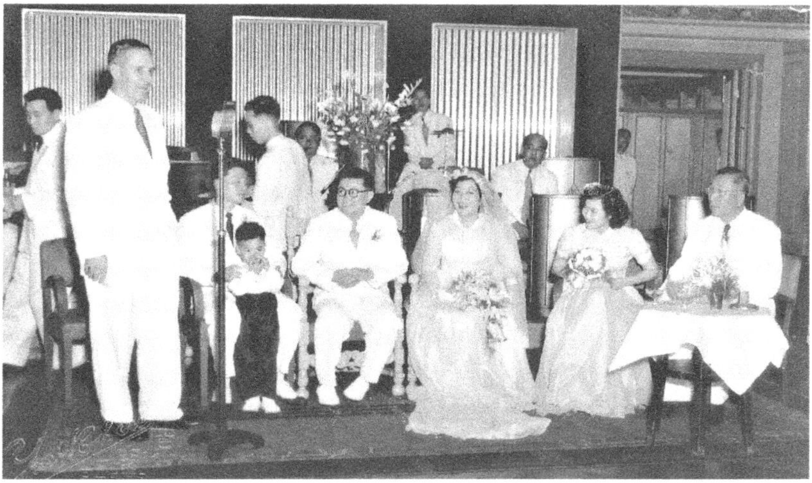

Figure 10.13 Dr. G. B. Ong and Dr. Christina Chow at their wedding reception (Professor Gordon King giving a speech) in 1950
Source: HKMMS with permission; photograph donated by Dr. Chua Sin Giap

In 1956, he was awarded the Harkness Commonwealth University Fellowship to go to Massachusetts General Hospital, Boston, and Bellevue Hospital, New York City. On his return to Hong Kong, he became surgeon-in-charge of Kowloon Hospital and oversaw Kwong Wah Hospital, a subvented hospital.[102] In 1964, his breakthrough came. He was appointed Chair of Surgery at HKU, the first Chinese to hold this post.[103] At the time, the department was poorly equipped with a budget of only HK$1,000.[104] From this humble beginning, he built over the next 18 years an empire with magnificent facilities that surgeons from other parts of the world would envy. Apart from Queen Mary Hospital, the empire had beds in three other hospitals, each with a special function: cardiac and thoracic surgery at Grantham Hospital, day surgery at Tung Wah Hospital, and general and breast surgery at Kwong Wah Hospital. Thus, from a small unit with only general surgery, he developed various areas of specialties to provide advanced services for Hong Kong and for training of staff.[105]

Ong rapidly developed a reputation as a master surgeon, bold and ground-breaking in his approach. The Surgical Department at Queen Mary Hospital became renowned as a center of excellence for innovative surgery of the esophagus, liver, biliary tract, and cancer of the head and neck. He pioneered a number of new techniques such as transsphenoidal approach to the pituitary gland, transoral approach to the upper cervical spine, transhiatal dissection of the esophagus and esophago-gastric anastomoses in the neck, Roux-en-Y choledochojejunostomy, and retroperitoneal approach to the common bile duct.[106] In 1966, Ong and his team conducted the first open-heart surgery operation. Their success led to similar operations in Hong Kong. Under his leadership, the Department of Surgery began using artificial kidneys for hemodialysis and kidney transplantation.[107]

Another major accomplishment of Ong was changing his department from one that only provided basic surgical training to an academic research-oriented institution. To facilitate surgical approaches and to discover the feasibility of certain new procedures that he had in mind, he tried them in the postmortem room or experimented on animals first. Moreover, he tested out the functions in animals after a new procedure before applying it to his patients. He left 250 scientific papers, more than 100 books and monographs, which must have been considered unusual for a surgeon in his era.[108]

His weekly staff rounds at Queen Mary Hospital, its large variety of complex surgical cases and an army of staff, never failed to impress visiting surgeons. A gracious host to visiting surgeons, to whom he introduced not only his impressive swift and bold techniques but also the best of Chinese cuisine, Dr. Ong and the Department of Surgery became a must for surgeons who traveled to East Asia to visit. He also became a much sought-after speaker at major international conferences and a visiting professor to leading medical schools.[109]

As a teacher, he established a special method of pedagogy by combining the use of seminars, weekly peer-reviews, and research on international development. He fostered links with leading international centers and established systems of visiting professorships and traveling fellowships to promote international exchange. In 1976, he founded the Asian Surgical Association as a forum for surgeons from all corners of the world to share their professional views.[110]

Ong introduced the surgical fellowship examinations in Hong Kong, first with the Royal College of Surgeons of Edinburgh and then other Royal Colleges, as early as the mid-1960s. His connection with the Royal College of Surgeons of Edinburgh was particularly strong. He was awarded the first John Bruce gold medal in 1970, appointed as Regent of the College in 1998, and received the award of the Pehin Aziz medal of the College in 2001. Ong was also a Hunterian Professor of the Royal College of Surgeons of England and a Moynihan Lecturer in 1974. However, his awards were not limited to the above. He was elected to the James IV Association of Surgeons Travelling Professorship in 1967 and was the Governor of the American Association of Surgeons from 1974 to 1979, and President of the International Society of Surgery from 1983 to 1985. He was awarded the gold medal from the College of Surgeons of Malaysia, and the Abraham Colles Medal from the Royal College of Surgeons in Ireland. He received the distinguished award OBE from the Queen of England, and PSM, the equivalent of a knighthood, by the King of Malaysia and was addressed as Tan Sri.[111]

There is no shortage of stories about Ong. The Royal College of Surgeons of England wrote about his imperialistic style, "Twice a week, on Wednesday and Saturday, this diminutive figure would sweep through the wards at Queen Mary Hospital like Napoleon leading the Grand Armee."[112] He was known to be bad tempered, and would shout, if not swear, should he encounter a challenge in the operating room.[113] He was particularly strict with the junior staff, who bore the brunt of his bad temper. One of them wrote,

> The professor was as cantankerous and autocratic as ever, and we each had to build our own defences against his abrasive style since we were too preoccupied to let this hinder our progress. To his credit, Professor O was an excellent surgeon. His dexterity and ability to master the trickiest situation was astounding—he had the greatest hand skills I had ever seen. Probably because of this technical mastery, he had a voracious appetite for the most difficult and dangerous operations.... His oft-repeated mantra was to stride forth with a "sharp knife and a stout heart."[114]

In class, he often said, "I'll stitch up your mouth if you utter incorrect answer," and the threat silenced the class immediately. Many thought that Ong, being a traditional Chinese, believed in discipline "only a strict teacher produces outstanding students."[115] Yet, Ong could engender such respect or fear, that when he entered an elevator, others in it would walk out.[116]

Ong was probably the only doctor then who could tell the press off, without worrying about the consequences. On the issue of patients who were receiving renal dialysis and were found to be hepatitis carriers, he refused to reply to the press. He told one of the staff of *SCMP*, "I am not going to give you any information; I am not on speaking terms with the press." Then he slammed down the phone.[117] He likened the nurses who took industrial action in 1979 for a higher wage "as terrorists who make innocent people their hostage."[118] This and his abrasive style did not endear him to nurses.[119] Fortunately, this style of leadership is no longer popular in the modern era and probably no longer tolerated.

However, Ong was known for his kindness and generosity to his colleagues and patients. He treated poor and wealthy patients alike and would never collect fees from patients who could not afford to pay. When his colleagues faced difficulties during an operation, Ong would always volunteer to help out. His work ethics was impeccable. In his working life at HKU and government service for over 30 years, he performed over 10,000 operations. He got up every morning at 5:00 and jogged for two miles before going to work. He said, "For a surgeon to work only 12 hours a day, what luxury!"[120]

Professor Tan Sri Guan Bee Ong retired in 1982, but he continued to work in private practice until 1999, when he was diagnosed with liver cancer. He succumbed to the illness in 2004, survived by his wife and his eight children (from two marriages). In 1984, HKU established a G. B. Ong Visiting Fellowship and Travelling Fellowship to enable visitors to come to Hong Kong to share their knowledge and experience and for the members of the Department of Surgery to undertake training overseas. The Royal College of Surgeons of Edinburgh named a room The G. B. Ong Room in his honor.[121] Professor Ong is remembered for his brilliant innovations and surgical skills, his impeccable work ethic, and his generosity to his patients and colleagues, and for putting the Surgery Department of HKU on the world stage.

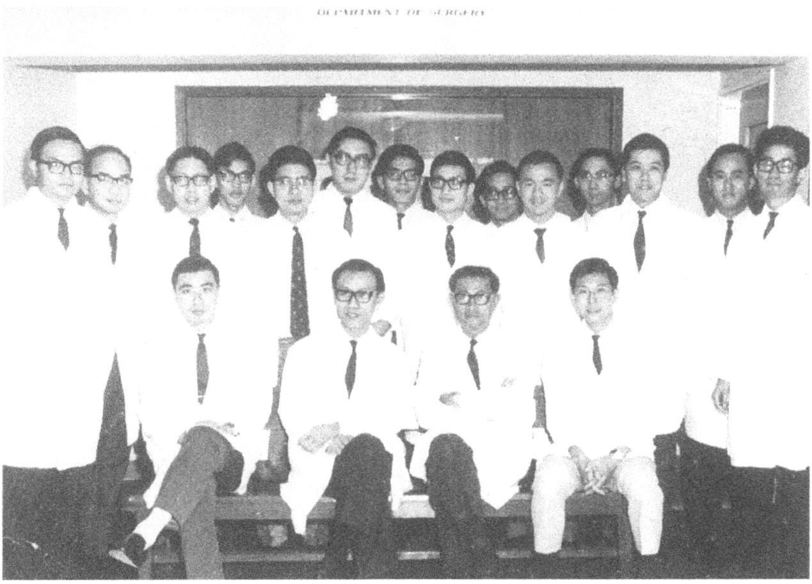

Figure 10.14 Professor G. B. Ong and the staff of the University Surgical Unit in 1970s

Standing L to R: Dr. Arthur Van Langenberg (L1), Dr. Frank Cheng (L2), Dr. Edward Leong Che-hung (L3), Dr. Paul Yue (L5), Dr. Michael Ma (L6), Dr. P. Wu (R3); Sitting L to R: Dr. Kwong Kwok-hei, Professor N. K. Yong, Profssor G. B. Ong, Dr. George Koo. Source: HKMMS with permission, photograph donated by Dr. Philip M C Wu.

11. Private Practitioners
Engaging in Politics to Improve Healthcare

Hong Kong has two medical and healthcare systems: the public system and the private system. Throughout the years, the proportion of registered doctors in the private sector was higher than in the public sector, about 70% to 30% in 1990. After the founding of the Hospital Authority in 1990, the conditions of service in public hospitals improved considerably, and the percentage of doctors in the public sector increased to around 47% in 2015.[1]

During the immediate postwar period, because of the poor economy in Hong Kong, funding for medical care had to compete with other social services such as education and social welfare. It was helpful to have members in the Legislative Council who would fight for more resources for medical services and recommend to the government the most effective way of managing the meager resources. During this period, the Medical and Health Department wisely spent its meagre resources on prevention and control of infectious diseases, which were the main killers at the time, leaving little to the curative portion of medical care. In the meantime, there was a marked increase in population, public medical services were overwhelmed. Government hospitals were congested, and outpatient clinics had long lines each day. By the early 1960s, with the improvement in economy and a higher budget for the Medical and Health Department, a 10-year plan was developed for the development of medical services.[2] The medical community was most fortunate to have two very knowledgeable and outstanding specialists in the private sector, Dr. Alberto Maria Rodrigues (legislator 1953–1958) and Dr. Fang Sin-yang, Harry (legislator 1974–1985) serving in the Legislative Council during the postwar period and guiding the government in developing medical and health services in Hong Kong. They also steered the NGOs to supplement the services delivered by the government.

At present, the private sector is providing about 80% of primary care in Hong Kong and government general outpatient clinics 20%. Until the arrival of the new millennium, general practitioners who provided primary care, both in private practice and in government, treated patients only for acute illnesses. They rarely found time for the essential work of prevention and health promotion. In the 1970s, communicable diseases were giving way to chronic noncommunicable diseases, which became major causes of morbidity and mortality. A medical system with good primary care often prevents or delays the onset of chronic disabling diseases and reduces the need for secondary and tertiary medical services. But Hong Kong has historically neglected primary healthcare. In addition, many doctors did not have the proper training to perform primary care services, and there was no primary care network to speak of. Family medicine and general practices as specialties were underdeveloped and undervalued, and they remained so in Hong Kong until the 1990s. In 1989, the government appointed the Working Party on Primary Health Care in Hong Kong chaired by Professor Rosie Young. The report's 102 recommendations were wide ranging and would require many new initiatives to implement.[3] Most of the recommendations were swiftly carried out by the Department of Health which was responsible for 20% of the primary healthcare in Hong Kong, but not the private sector. Primary reform in the private sector took place much later and not until there were more trained general practitioners in Hong Kong.[4]

One of the exceptional private physicians in this chapter is a general practitioner who recognized the problems of his colleagues in general practice as early as the 1970s and took it upon himself to do something about it. He was Dr. Lee Chung-yin, Peter, who formed the Hong Kong College of General Practitioners long before the government's primary care reform. He promoted family medicine and brought about a new breed of family physicians in Hong Kong.

Alberto Maria Rodrigues 羅理基 (1911–2006)

MBBS, JP, Military MBE, OBE, CBE, Hon LLD (HKU), Officer of the Order of Christ, Chevalier de la Legion d'honneur

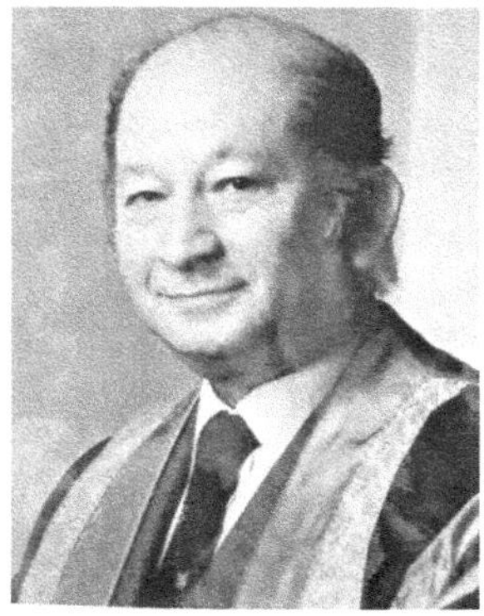

Figure 11.4 Sir Alberto Maria Rodrigues
Image courtesy of Dr. A. E. Rodrigues (son of Sir Albert)

Sir Alberto Maria Rodrigues (often anglicized as Albert) was born in 1911 in Hong Kong. His mother died shortly after his birth and sadly, his father also passed away when he was at a tender age of nine. Fortunately, his uncle, who had seven children of his own, brought him up, and he had a relatively happy childhood. Rodrigues had a long association with Macau, because his grandfather was a ship captain, and his boat traveled the Hong Kong-Macau-Guangzhou route. He attended St. Joseph's College, and his will to succeed turned him into a prize student. He was admitted into the medical school of HKU on a scholarship. As an undergraduate, he excelled in sports, especially in badminton, football, and hockey. However, it was cricket that he enjoyed most, having competed in and later captained the First Eleven successfully. He also played piano in a band, and later was taught by a Canadian internee to play guitar in the POW camp.[5] He received an MBBS degree in 1935.

Further training in obstetrics and gynecology took him to England. He then spent about one year in Lisbon, where he practiced medicine before returning to start his private practice in Hong Kong. When the Second Sino-Japanese War began in 1937, Rodrigues joined the Portuguese Company of the Hong Kong Volunteer Defense Corps. During World War II, he served as a medical officer in the Field Ambulance Unit under Dr. Lindsay Ride. After Hong Kong surrendered, he and the whole garrison were imprisoned as POWs in the wretched Sham Shui Po barracks. There, Rodrigues distinguished himself as the medical officer in charge of the dysentery ward. At one time the ward was packed with 800 patients. Both bacillary and amoebic dysentery were common then, but he was only given a small supply of sulphur drugs. The other deadly infectious disease at the camp was diphtheria. As the camp had only a small amount of anti-toxin brought in by Dr. Percy Selwyn-Clarke, many died. Although Rodrigues marveled that so many patients recovered from these horrendous infectious diseases despite the lack of medications, most patients believed that it was due to his expert care that they survived. Malnutrition and vitamin deficiency were the other prevalent afflictions at the time. Rodrigues ingeniously solved the problem of vitamin C deficiency by growing tomatoes in the campsite from seeds of tomatoes from cans. But he was not able to cure beriberi and pellagra, which were widespread. Despite the desperate situation, he organized a band and entertained the camps in the evenings to sustain the inmates' morale.[6] For his outstanding work in the camp, he was promoted from Lieutenant to Major after the war and was awarded a member of the British Empire (MBE) in 1948[7] and an Officer of the Order of Christ in 1949.[8]

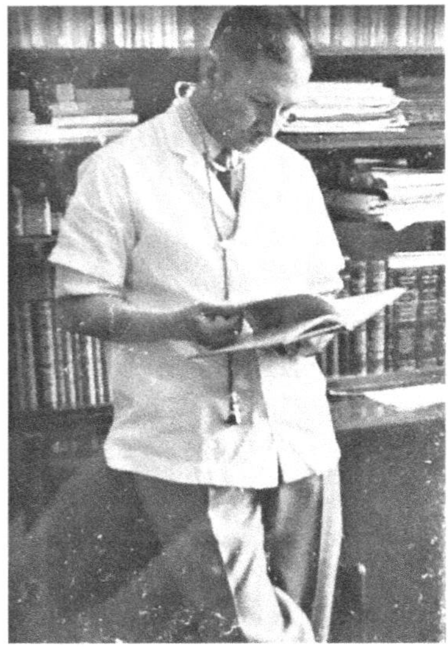

Figure 11.5 Young Rodrigues in the clinic
Image courtesy Dr. A. E. Rodrigues

After the war, Rodrigues returned to private practice. He became Medical Superintendent of St. Paul's Hospital in 1953, representing the hospital in medical affairs to the government; he was also Chairman of the Hospital Advisory Board.[9] He delivered more than 2,000 babies in the postwar baby boom era. Because of his meticulousness, he was responsible for low infant mortality and earned the gratitude of thousands of mothers.[10] A devout Catholic, Rodrigues was dedicated to his church and to the hospital. He was made a Chevalier of the French Legion of Honor in 1962 and a Knight Grand Cross of the Roman Catholic Order of St. Sylvester in 1966.[11]

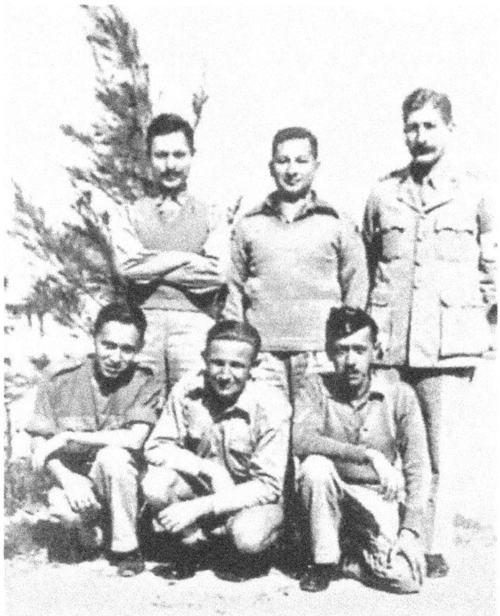

Figure 11.6 Dr. Rodrigues (standing center), Dr. Solomon Bard (Standing L1), and other POWs

Image courtesy of Dr. A. E. Rodrigues

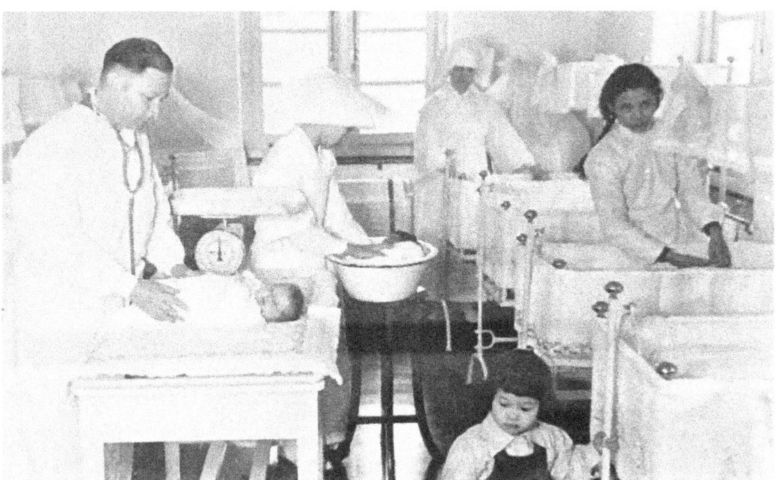

Figure 11.7 Dr. Rodrigues at St. Paul Hospital's nursery 1949

Image courtesy of Dr. A. E. Rodrigues

Even as a young man, Rodrigues had a great interest in public service. He was first elected to the Urban Council in 1940, at the young age of 29—a remarkable achievement, as he did not belong to any organization with a political platform.[12] After the war, he resumed his work in the Urban Council. But in 1950, he left for postgraduate studies in the US. On his return, he served in the Legislative Council from 1953 to 1959, when he was appointed to the Executive Council. He served as a Senior Unofficial Member in the Executive Council until his retirement in 1974.

Rodrigues's appointment as an Unofficial Member of the Legislative Council and later the Executive Council likely influenced the development of medical and health services during this period. Immediately after the war, most of the limited budget for medical and health services was spent on prevention of infectious diseases with little left over for curative care. The government encouraged voluntary agencies to build hospitals and to deliver the more expensive inpatient services. Even with the progressive rise in economy in the 1960s to the 1970s, the government aimed at delivering outpatient care to 50% and hospitalization to 80% of the population, unable to provide a comprehensive medical service to the whole population.[13] It planned to build outpatient facilities according to the size of the population. For example, there would be a standard dispensary for a 100,000-person urban population and a 50,000-person rural population. A standard outpatient center then was defined as one with a general outpatient clinic, a maternal and child health center, and maternity beds, varying from six in rural health centers to 24 in urban health centers.[14] Such a plan of medical development for a developing region such as Hong Kong at the time when the budget was limited was sensible and satisfied Rodrigues's wish to keep low maternal and infant mortality.

Rodrigues's public services, in addition to serving in the two councils, Legislative and Executive, were extensive. Drug addiction was a widespread problem in the 1950s and 1960s. He believed that drug addicts should not be treated as criminals, which was the government policy at the time.[15] In 1959, the government published a White Paper on the "Problem of Narcotic Drugs in Hong Kong,"[16] outlining its anti-drug measures. In addition to combating drug trafficking, it planned to establish treatment centers for drug addicts, but there was no facility for rehabilitation. In 1961, Rodrigues and Brook Bernacchi, Chairman of the Reform Club in Hong Kong, founded the Society for the Aid and Rehabilitation of Drug Abusers (SARDA),[17] a voluntary organization, aiming to treat and rehabilitate drug addicts and to promote public education against drug abuse and to make recommendations to the government.[18] In 1963, SARDA established the Shek Kwu Chau Treatment Center, on a remote island, for addicts.[19] It was so successful that a new hospital and a reservoir were added three years later to increase the accommodation from 200 to 500 subjects.[20] SARDA carried out several very effective anti-drug campaigns with an intensive public education program and wide publicity through the newspapers, radio, and television.[21] In 1965, Rodrigues took over the overall responsibilities on anti-drug addiction in becoming Chairman of the Action Committee Against Narcotics (ACAN), which advised the government on the overall policy and strategy against drug abuse in Hong Kong and coordinated several government departments, such as Health, Police, Customs and Excise, Correctional Services, Social Welfare, Educational and Information Services, and various voluntary organizations such as SARDA, and the Hong Kong Council of Social Service, so that there would be a unified approach and no duplication of services.[22] For his dedicated and effective role in anti-narcotics and other public services, Rodrigues was knighted by Queen Elizabeth II in 1964.[23]

In 1962, Rodrigues was appointed chair of a working party to establish the School Medical Service[24] which would take over the medical function of the School Health Program.[25] When it was formed, he served as its chair.[26] The School Medical Service was operated by private practitioners under the auspices of the Hong Kong Chinese Medical Association on a per-capita contributory basis. The School Health Program continued to assume responsibility for environmental sanitation, control of communicable diseases, immunizations, and health education for all registered schools in Hong Kong. Rodrigues served on the School Medical Services Board until his retirement in 1974. Although only around 25% of school children participated in the School Medical Service in the beginning,[27] the number increased when the terms improved for the participants, allowing an unlimited number of visits to the medical practitioners.[28] An avid sportsman, Rodrigues promoted sports in schools whenever he had an opportunity. He was President of Hong Kong Badminton Association and supported students' participation in competitions outside the colony.[29] He was the founding board chairman of the Jubilee Sports Center which was established in 1977 to improve sports standards and nurture local elite athletes. The center was renamed Hong Kong Sports Institute in 1991.[30] Five Rodrigues Awards were donated by Dr. Mary Gray Rodrigues, Sir Albert's daughter-in-law, in his honor for HKU Sports Scholars.[31]

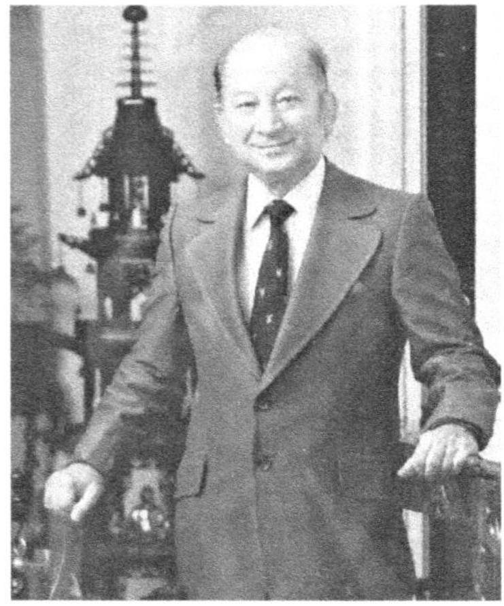

Figure 11.8 Dr. Rodrigues at home
Image courtesy of Dr. A. E. Rodrigues

Rodrigues had a long association with his alma mater. In 1962, he received an honorary degree of Doctor of Laws from HKU.[32] His long service to the University only began in 1967, when he was appointed Chairman of the Council of HKU. He was the first lay member of the university to succeed the Vice-Chancellor as Chairman of the University Council.[33] A year later, he broke another tradition and was appointed the first Pro-Chancellor of HKU by Governor Sir David Trench.[34] This position enabled him, in the absence of the governor who was the Chancellor, to be the head of the university. He continued as Chairman of the University Council until 1985 and Pro-Chancellor until 1994. He claimed his proudest moment was to confer an honorary degree on Mother Teresa in 1993.[35]

Sir Alberto Maria Rodrigues died in 2006, at the ripe old age of 95. An altruistic man, Sir Alberto spent the longest time in voluntary public service, starting at the age of 29, engaging in distinguished war service, acting enthusiastically as Unofficial Member of the Legislative and Executive Councils, leading highly effective campaigns against narcotic addiction, actively promoting sporting activities and School Medical Service, and served his alma mater with dedication until he turned 82, a total of 53 years. His public service was associated with progressive advances in medical and health services and education in Hong Kong. Such a long record of service has yet to be surpassed. His selflessness and his devotion to Hong Kong will long be remembered.

Fang Sin-yang, Harry 方心讓 (1923–2009)

MBBS, Hon MD(Liverpool), JP, Hon LLD (HKU, CUHK), DSSc (Poly U), DSc (OUHK), GBM, CBE

Sir Sin-yang, Harry, Fang was a renowned orthopedic surgeon and a thoughtful and effective legislator. He was known as the "Father of Rehabilitation" in Asia, leading the campaign for the welfare of people with disabilities, fostering equal opportunities and changing the public's opinion about them. He also contributed enormously to improving the medical and healthcare system in Hong Kong.

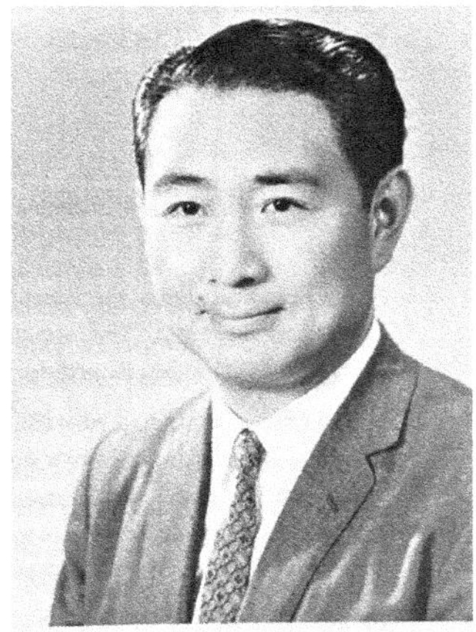

Figure 11.9 Dr. Fang Sin-yang, Harry
Image courtesy of Christine Fang

Fang was born in Nanjing, China. After the family moved to Hong Kong to escape political tumult and instability, he attended King's College, where he worked very hard to become matriculated, because he had to learn to speak English and Cantonese. Yet he graduated in 1940, one year earlier than most students, and was admitted to the HKU medical school. At that time all students had to live in residence, and Fang was unable to find a spot. Thanks to Father Kelly's ingenuity, the pantry of Ricci Hall became Fang's living quarters.[36] This, and other acts of kindness of the Catholic Church to his family, led to his conversion to Catholicism.[37]

In 1941, Japan invaded Hong Kong. Like many other students, he escaped to Free China and continued his studies in Chongqing, where the Shanghai Medical College had moved during the war. He graduated in Shanghai in 1947 and returned to Hong Kong, where he began his career as a surgeon. When he became the first assistant to Professor Arthur Hodgson of the Orthopedics Unit at Queen Mary Hospital, he took to it "like a fish to water," and it did not take long before he became one of the most brilliant orthopedic surgeons in Hong Kong.[38] He won the first scholarship awarded by the Sino-British Fellowship Trust in 1952, which enabled him to study further in the most prestigious training centers in the UK. He was impressed with the origin of the Sino-British Fellowship Trust, as the funds were collected by one person, Bishop Ronald O. Hall. This likely inspired him to raise funds for charitable purposes at a later date.[39] In Liverpool, he completed a dissertation on what happened to the cervical spine at the final moment of dispatch of convicted murderers executed by hanging.[40] In 1958, he was appointed the Hong Kong government's first orthopedic specialist.[41] Although he was posted in Kowloon Hospital, he covered services at Grantham Hospital, Tung Wah Hospital, and Ruttonjee Hospital as a consultant. In these four hospitals, he trained staff to become the next generation of orthopedic surgeons in Hong Kong.

In the 1950s and 1960s, tuberculosis of the spine was prevalent. Although the disease affects the anterior spine, surgery was carried out using the posterior approach. Fang suggested the anterior approach to the spine for debridement and spinal fusion. The first such operation was carried out in 1955, when Professor F. E. Stock performed a thoracotomy to expose the thoracic spine, and Fang and Professor A. R. Hodgson carried out the debridement and spinal fusion using bone graft. This operation was dubbed "the Hong Kong Operation."[42] Fang's detailed knowledge of the cervical spine came in handy for the transoral approach for lesions of the cervical spine,[43] when he and Prof G. B. Ong formed a team for this operation. Soon Fang's reputation soared in Hong Kong.

In 1961, Fang began private practice. He worked at St. Paul's Hospital and Hong Kong Sanatorium and Hospital, but he also acted as an honorary consultant to the orthopedic units in Tung Wah Hospital, Grantham Hospital, and the Children's Convalescent Home at Sandy Bay. He soon realized that although the surgeon can repair, renew, and save life, many patients are not restored to a good quality of life in a world often intolerant of disability. He claimed that his interest in rehabilitation was a response to the needs of his patients.[44] He and Professor Hodgson formed The Hong Kong Society for Rehabilitation and The Society for the Relief of Disabled Children. He learned to be very good at raising funds from wealthy benefactors and was able to raise funds to establish Margaret Trench Medical Rehabilitation Center in 1963. Since rehabilitation alone could not solve other social issues of the disabled, Fang formed the Joint Council for the Physically and Mentally Disabled in 1964, which later merged with the Hong Kong Council of Social Services to provide more comprehensive services for people with disabilities.[45]

In 1980, Fang made a request to Governor MacLehose for a piece of land in Sandy Bay and funds to build a rehabilitation center in Hong Kong. It was approved on condition that Fang had to raise 20% of the cost privately. Fang had no difficulty in raising the funds required, and in 1984, MacLehose Medical Rehabilitation Center was completed, to which the governor kindly agreed to lend his name. The rehabilitation center differs from others, as it is also a center for training thousands of healthcare professionals of Hong Kong and China and is recognized as a center of excellence by the WHO.[46]

Fang took the lead to develop Hong Kong Sports Association for the Physically Disabled in 1972. Hong Kong Sports Association for the Mentally Disabled was established later in 1976. This led to athletes with disabilities being able to compete in sports locally and internationally. Thanks to his successes in rehabilitation, Fang was invited by international leaders to play a leading role in developing international organizations which would lead to equal opportunities and full community participation for people with disabilities. He founded the Far East and South Pacific Games Federation with Japan in 1974. The first game was held there in 1975. He brought the third game to Hong Kong in 1982 and the Abilympics in 1991.

Fang's contributions to rehabilitation were not limited to Hong Kong. He was instrumental in introducing the concept of rehabilitation to China. By establishing the World Health Organization Collaborative Center in Wuhan, over 1,000 rehabilitation doctors were trained and distributed throughout China. He helped Deng Pufang, son of Deng Xiaoping, to develop the infrastructure and various programs for people with disabilities in China.[47]

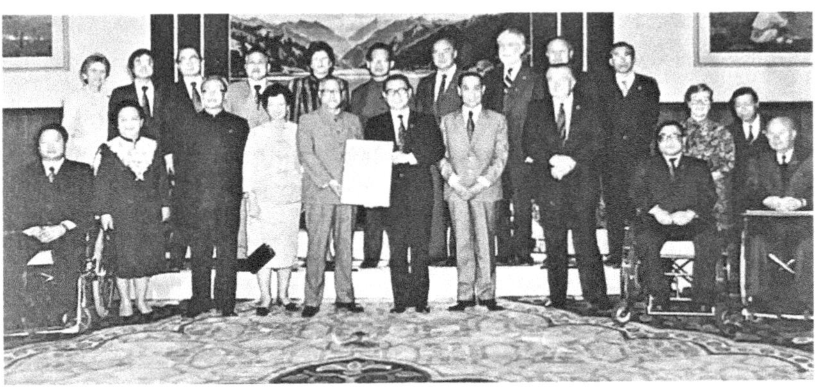

Figure 11.10 Dr. Fang presenting the Charter for the Disabled to Premier Zhao Ziyang in 1984, Deng Pufang in a wheelchair on the right side
Image courtesy of Christine Fang

In 1974, Fang received a telephone call that changed his life and made his work on rehabilitation much more widespread and effective in Hong Kong. The call came from Governor Murray MacLehose, asking for advice for his five-months pregnant daughter who became paralyzed after a car accident. Fang had been working on rehabilitation of these individuals to return to them better function and quality of life. Happily, Sylvia, MacLehose's daughter had an excellent outcome: a healthy baby delivered by Caesarean section at term. She carried on living a near-normal life due to early rehabilitation. In the fall of 1974, Fang was appointed to the Legislative Council as an Unofficial Member (1974–1985).[48]

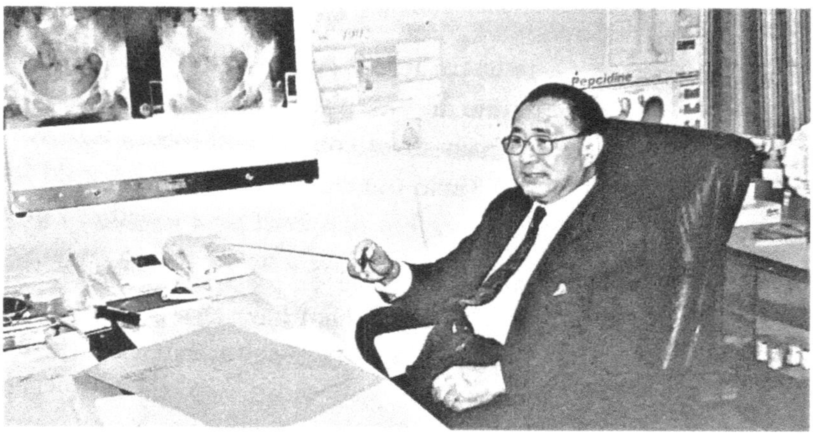

Figure 11.11 Dr. Harry Fang in his office
Image courtesy of Christine Fang

Fang believed that the governor appointed him to the Legislative Council to agitate for changes in the healthcare system, and he did not disappoint the governor. In 1977, Fang and his colleagues were able to produce the first White Paper on Rehabilitation, "Integrating the Disabled into the Community: A United Effort," aiming at delineating the official policy for rehabilitation and presenting the policy proposals.[49] It was a comprehensive document covering diagnosis, prevention, screening, assessment, medical treatment, social rehabilitation, and rehabilitation services. The program proposed was to be reviewed every three years. In 1991, the government appointed a Working Party on Rehabilitation Policies and Services under the chairmanship of the Secretary for Health and Welfare, to review the status of rehabilitation and to develop further policy. A White Paper, "Rehabilitation. Equal Opportunities and Full Participation: A Better Tomorrow for All," was published. Although Fang had retired from the Executive Council by then, there is no doubt that he had considerable input in the preparation of the document, as the title bore his motto for the disabled: "Equal Opportunities and Full Participation for all."[50]

From 1978 to 1983, in addition to being a member of the Legislative Council, Fang was concurrently an Unofficial Member of the Executive Council,[51] making it easier for him to make some fundamental systemic changes to the whole healthcare system in Hong Kong. He proposed that the Medical and Health Department should be divided into two separate entities: the Hospital Authority and the Health Department. He believed that it was largely the result of his behind-the-scene efforts that the Hospital Authority was created in 1990.[52] Around the same time he also called on the government to appoint a Working Party on Postgraduate Medical Education and Training, which gave birth to the Hong Kong Academy of Medicine Preparatory Committee. He addressed the problem of shortage of doctors, proposing to allow non-Commonwealth doctors to practice in Hong Kong,[53] giving higher salaries to doctors,[54] and supported the establishment of a dental school.[55] In addition to medical and health issues, Fang raised important issues related to education and housing, such as establishing a senior secondary school for children with disabilities[56] and initiating a home ownership scheme in association with private building concerns.[57]

In his autobiography, Fang wrote about his success as a fundraiser. He used many novel methods of fundraising, and he estimated that he had raised a total of HK$1.5 billion. He managed to persuade The Royal Hong Kong Jockey Club to donate HK$300 million to the Institute of Radiotherapy and Oncology at Queen Elizabeth Hospital, HK$300 million to CUHK and the University of Science and Technology for biotechnology, HK$270 million to HKU for redevelopment of the Faculty of Medicine, and HK$165 million to Hong Kong Academy of Medicine for the Jockey Club Building.[58] Apparently Fang's biggest requests were always accompanied by a big smile, which charmed the most intimidating, and "no" was seldom the answer.

Happily married to his teenage sweetheart, Laura, they were blessed with six children. However, he had an extended family of 14 children due to the early death of his two brothers. He cared for every one of them

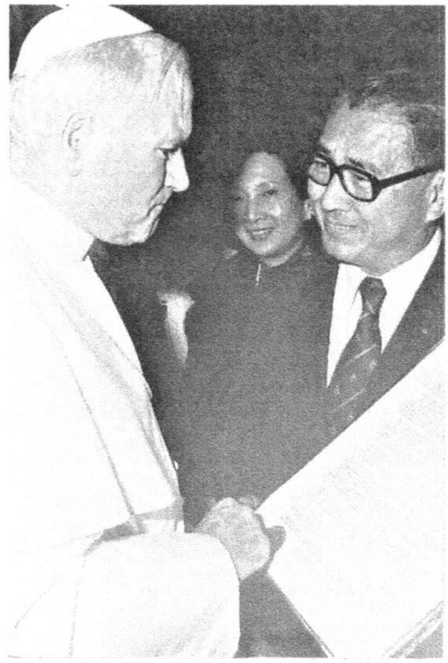

Figure 11.12 Dr. Harry Fang presenting the International Charter for the Disabled to Pope John Paul II at Vatican, 1981

Image courtesy of Christine Fang

and ensured that they received an excellent education. According to David Fang, his nephew, "He (Harry) ate heartily, never fussy about his food or drink. He had boundless energy and enthusiasm, taking all tasks large and small with his stride. Fatigue only appeared when he was injured once falling on the tramway, rupturing his quadriceps tendon and another time when he caught pneumonia on a trip to Africa.... Mahjong with family friends provided regular relaxation, while his steward's box at the races was fully utilized for entertaining guests, with occasional jubilation."[59] It is likely that his enjoyment on these occasions was mixed with fundraising.

Professor Sir Harry S. Y. Fang passed away in 2009, at the age of 86. In his lifetime, he received many honors. He was elected a fellow of a number of colleges: the Royal Colleges of Surgeons of Edinburgh, American College of Surgeons, and the Royal Australasian College of Surgeons. He was awarded honorary doctorates by both HKU and CUHK; the Citizen of the Year and Man of the Year in the UK in 1981; Rehabilitation International Man of the Year in 1984, and the same organization's President Award for outstanding and distinguished service in 1988. In 1990, the US awarded him the Preminger Medallion, a medal of distinction of the People-to-People Committee for the Handicapped, and the United Nations presented him with a special award the following year. He was appointed an OBE in 1969, CBE in 1980, and was knighted in 1996.[60]

In his eulogy, Dr. York Chow said, "Human greatness is not measured by one's power or wealth. It is measured by the number of people one can inspire and motivate to render help, support, care and love to other fellow men. Harry is an international giant and a Hong Kong legend in this regard, and we are blessed to have been associated with him ... "[61] Professor Sir Harry S. Y. Fang's charisma, vision, creativity and resourcefulness and ability to make things happen will long be remembered and admired by his family, his colleagues, and his friends.

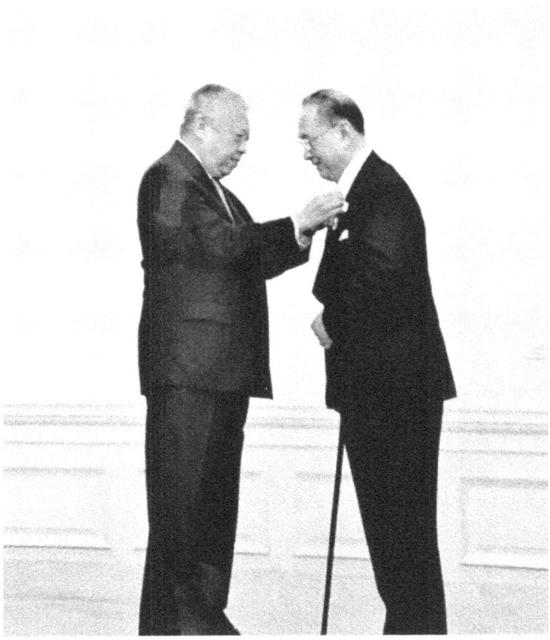

Figure 11.13 Sir Harry Fang, receiving the Grand Bauhinia Medal from Chief Executive Tung Chee-hwa in 2001

Image courtesy of Christine Fang

Lee Chung-yin, Peter 李仲賢 (1926–2013)

MBBS, JP, Hon LLD (HKU)

Dr. Lee Chung-yin, Peter was a family doctor with a vision. He founded the Hong Kong College of General Practitioners/ Family Physicians making general practice into a discipline that required strict training and of high standard in Hong Kong.

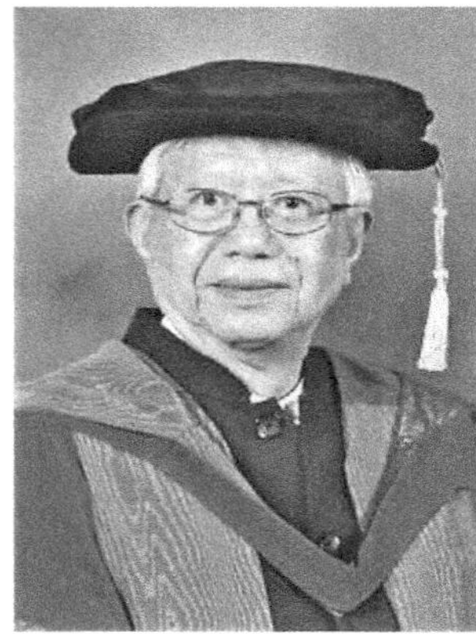

Figure 11.1 Dr. Lee Chung-yin, Peter

Source: Hong Kong College of Family Physicians, reproduced with permission

Lee attended St. Joseph's College and graduated when the war broke out in 1941. He entered medical school in 1947. His father, Mr. Li Chi-hung, established Sun Hing Hong Company after the war, and it developed into a very successful shipping company.[62] While an undergraduate, Lee organized the HKU Student Society, the precursor of the HKU Students' Union, and persuaded others to cooperate and revive student involvement in the university. Soon after graduation, Lee became Clerk of Convocation of HKU. In 1968, he was elected Chairman of Convocation and served for two other terms (1971, 1974), demonstrating fully his spirit of public service and organizing abilities.[63] On several occasions, Lee spoke out on behalf of his alma mater on issues such as urging the government to give loans to university students in need[64] and proposing a department of music for HKU.[65] He was a member of the University Council for 35 years. He contributed so much to the university that the campus has a road named after him, Chung Yin Road, extending from East Gate to Loke Yew Hall.

Edmund Blunden, Professor of English and a world-renowned poet and author, recognizing Lee's talents, dedicated a sonnet to him in 1960:[66]

> Peter, whose public spirit all men know
> And still whose good deeds oft escape our eye,
> Veiled by your modest manner. Passing by,
> I just called in quiet and brief although
> Devising, drafting, doing so much—and so

You smoothed our path among the rest—we try
To offend you with good will. O do not sigh
So deeply. Six more line, that's all, you know.
Musical Medical Man! Observer hold
Of human ailments, conqueror of the same
From masqueritis to the common cold,
May fortune bring you more than merely fame,
Dear giver, may you gather tons of gold ...
For which, in due course, you'll receive the Masquers' claim.

Lee began his private practice after graduation in early 1950, a time when the city was inundated with refugees from the mainland, resulting in a shortage of housing, medical and health services, and education. Lee co-founded the Hong Kong Civic Association with a group of teachers, entrepreneurs, and professionals, and was Secretary-General of the association between 1958 and 1964.[67] In 1960, he led the association to form a coalition with the Reform Club,[68] and the coalition sent a delegate to London to press the British government for constitutional reform. The demands were rejected.[69] Lee spoke out on several issues to improve the living conditions in Hong Kong, calling on the government to encourage the formation of non-profit-making housing cooperatives by releasing suitable sites at low cost.[70]

In 1968, Lee was elected President of the Hong Kong Medical Association (HKMA) and served for three terms. Again, he spoke on important issues, such as urging private doctors to help with the shortage of staff in the public sector,[71] and for the control and regulation of the proliferating private laboratories.[72] Lee's most important accomplishment as President of HKMA was to canvas successfully for the association to be accepted as a member of The World Medical Association (WMA), whose mission is to promote the highest possible standards of medical ethics.[73] Inspired by the existence of colleges and academies of general practitioners/family physicians in Western countries and their missions,[74] Lee wanted to establish a similar college in Hong Kong.

As noted in the 1950s and 1960s, infection and infectious diseases were responsible for 60% to 70% of all deaths. The most common complaints in outpatient clinics were upper respiratory tract infections and gastrointestinal problems. As Hong Kong's economy improved, the pattern of diseases altered. Since the 1970s, doctors began to attend more patients with chronic noncommunicable diseases, such as heart diseases, stroke, diabetes, cancer, dementia, and degenerative joint disease and these diseases accounted for about 60% of all deaths in Hong Kong.[75] Most general practitioners in Hong Kong at the time had little previous experience in treating and preventing these diseases.

Having traveled around the world and attended several international conferences, Lee was acutely aware of the defects of the medical system and the lack of training in treatment and prevention of chronic noncommunicable diseases among general practitioners in Hong Kong. He perceived that most of them were not inclined or did not have the opportunity to update or upgrade their skills. As Hong Kong people tended to shop around for doctors and did not have the idea of having a family doctor, it was difficult to become a family doctor in Hong Kong. Lee observed that the general practitioners were at risk of becoming "tradesmen with medical degrees," he aspired for a new breed of family physicians who would be specifically trained for the task by receiving appropriate postgraduate clinical training.[76] In 1973, he sought the HKMA Council on the advisability of establishing the Hong Kong College of General Practitioners (HKCGP). By 1977, the college was established with Lee as founding president. Lee donated generously to the college, a lease of 75 years for half a floor of Duke of Windsor Social Service Building on 15 Hennessy Road, Wan Chai, to serve as the headquarter of the College.[77] The first general meeting was held in 1979 in City Hall Theatre.[78]

Once the College was formed, it set about to define the discipline, the core knowledge, and the professional skills of a general practitioner, which became the academic content of the specialty of general practice. A journal was then produced by the college and widely distributed throughout Hong Kong to provide information to its readers about the discipline of general practice and clinical information. The college then established a program of continuing medical education, which attracted general practitioners who were keen to learn about their discipline and provided information on how to apply the latest advances in medicine to care for their patients. A vocational training program was initiated on a small scale in two hospitals: Evangel Hospital and Our Lady of Maryknoll Hospital. It gradually expanded to involve more hospitals and was based on the services of volunteers (both trainers and trainees). Even when more hospitals were involved, the program was inadequate. The college

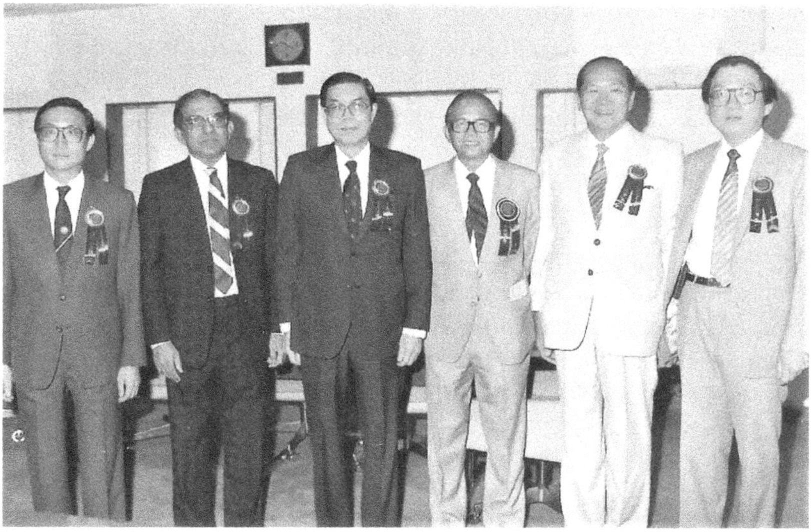

Figure 11.2 The unveiling of the HKCGP premises on the 8/F of Duke of Windsor Social Service Building on 18 May 1985 (Dr. Peter Lee, L4)
Source: Hong Kong College of Family Physicians, reproduced with permission

donated generously for the establishment of Visiting Professorships in HKU and CUHK in 1982 and 1984, respectively. In 1984, a Family Medicine Unit in the Department of Community Medicine was formed at CUHK, and in 1985, a General Practice Unit was set up in the Department of Medicine at HKU. Initially situated at Violet Peel Clinic, the General Practice Unit of HKU was later moved to Ap Lei Chau and renamed Ap Lei Chau Family Clinic.[79] The two universities finally took up the responsibility of training family doctors.

In the meantime, the attitude of the rest of the world was changing in relation to primary care, because studies have shown that healthcare systems that rely on primary care produce better health outcomes, reduce disease mortality, and result in higher patient satisfaction and lower healthcare costs. Furthermore, the WHO published a document in 1981, "Global Strategy for Health for All by the Year 2000," promoting the primary healthcare approach as the key to achieving the goal.[80] The Hong Kong government began to pay more attention to primary healthcare. In 1989, it established a Working Party on Primary Health Care, and the report was published in 1990.[81] The recommendations were numerous and carried out rapidly in the government outpatient services but not in the private settings. Recognizing the importance of primary care, in the same year, the Hong Kong Medical Council recognized the postgraduate diploma of the Hong Kong College of General Practitioners (HKCGP) as a quotable qualification. Having achieved the first objective, the HKCGP changed its name to the HKCFP in 1997.

The next objective in Lee's agenda for the college was to secure "specialty status" for the discipline. The intention was to ensure that the discipline of general practice/family medicine would, in the future, require the same stringent training and achieve the same high professional standard as other disciplines. When the Academy of Medicine Ordinance was enacted in 1992, the HKCGP was listed as one of its colleges. The third objective for Lee was to elevate the standards of continuing education and vocational training to achieve academic excellence and prestige of the fellowship degree (FHKCGP/FHKCFP). A conjoint fellowship examination of the Royal Australian College of Family Physicians and the Hong Kong College of General Practitioners was carried out in 1987. The results authenticated the standing and reputation of the HKCGP fellowship degree, which was henceforth internationally recognized.[82] The last objective of the college, and an ambitious one, was to persuade and assist the government to transform the healthcare delivery system of Hong Kong Special Administrative Region from hospital-based to community-based. This was an uphill battle, and Lee was unable to see its achievement in his lifetime, as he passed away in 2013.

During his terms of presidency of HKCGP, Lee established important links between the college, the government Medical and Health Department, and the medical faculties of both universities for the training program to be established, and for the HKCGP to be included in the Academy of Medicine. To bring this about, Lee did all the entertaining associated with conferences and meetings necessary through his own personal expenses. As he became well known internationally, he was made President of the World Organizations of Family Doctors (WONCA) from 1992 to 1995. He successfully bid for the Regional Asia-Pacific WONCA Conference and the World WONCA to take place in Hong Kong in 1987 and 1995 respectively—a most useful step in impressing on the local government the importance of family medicine.[83]

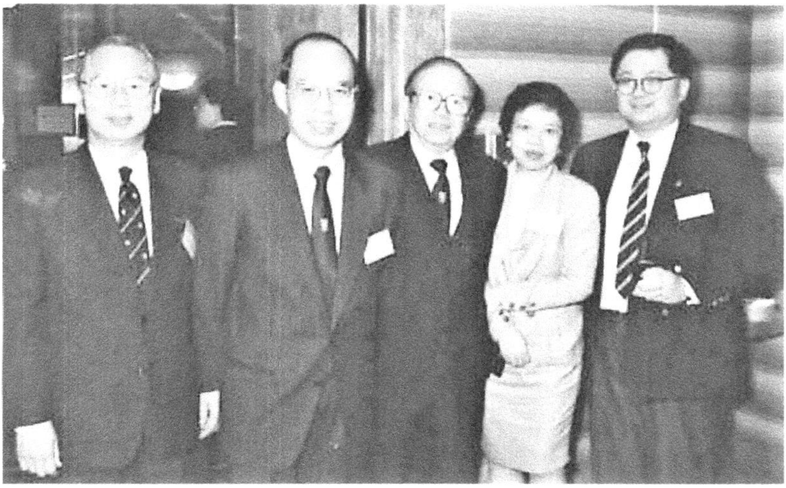

Figure 11.3 The inauguration of the Hong Kong Academy of Medicine in 1993, Dr. Peter Lee in center, Professor David Todd on far left
Source: Hong Kong College of Family Physicians, reproduced with permission

When the People's Republic of China opened its doors in the late 1970s, HKMA visited the Chinese Medical Association in Beijing in 1979. Lee took the opportunity to introduce the new medical discipline of general practice / family medicine to their hosts and generated considerable interest. Lee, as President of the HKCGP went to Beijing again in 1986 and met with the Minister of Health to publicize the concepts and principles of general practice. As a result, the Beijing Society of General Practice was formed in 1989 and was accepted as an associate member of WONCA.[84]

Dr. Lee Chung-yin, Peter brought about a new breed of family physicians in Hong Kong and introduced the concept of general practice in China. He was, indeed, "a towering icon of the medical profession and a role model for all young professionals," as described by Dr. Stephen Foo, a past president of the Hong Kong College of Family Physicians.

12. The First Two Female Professors
Trailblazing Women Doctors in Hong Kong

Before World War II, it was not common for girls to obtain higher education in Hong Kong, for many reasons. The traditional Chinese custom that girls should be homemakers and need not go to school prevailed. The only university in Hong Kong did not admit females until 1921, ten years after it was founded, and only a small number of female students were admitted each year after 1921. Education was expensive then and was usually paid for by the family.

During the immediate postwar period, most families in Hong Kong were poor. These families struggled to send their boys to school while their girls stayed home to look after their younger siblings and to do housework. In the late 1950s, as Hong Kong's economy gradually improved, the government began to expand primary education. By 1971, the government was able to provide free and compulsory primary education to all children. As a result, all girls received primary school education. In 1978, the government implemented free and compulsory education up to nine years and expanded senior secondary education and tertiary education. The growth of secondary schools resulted in a rapid increase in the percentage of full-time students aged 12 to 16, from 37% in 1961 to 70% in 1976. The target of 100%, boys and girls alike, was finally reached in 1981.[1] In 2008/2009, Hong Kong began to provide 12 years of free and compulsory education.

As Hong Kong gradually transformed into a financial and service center, there was a need for the government to develop and expand tertiary education to satisfy local demand. In the early 1980s, there were only two universities in Hong Kong, The University of Hong Kong and the Chinese University of Hong Kong. By the mid-1990s, Hong Kong had ten degree-granting institutions, eight of which were under the University Grants Committee, offering young people a variety of choices in higher education.

In 1996, an equal proportion of boys (21.9%) and girls (22%) received matriculation or university education in the 19 to 24 age group in Hong Kong.[2] The increase in the number of girls receiving higher education took place because since 1974, women were able to work outside the home as a result of the government permitting domestic workers from other Asian countries to work in Hong Kong and the government policy of compulsory free education. In other parts of the world, social changes were also occurring. In 2017, there were 30% more girls than boys in universities in the UK, and girls did better than boys by about 8 percentage points at the General Certificate of Secondary Examination.[3]

To enter the Faculty of Medicine at HKU or CUHK, two science subjects, physics and chemistry, are required. In the past, girls did not take science subjects because they thought the subjects were too difficult and uninteresting. As more science-related job opportunities opened up, more science-trained graduates were required. In schools, science subjects were made more interesting by curriculum reforms in the 1990s.[4] As a result, more girls took science subjects and entered the Faculty of Medicine or Science in HKU. Table 12.1 shows that in 1961, males dominated the new entrants to the university, especially in the Faculty of Medicine, but by the year 2020, the situation was reversed.

Table 12.1 Male to female ratio of all first-year students in the Faculty of Medicine and non-medical students at HKU

Students	1961	1990	2020
Year 1 undergraduates other than medicine	1:0.61	1:0.73	1:1:26
Year 1 medical students	1: 0.18	1:0.32	1:1.18

Source: Courtesy of Faculty of Medicine, HKU

During the last few decades, the number of females in the faculties of HKU, medical and non-medical, has also increased. The process has been very slow. In 2021, males still dominated in the professorial rank at HKU with male to female at 2.6:1, but in the lower academic level, the ratio was reversed.[5]

The stories of the first two female professors in the Faculty of Medicine at HKU, Professor Chun Wai-chan, Daphne, and Constance Elaine Field, will be told in this chapter, not so much of their struggle to be promoted but their achievements during their tenure as professors of their respective departments, obstetrics and gynaecology and pediatrics—the traditional fields for women doctors.

Chun Wai-chan, Daphne 秦惠珍 (1912–1992)

M.B.B.S., F.R.C.O.G., F.R.C.S., DSSc, CBE

Professor Chun Wai-chan, Daphne was a female doctor with many firsts: the first Chinese woman to gain a fellowship in the Royal College of Obstetricians and Gynecologists and the Royal College of Surgeons of Edinburgh. As the first Chinese woman professor (1957–1972) at HKU, Chun paved the way for women in the Medical Faculty.

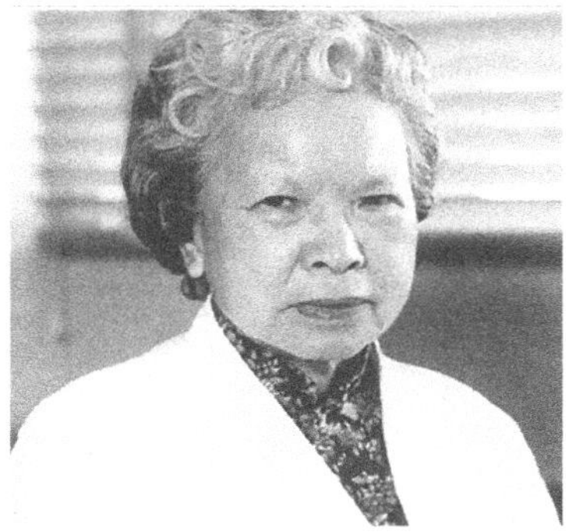

Figure 12.1 Professor Chun Wai-chan, Daphne
Image courtesy of Department of Obstetrics and Gynecology, HKU

Chun was born in Hong Kong and educated at St. Stephen's Girls' College. She graduated from HKU with an MBBS in 1940, winning several prizes. She became the second assistant in the Department of Obstetrics and Gynecology in HKU. After the Japanese invasion in 1941, she helped Professor Gordon King to escape from Hong Kong. Later she, too, succeeded in making her way into Free China, where she worked for a while in Chongqing Maternal Hospital. To obtain further training, she left for England, where she held posts in various London maternity hospitals, including Queen Charlotte's Hospital, and received first-class training in the specialty. She became the first Chinese woman to be admitted as a member of the Royal College of Obstetricians and Gynecologists, and in 1957, she became a Fellow of the college. She was also the first Chinese woman to be made a Fellow of the Royal College of Surgeons of Edinburgh.[6] In 1949, Chun returned to Hong Kong and was appointed Lecturer at HKU. In 1950, she was promoted Senior Lecturer, and in 1957 she succeeded Professor Gordon King on his retirement to the Chair of Obstetrics and Gynecology.[7] Her appointment was a milestone in the history of the university.

As head of the department, she spent her time between Queen Mary Hospital and Tsan Yuk Hospital. Since the time of Professor Tottenham, the training of obstetrics for medical students, interns, and residents took place at Tsan Yuk Hospital. Her term as head of department was associated with a marked reduction in neonatal and maternal mortality in Hong Kong. In 1972, when she retired, the very low perinatal (16/1,000) and maternal mortality (0.2/10,000) at Tsan Yuk Hospital was unrivalled by other hospitals in the world. During that year, Tsan Yuk also celebrated its golden anniversary. Sir Murray MacLehose unveiled a plaque to commemorate the occasion and praised the maternity hospital as one of the world's best.[8]

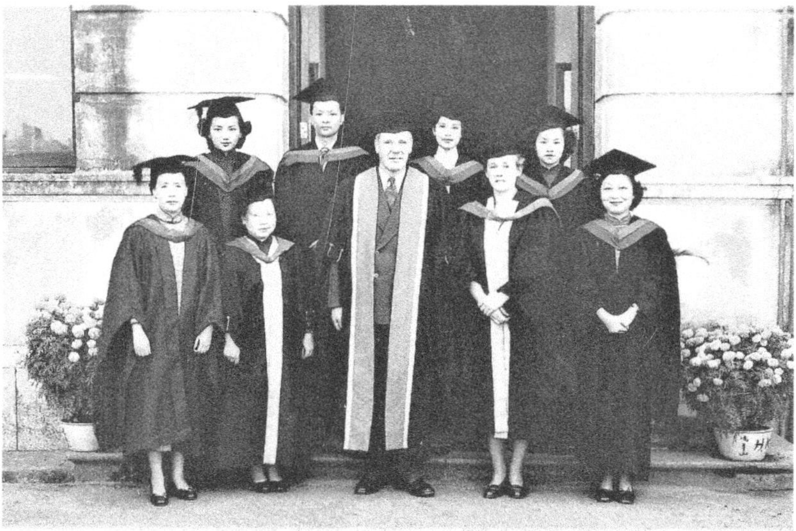

Figure 12.2 Professor Daphne Chun (front, L2) and Professor Gordon King (front, center) and graduates of 1951
Source: HKMMS, reproduced with permission

Chun was well known as one of the most outstanding pelvic surgeons in the world. Han Suyin, in her book, *My House Has Two Doors*, described Chun's extraordinary ability as a surgeon:

> ... Gordon King was in love with his profession and would rear extremely good gynecologists such as the small and wonderful Daphne Chun. Daphne's hands were a marvel, tiny and so able, so nimble! She was quite happy operating the whole day and I both envied and resented her enthusiasm, and the beam on her face when yet another belly had to be opened ...[9]

She was described by her trainees as "fearless" in carrying out operations, and she trained a number of excellent pelvic surgeons. The Caesarean section rate in Tsan Yuk Hospital gradually increased from 0.88% of all pregnancies in 1951 to 2.32% in 1956, as the operation was made safer and carried out with well-defined indications. There were no maternal deaths in Tsan Yuk during this period.[10]

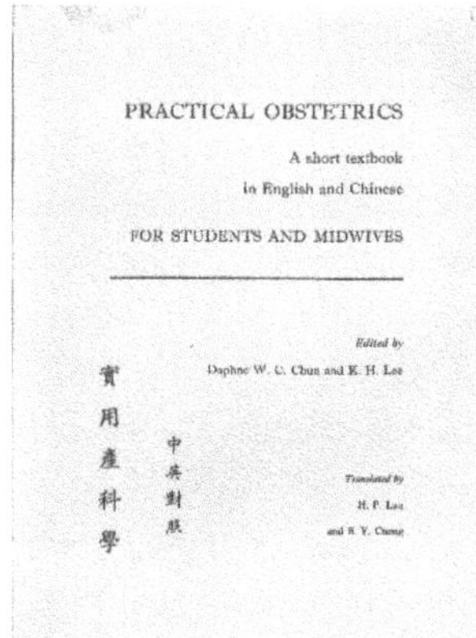
PRACTICAL OBSTETRICS
A short textbook
in English and Chinese
FOR STUDENTS AND MIDWIVES
Edited by
Daphne W. C. Chun and K. H. Lee
實用產科學
中英對照
Translated by

Figure 12.3 ***Practical Obstetrics*** **by Professor W. C. Chun and Dr. K. H. Lee**
Source: HKMMS, reproduced with permission

After World War II, the number of hospital confinement beds was limited, and the birth rate was high. Most of the deliveries were carried out in private maternity homes by registered private midwives or government midwives in government clinics.[11] In 1961, Chun was appointed a member of the Midwives Board, and she insisted on a high standard for the profession.[12] In the 1970s, as women came to realize the safety of hospital deliveries, the number of hospital confinement beds increased while those in private maternity homes declined. By the late 1980s, private maternity homes disappeared in Hong Kong.[13]

Academically, Chun was an internationally acknowledged leader in gestational cancers, such as choriocarcinoma and other trophoblastic tumors and their prevention, as well as in hormonal disorders of pregnancy, neonatal jaundice, and fetal distress. As a teacher, Chun encouraged her students to see obstetrics and gynecology as an integral part of medicine and not as an esoteric field. She worked hard to provide them with good practical experience. She published a book with members of her staff, based on the experience in Hong Kong, entitled *Practical Obstetrics: A Short Textbook in English and Chinese for Students and Midwives,* for medical students and midwives.[14]

Her other major contribution to Hong Kong was in family planning. The population in Hong Kong increased very rapidly, by about one million in each decade from 1950 to 1980, due to the postwar baby boom and refugees from the mainland. In 1952, the Hong Kong Eugenics League was reestablished by Professor Gordon King and renamed The Family Planning Association of Hong Kong. Chun, who had joined the league in 1940, became an active member of the association, serving as president from 1957 to 1962.[15] She led the fight against population increase and frequently gave lectures and talks on radio and television on family planning,[16] never losing a chance to emphasize the advantages of a smaller family.[17] She was responsible for introducing the intrauterine device for birth control and found it safe and effective.[18] She urged the public to support the Family Planning Association and their clinics.[19] As a result of her efforts and efforts of others, the crude birth rate in Hong Kong decreased from 37 live births per 1,000 in 1958 to 19.5 live births per 1,000 in 1972.[20]

As the activities of the Family Planning Association expanded, Chun called on the government to take over its activities rather than leaving them to an NGO.[21] In 1974, the government finally amalgamated the 32 Family Planning Clinics with Maternal and Child Health Centers to become Family Health Service.[22] The crude birth rate continued to decline and reached the lowest level of 6.9 live births per 1,000 in 2003.[23]

After her retirement, Chun remained active with family planning work both in Hong Kong and China. She called for a "drastic" population program in Hong Kong[24] and a "Commissioner for Population." She traveled to China several times to promote family planning programs and to share her experience with her counterparts.[25]

In 1959, Professor Chun was honored with appointment as CBE.[26] On her retirement in 1972, she became an Emeritus Professor and was conferred Doctor of Social Sciences from HKU.[27] Professor Chun is remembered for her "basic toughness of fiber.... mingled with a humanity of approach," which made her a determined and dedicated surgeon, stern but respected by her students, colleagues, and patients, and an inspiration to many female doctors.[28]

She emigrated to Canada in the 1980s and passed away in 1992.

Constance Elaine Field (1911–2002)

MBBS, MD, MRCP, FRCP

Professor Constance Elaine Field was the first Professor of Pediatrics (1962 to 1971) in HKU. But she had to fight hard to have a dedicated Department of Pediatrics. She built a strong foundation for the department to grow, and organized and launched the first much-needed longitudinal growth and development study of 800 Chinese children in Hong Kong.

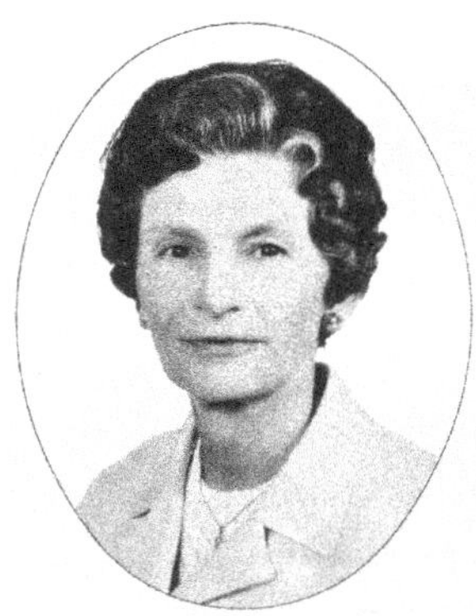

Figure 12.4 Professor Constance Elaine Field
Source: Department of Pediatrics and Adolescent Medicine, HKU, reproduced with permission

Field was a graduate of London University in 1934 and obtained her Doctorate in Medicine in 1937. She received postgraduate training at University College Hospital with Dr F. J. Foynton, one of the great English pioneers in children's diseases, obtained an MRCP after four years. She was interested in bronchiectasis, which was then a common disease in overcrowded communities, and began a longitudinal study of children with bronchiectasis to assess the long-term results of either radical (removal of diseased lobes of the lung) or conservative treatment. Chronic chest diseases in children became her expertise, on which she published many books and papers.

She had a series of appointments at the Hospital for Sick Children in Great Osmond Street. After World War II, she became Assistant Director of the Institute of Child Health in London. She received a Nuffield Fellowship in Child Health to visit institutions in the US, Scandinavia, and Finland. Although she had a good chance of securing a teaching post in England, she chose to offer her services in Malaya, a community without the advantages of a national health service. In 1949, she was appointed Specialist in Child Health in the Federation of Malaya (now known as Malaysia), where she developed a rudimentary service for underprivileged children. In 1955, she moved to Singapore and headed the pediatric unit at Singapore General Hospital and was Second Master of the Academy of Medicine of Singapore for one year (1959–1960). In Singapore, she was the prime mover in forming voluntary associations for children care, notably Singapore Pediatric Association and Spastic Children Society.[29]

During the immediate postwar years, there was no pediatrics specialty in East Asia. Children's wards were rare and infant mortality was high. When Field was appointed the first Professor of Pediatrics at HKU in 1962, there was no department of pediatrics but a pediatrics unit within the Department of Medicine. A senior member of the Department of Medicine headed the unit. Most of the time, the senior member did not serve for long, as he or she moved on to something else because their interest was not in pediatrics or in academic medicine.[30]

When Field arrived in 1962, she found the disease in children in Hong Kong "was gross, advanced and some of it preventable." She was referring to tumors of all varieties, late stages of blood or kidney disease, and advanced nutritional rickets.[31] She drafted a few medical officers, including Drs. Alice Chau and Paul Yue, with interest in pediatrics from the Government Medical and Health Department. With funding support from the Li Shu Fan Medical Foundation, she appointed Dr. Tsao Yen-chow as the first lecturer.[32] With this skeleton staff, she provided clinical care and teaching of undergraduates with little time for research. She spent the next two years negotiating for a dedicated pediatrics department. Finally with the support from the Vice-Chancellor and Senate, the Pediatric Department was officially established on 1st July 1964.

In the beginning, Field spent a great deal of effort in establishing a pediatric identity. Pediatrics became a subject in the final MBBS examination in 1965.[33] She established certain clinical practices at Queen Mary Hospital, to avoid cross-infection, as infectious diseases were common then. Field's policy was to "keep children's admissions to a minimum" and to "provide ambulatory service as far as possible." The Pediatric Department at Queen Mary Hospital had two wards: Children's Wing and Head Ward. Pediatric medical officers were required to attend all sick children at Casualty (Accident and Emergency Department) who needed admission according to the assessment of the casualty officers. These children were screened for potential infectious diseases before admission to Children's Wing, where they were further observed for these diseases, that could have been missed during the initial assessment. Only those who required continuing hospital care and who had no evidence of infectious disease would be admitted to Head Ward. In addition, semi-micro laboratory services were developed, to avoid an excessive amount of blood taken from children for various laboratory tests. Realizing the importance of training doctors for improving the care of children, Field began to train future pediatricians.[34]

Soon after her arrival, she founded the Hong Kong Pediatric Society for practitioners interested in pediatrics to meet and discuss their problems and to learn from each other. It was inaugurated with the first annual meeting in 1963.[35] Through the Pediatric Society, she promoted good healthcare practices among childcare workers.

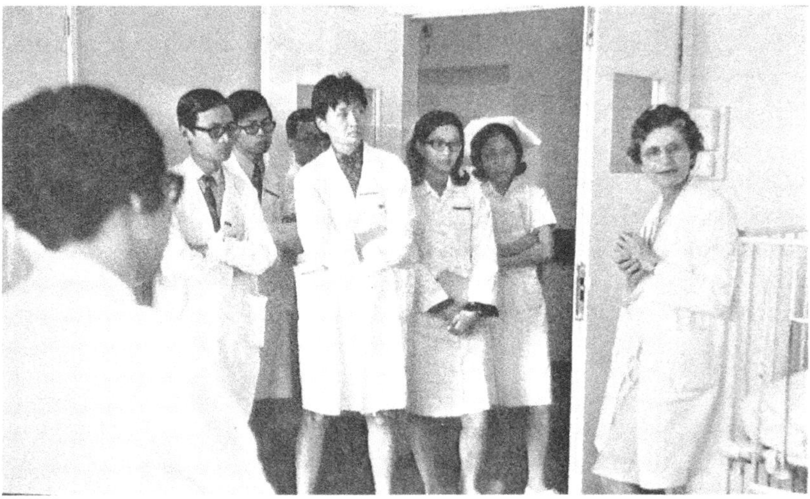

Figure 12.5 Professor Field (R1), Dr. Leung Nai-kwong (front L1), and Dr. Anita Li (front L2) during ward round

Source: Department of Pediatrics and Adolescent Medicine, HKU, reproduced with permission

Field made special efforts, reaching out to the community to arouse interest and to promote child health issues. At the time, there was no provision for remedial care and education for children with cerebral palsy and those with mental disabilities in Hong Kong. She founded the Hong Kong Spastic Children's Association and the Association for the Mentally Handicapped with the aim of organizing special educational and training facilities for these children. Funds were raised by the Spastic Children's Association, together with a generous donation from an American philanthropist, resulting in the building of Hong Kong Red Cross John F. Kennedy Center to provide therapeutic, nursing, education, and residential services for children with disabilities. She also organized the first special assessment service for children with disabilities and promoted the establishment of special schools for these children for the first time in Hong Kong.[36] In 1973, a school was established by the Spastics Association of Hong Kong (SAHK) for children with physical handicap and was known as the Sau Mau Ping Training Centre. In 1979, it was formally registered as Elaine Field School.[37]

Field obtained a grant of £40,000 from Britain's Nuffield Foundation for a longitudinal study of growth and development of Chinese children in Hong Kong and the influence of home conditions. Although cross-sectional studies and longitudinal studies had been done on the physical growth of Chinese school children by Professor Francis Chang and his colleagues in the Department of Anatomy of HKU, no one had investigated the growth of infants and preschool children or their psychological development and influence of home environment—a topic important for local pediatricians. The study involved 800 Chinese children recruited between 1967 and 1972. They were examined every year for physical and behavioral development, presence and absence of illness, as well as their feeding pattern.[38] The results of the study were published in a book that she coauthored with Flora M. Baber, *Growing up in Hong Kong* (Hong Kong: Hong Kong University Press) in 1973. It became a classic in its field and provided data of normal growth and development for Chinese children. Longitudinal studies are notoriously difficult to carry out and require considerable personnel and funding. In addition to the Nuffield Foundation of England, Field was able to obtain financial support from Li Shu Fan Medical Foundation and later from the Hong Kong Government Social Welfare Department Lotteries Fund.[39]

She was nicknamed "Old Granny" by her students, because she was already 51 years of age when she was appointed although now, 51 probably just marks the beginning of middle age. They admired and respected her because she was kind and hard working. She could be found in hospital wards late into the evening on most days. Unlike most teachers in those days, she was always soft spoken and did not shout or ridicule students. It is also known that her advice was always sound and sensible. Lady Peggy Templer, wife of the distinguished Field Marshal Sir Gerald Templer, met Field when her husband was posted in Malaya as High Commissioner and Director of Operations. Lady Templer was told by Field to do something useful and help those with hearing impairment. As a result, the Commonwealth Society for the Deaf was created, resulting in countless schools, teacher training, and rehabilitation programs for the deaf, including those in Hong Kong.[40]

Professor Elaine Constance Field retired in 1971 and returned to the UK to look after her elderly mother. Her popularity can be seen by the number of visiting students and ex-colleagues she warmly received every year. Although Professor Field was professor at HKU for only nine years, she laid a strong foundation for patient care and clinical research for the department and allowed it to grow.

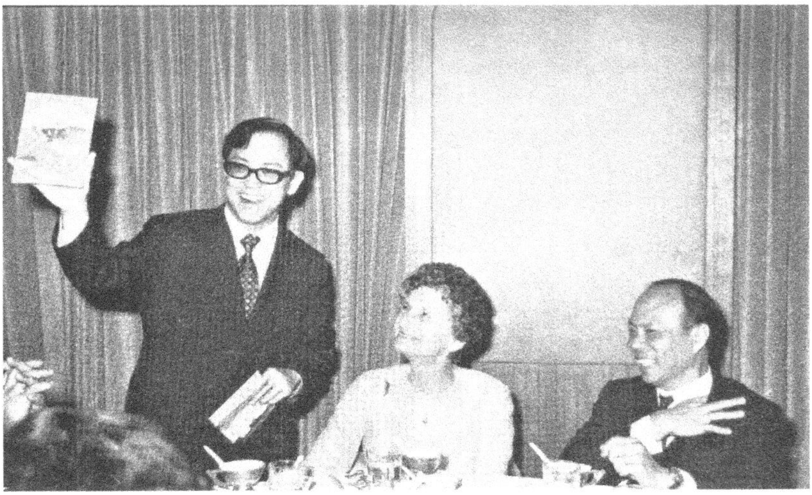

Figure 12.6 Farewell dinner to Professor Elaine Field (center) with Dr. Tsao Yen-chow (standing) on her left

Source: Department of Pediatrics and Adolescent Medicine, HKU, reproduced with permission.

13. The Last Medical Missionaries
Spreading the Gospel in Action in Hong Kong

Throughout the years, medical missionaries arrived in Hong Kong and China to "heal the bodies, and save the souls." Clinics and hospitals were built and sponsored by both Protestant and Catholic missionary societies. They provided the necessary medical services to the impoverished in Hong Kong during the latter part of the nineteenth century and the first half of the twentieth. After World War II, the government depended on nongovernmental agencies, especially the medical missionaries, to provide medical care. However, during the latter half of the twentieth century, there were fewer and fewer medical missionaries in Hong Kong. Within medical missions, there were debates regarding the efficacy of medical practice as a means of evangelism. The medical missions were also criticized because the perceived superiority of Western medicine perpetuated the stereotypes that Western societies were the "gold standard" of civilization. Moreover, by the 1970s and 1980s, Hong Kong's economy was flourishing. The government greatly expanded its medical and health services and was no longer dependent on nongovernmental agencies.

The LMS had a long history of sending medical missionaries to China and Hong Kong to spread the gospel through providing education and medical care. Soon after Hong Kong became a colony, the LMS moved their base from Macau to Hong Kong, and on 1 June 1843, opened Medical Missionary Society Hospital, which was closed around 1853 because of funding difficulties. After a hiatus of almost 30 years, the LMS and the Chinese elite built Alice Memorial Hospital, which also served as the teaching hospital for HKCM in 1887.[1] Additional small hospitals sponsored by the LMS were added to meet the increasing demand in the following decades. These hospitals were built next to each other, and in 1954, the complex was renamed Alice Ho Miu Ling Nethersole Hospital and was incorporated by an ordinance of the Legislative Council.[2] Dr. Edward Hamilton Paterson was the last in the line of the LMS medical missionaries sent to Hong Kong when he joined the Alice Ho Miu Ling Nethersole Hospital in 1951.

The Catholic missions arrived in Hong Kong soon after the establishment of Hong Kong as a British Colony. As early as 1845, the building of a hospital for the sick sailors from Goa and the Philippines was proposed by the mission but it was not realized. In 1852, a small hospital, St. Francis' Hospital, was built in Wan Chai, but this lasted for only seven years because of difficulty in sustaining the operation from lack of funds.[3] Other missions also landed in Hong Kong. The Canossian Missions, whose goal was to provide education for girls, soon found that they were also running an orphanage for a large number of abandoned children.[4] Then, out of necessity, they branched into providing nursing care for the sick and poor children and women. As more Canossian Sisters arrived, they formed a small community in Wan Chai. In 1869, they took over the running of the reconstituted St. Francis' Hospital and continued to operate the hospital until 1959, when a new Canossa Hospital was opened in Old Peak Road, and the old St. Francis' Hospital was finally closed down.

The story of St. Paul's Hospital in Hong Kong is similar. When the Sisters of St. Paul de Chartres arrived in 1848, their main task was to take care of foundlings. The sisters established an orphanage, "Asile de la Sainte Enfance," in Wan Chai for abandoned children, mainly girls. When plague ravaged Hong Kong in 1894, many poor children and elderly women came to the orphanage looking for shelter and care. As a result, the sisters established a hospital for Chinese women and babies in Wan Chai, which was equipped with an operating theatre and a dispensary for outpatients.[5] In 1915, the facilities in Wan Chai were gradually moved in stages to the new premises in Causeway Bay—the new modern St. Paul's Hospital, which was finally completed in 1918. It continues to operate today.[6] A branch hospital, St. Teresa's Hospital, was opened on the Kowloon side in 1940.

The last Catholic mission to start providing medical care before World War II was the Chinese Sisters of Precious Blood. In the 1920s, the sisters began operating an orphanage in Sham Shui Po, one of the poorer districts in Hong Kong. In 1936, they extended their operation, adding a hospital for orphans and impoverished children in the neighborhood—Precious Blood Hospital. Later, this hospital turned into a general hospital for the sick and poor in the district.[7]

After the war, a huge influx of refugees to Hong Kong created a great demand for social and medical services. Many religious bodies responded by opening clinics and planning to build new hospitals. In 1955, the Protestants opened Haven of Hope Sanatorium for TB patients in Junk Bay. In 1961, the Maryknoll Sisters opened Our Lady of Maryknoll Hospital in Wong Tai Sin. Caritas Hong Kong, the Catholic Diocese's social services organization, established the Caritas Medical Centre in 1964 in Sham Shui Po. As of December 1963, in Hong Kong, there were 2,082 beds in government hospitals and 1,893 beds in the hospitals sponsored by NGOs such as religious bodies. NGO hospitals played an important role in providing the much-needed inpatient care for the public during the first few postwar decades. In the 1970s, most of the NGO-sponsored hospitals received subvention from the government because of the high cost of running hospitals, and in 1990, most were absorbed into the public hospital system under the Hospital Authority. However, some remain as private hospitals; for example, the French hospitals (St. Paul and St. Teresa) and Baptist Hospital.

Unlike other Catholic orders that ventured into Hong Kong to provide healthcare and to build hospitals and clinics, the Missionary Sisters of St. Columban came to Hong Kong in 1949 to be responsible for operating Ruttonjee Sanatorium for TB patients. They came with a complete team of doctors, nurses, and radiographers. The Missionary Sisters of St. Columban was formed in 1922 in Ireland as women collaborators of the Columban Fathers, who had just started a mission in China. In 1926, the first batch of Columban Sisters arrived in Hanyang to start their ministry in healthcare and education.[8] Life was not easy for the missionaries then, as China was plagued by civil wars and at times famines and epidemics. The situation became increasingly difficult in the 1930s, when Japanese invasion in China culminated in the Second Sino-Japanese War. After World War II, on the establishment of the People's Republic of China, the political situation changed. Foreign missionaries were forced to leave the country. Thus, it was most opportune for the people of Hong Kong when the Superior General Mother of the Columban Sisters visited Hong Kong in 1947 and the Director of the Medical Department requested her team to run Ruttonjee Sanatorium.[9] The invitation was accepted, and in 1948, the first batch of sisters from Hanyang arrived in Hong Kong, marking the beginning of a long association between the Columban Sisters and Ruttonjee Sanatorium. At the time, Ruttonjee

Sanatorium was being converted from the old Royal Naval Hospital and the sisters took part in the refurbishing and equipping of the sanatorium. In preparation for their work, two sisters from Hanyang went to Brompton Hospital in London for special TB nursing training.[10]

Ruttonjee Sanatorium was situated on a hill in Wan Chai, on the original site of Seamen's Hospital by the sea, which was first constructed in 1842. From 1843 to 1873, Seamen's Hospital served sick sailors, supported by subscriptions from private firms and ship companies. The hospital was rebuilt by Jardine, Matheson & Co. in 1866. In 1873, when the hospital ran into financial difficulties, it was sold to the Admiralty to become Royal Navy Hospital, to replace the hospital ships.[11] During the Battle of Hong Kong in 1941, Royal Navy Hospital was hit by many shells and was deemed beyond repair by the navy. When it was acquired by the Hong Kong Anti-TB Association, extensive rehabilitation of the buildings was made possible by a donation from Mr. Jehangir Hormusjee Ruttonjee, a prominent entrepreneur in the Parsee-Indian community in Hong Kong, in memory of his daughter who died from TB.[12]

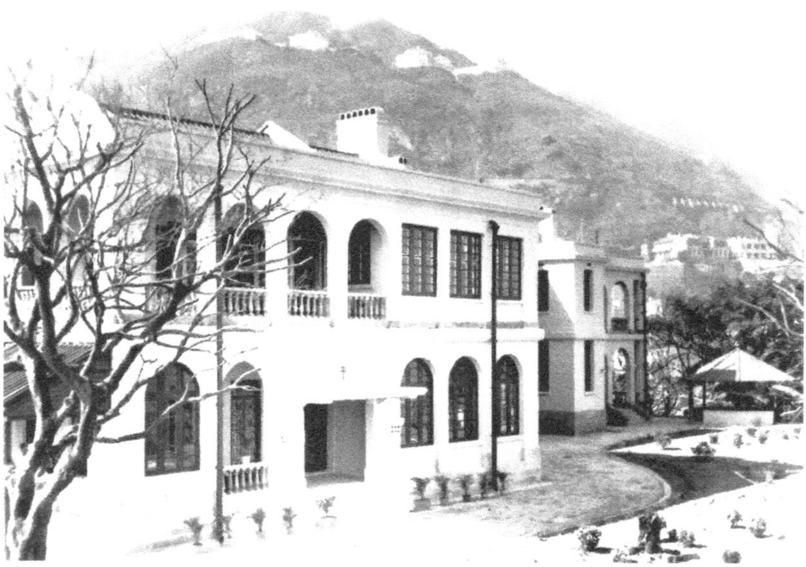

Figure 13.1 Ruttonjee Sanatorium (1949–1991)
Image courtesy of Hong Kong Tuberculosis, Chest and Heart Diseases Association

In the early 1950s, TB proliferated in Hong Kong among the poor living in overcrowded conditions. An English nurse who was working in Ruttonjee Sanatorium wrote about the financial and other difficulties encountered in the hospital:

> In the early days at the hospital there was very little money, and furniture like bedside lockers was made from ordinary boxwood painted white. Medical equipment was very scarce, blood pressure apparatus etc. was loaned from ward to ward. The mattresses were filled with wood shavings and in fact the nuns themselves slept on those for many years, and they did not complain. We had many problems with water supply in Hong Kong ... This had consequences which made working in an infectious disease hospital very problematic, but no one complained.[13]

Despite the limitation of resources, services to patients expanded. In 1954, an operating theatre was opened where well-known surgeons of Hong Kong regularly performed surgery on the patients. For example, Dr. Kenneth Hui, a leading surgeon in Hong Kong, performed thoracoplasty to collapse the lung, and Professor Arthur Hodgson of HKU carried out his world-renowned "Hong Kong Operation" for TB spine.[14] Ruttonjee Sanatorium, together with the Government Chest Service, collaborated with the British Medical Research Council (MRC) in various clinical trials of drug regimens in treatment of TB.

Dr. Edward H. Paterson, Sister Mary Aquinas Monaghan, and Sister Mary Gabriel O'Mahony were the last few medical missionaries in Hong Kong. Their work had a lasting influence on the health of the population and medical services in the region. The people of Hong Kong are grateful for their selfless sacrifice and for their love-in-action.

Edward Hamilton Paterson 巴治安 (1920–2013)

OBE, FRCS, Hon. DSSc (HKU)

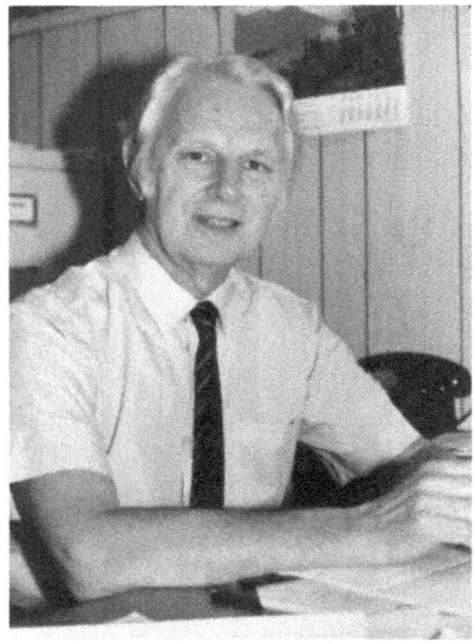

Figure 13.2 Dr. Edward Paterson, 1986

Image courtesy of Alice Ho Miu Ling Nethersole Charity Foundation

Dr. Edward Hamilton Paterson was born in 1920 in Lushan, Jiangxi province, to a very religious Scottish family. His father was a medical missionary of the LMS, who was posted to hospitals in Hubei. Paterson's three uncles were also ministers of the church. After spending his childhood in rural China, Paterson obtained his primary education in Shanghai, where the family relocated. In 1931, he was sent back to London for secondary education, followed by university education at Middlesex Hospital Medical School, where he graduated in 1943. After graduation, he received postgraduate training at Hammersmith Hospital and Harrow Hospital and then served in the Royal Army Medical Corps. In 1947, he joined Middlesex Hospital and St. James's Hospital in Balham. After receiving his FRCS in 1948, Paterson became a medical missionary of the LMS and was posted to China in 1950. In Beijing, he spent the first six months learning the Chinese language and was then sent to Mackenzie Memorial Hospital in Tianjin. When the Korean War broke out and foreign missionaries were no longer welcome, Paterson was relocated to Nethersole Hospital (Alice Ho Miu Ling Nethersole Hospital) in Hong Kong as a senior surgeon in 1951. The following year, Paterson married Barbara Knight, an LMS missionary teacher.[15]

Dr. F. R. Ashton was the Medical Superintendent of Nethersole Hospital when Paterson arrived. Dr. Ashton had served before the war as Medical Superintendent and resumed his position after Japan surrendered. Ashton recognized the need for the hospital to have more specialization and to have a postgraduate training program. In 1951, the operating theatre of Nethersole Hospital had little modern equipment, and its ward procedures were old-fashioned. There was no anesthetic apparatus, and only four types of anesthetic were available: open ether with a Schimmelbusch mask, intravenous thiopentone, spinal procaine, and local procaine, all of which had to be carried out by the surgeon himself. With a small budget, Paterson improved the equipment in the theatre and introduced modern surgical treatment. He bought a laryngoscope and some endotracheal tubes, along with a home-made ether vaporiser, and improved the process of anesthesia. But the surgeon still needed to induce anesthesia himself before scrubbing up for the operation. However, after a few years, Paterson was able to report that "major lung resections were being done in this theatre and what was probably Hong Kong's first right lobe hepatectomy, in 1957."[16] Paterson was trained as a general surgeon, but he excelled in the repair of cleft lips and palates. In the 1950s, many babies with such deformities were abandoned by their parents. From 1955 to 1976, Paterson operated on 1,800 such patients and developed a "Cleft Team" to provide comprehensive care for these children and improved the lives of many.[17] In fact, it was reported that over 80% of such cases in Hong Kong were treated by his team in 1976.[18] He also pioneered the "heptagon operation"[19] for correcting severe bilateral cleft lips.

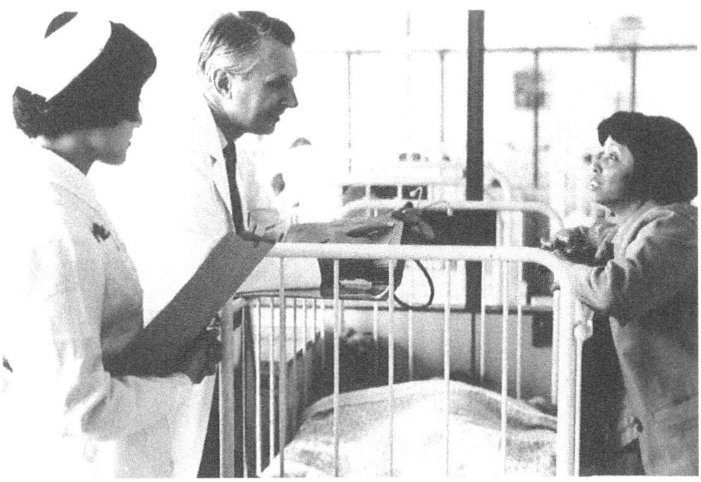

Figure 13.3 Dr. Edward Paterson, conducting ward rounds at United Christian Hospital, talking to the mother of a child

Image courtesy of Alice Ho Miu Ling Nethersole Charity Foundation

Paterson was elected President of the Hong Kong Branch of the International College of Surgeons in 1963, and President of the Hong Kong Surgical Society in 1966, reflecting his high standing as a surgeon.[20] In 1963, Ashton retired and Paterson succeeded him as Medical Superintendent of Nethersole Hospital. Besides his role as Senior Surgeon of Nethersole Hospital, Paterson oversaw the building of new staff quarters and an East Wing for the Hospital.

In the 1950s, the rapid rise in population led to a great demand for medical services. Because of this, the Hong Kong Director of Church World Service called a meeting of overseas missionaries, including Paterson and local Christian representatives, to discuss the idea of a new hospital to meet the increasing demand. However, no follow-up action was taken.[21] In 1963, the Hong Kong Christian Council decided to build a new hospital in Kowloon, and in the following year, Nethersole Hospital agreed to participate in the project by helping train staff.[22] During the following year, the 1964 White Paper on the Development of Medical Services was published. In it, the government estimated that 3,500 acute general beds were needed by 1972 to meet the ratio of 2.5 acute beds per 1,000 population. More beds were planned for Kowloon, to redress the imbalance between Hong Kong Island and the rest of Hong Kong.[23] After some negotiation with the government, the Hong Kong Christian Council decided that the new hospital would be built in Kwun Tong, Kowloon.[24] A governing body for the new hospital, United Christian Medical Service, was formed in 1970, to oversee the project.

This new hospital was to be Paterson's dream hospital. In 1968, Kwun Tong had a population of around 380,000 and about 1,200 factories in a densely packed area. There was only one government clinic, and the closest public hospital, though only five miles away, could take an hour to reach because of heavy traffic.[25] Given the rapidly growing population, the new hospital would unlikely meet the demand even if it had 540 beds—the highest number of beds permitted according to the size of the lot assigned to the new hospital. Paterson reckoned that he would need to build a "hospital without walls": the medical and health services would have to be delivered to the community to improve the health of the people, so as to reduce the demand for hospital services. He planned two projects—community nursing and community health—to integrate them with hospital services.[26]

Community nursing was not totally new in Hong Kong. Yang Social Service Center had home nursing since 1967, and Our Lady of Maryknoll

Hospital nurses had started home nursing in 1970.[27] Many people, including the government, did not believe home nursing was feasible due to the cramped living conditions.[28] Paterson invited an experienced nurse, Ms. Joan Gray, from London, to lead a postgraduate course in community nursing in 1972 at Nethersole Hospital. This was followed by a trial community nursing program in Sau Mau Ping Health Center, when it began providing service in October 1972. The demand for community nursing service increased with the opening of United Christian Hospital (UCH) in 1973. Besides nursing care, the community nurse performed roles such as exercise therapist, health advisor, and case finder. Paterson won a small victory when the government finally agreed to subsidize the community nursing service of the community health project of UCH in 1977. The effectiveness of community nursing was further acknowledged when the government started its own community nursing program in 1979.[29] Today, the community nursing program is an important component of nursing service in Hong Kong.

A community health project, which is based on a hospital in an urban setting, was a new concept in Hong Kong. The basic philosophy of the project was that residents in a district, such as Kwun Tong, should assume responsibility for their own health and that of their neighbors.[30] In Kwun Tong, one of the first steps toward a "hospital without walls" was the establishment of community health centers where community nursing teams were based in Kwun Tong itself. They served the residents at different levels. At the first level was the routine clinic service concerning diagnosis and treatment of illnesses. At the second level was the prevention of disease and health education. A number of different health maintenance programs for prevention were rolled out in stages, targeting different groups: 1) An infant health maintenance program was started in 1976 enrolling mostly babies born in UCH. It provided a more comprehensive service than that offered by the government Maternal and Child Health Center, and the program was very popular. 2) A schoolchild health maintenance program was introduced riding on the government School Medical Service. Schools, rather than individual students, were enrolled, and health education was provided to the participating schools. School children received medical treatment and health checks. 3) An occupational health maintenance program targeting factory workers in the district began in 1977. This included clinic service, assessment of workers before employment and fitness to return to work after injury. First aid and accident management education were offered to the participating factories. 4) An adult program began in 1979, providing annual screening and health advice for common problems such as hypertension and diabetes. 5) A geriatric health maintenance program was initiated the same year, which offered health examinations, advice on physical fitness, and a social club. Health education to the community was led by the Health Education Unit, which produced educational materials in the form of posters, leaflets, displays, and books. Exhibitions and seminars were organized, often in collaboration with local government and welfare bodies. A monthly newspaper, the Voice of Community Health, was distributed free in the centers.

To promote a higher level of health consciousness, social workers with community development skills were employed to engage local residents to take responsibility for the health of the community. Program such as people's health committees were set up based at the health centers to discuss local health issues. A Good Neighbor's program to encourage members to look after their neighbors was also attempted. Activities such as health weeks and senior citizens weeks were organized from time to time.[31] Volunteer recruitment and training were important aspects of community engagement. The community health project, though extensive and involving many people, was not supported by the government.

It is difficult to assess the overall effect of the Kwun Tong Community Health Project on the health of the residents in the district, as no study is available. Community nursing service had been shown to be cost-effective in relieving pressure in hospital beds,[32] but the effects of the health maintenance programs are less clear. Paterson disagreed[33] with the emphasis to expand the hospital beds as proposed in the 1974 White Paper on the Further Development of Medical and Health Services.[34] Paterson's idea of community health was in line with the ethos of the Declaration of Alma-Ata of 1978, which advocated "maximum community and individual self-reliance and participation in the planning, organization, operation and control of primary health care..."[35] The 1990 report of the government's Primary Health Care Working Party recommended a district health system approach to reorganize primary healthcare. Each primary healthcare district would provide services including medical care, family health, student health, community nursing, health promotion, and education. The organization is quite similar to that of the Kwun Tong Community Health Project, except there was less emphasis on integration with the district hospital.[36] Paterson was indeed a visionary in the concept of community health service to maintain health in order to reduce hospitalization. A new combined United Christian Nethersole Community Health Service was launched in 1997, when the "old" Nethersole Hospital was relocated to Tai Po.[37] The spirit of the Kwun Tong Community Health Project lives on.

Paterson was also an innovator. UCH scored many firsts in Hong Kong when it opened in 1973. It had the first Accident & Emergency Department with observation beds when other public hospitals were still using the archaic term "Casualty" Department. It also had the first psychiatric unit within an acute general hospital, a setup that led to less stigma for psychiatric patients. It opened a geriatric unit before any government hospitals did. Paterson proposed the training of nurse physician assistants in 1975, and eight nurses were trained in 1978—an idea more than two decades ahead of the Advanced Practice Nurse Program introduced by the Hospital Authority in 2000. The hospital also operated a volunteer's department and ran a nursery for children of its staff.[38] In 1985, Paterson stepped down as Medical Superintendent of UCH in order to focus on planning the extension of the hospital.

Paterson served as a member of the Medical Development Advisory Committee of the government for six years.[39] He was the "white knight" who delivered UCH as an interim teaching hospital to CUHK in 1983, when Prince of Wales Hospital was not yet ready to take clinical students.[40] In recognition of his contributions to Hong Kong, he was appointed Justice of the Peace in 1978 and OBE in 1979. In 1985, he was awarded an honorary degree of Doctor of Social Sciences by HKU. He retired in 1989 and was engaged by the WHO as a consultant on the subject of hospital in community.[41] In his retirement, he wrote a book on the history of UCH—Dreams and a Hospital—a sequel to his previous work, A Hospital for Hong Kong, on the centenary history of Alice Ho Miu Ling Nethersole Hospital. He died on 12 January 2013 and is survived by two of his three sons.[42]

Professor Francis Moore, at the conferment ceremony of honorary DSSc, described him as "a man of rectitude but humility, imagination but patience, humane physician ..." As a medical missionary, perhaps he would be better remembered by the motto of the hospital he established:

> "With Christian love we care,
> With excellence we serve."

Sister Mary Aquinas Monaghan
亞規納 / 區貴雅 (1919–1985)

Hon. DSSc (HKU), OBE, FRCP

Sister Mary Aquinas was born Kathleen Gertrude Monaghan on 30 August 1919 to a devout Catholic farming family in County Galway, Ireland. She was the second child of a family of nine. Soon after graduating from high school, she joined the Missionary Sisters of St. Columban at Caheracon, County Clare in 1939, taking the name Sister Mary Aquinas. World War II prevented her from joining the mission in China. Instead, she was sent to study medicine at University College Dublin. She had the rare honor, together with Sister Gabriel O'Mahony, to be among the first four nuns in Ireland graduating as physicians in 1947, after the ban for nuns to practice medicine was lifted by the Vatican in 1936. She did her residency training in Our Lady of Lourdes Tuberculosis Sanatorium, Dublin, and Coombe Maternity Hospital, Dublin. Because China no longer welcomed foreign missionaries, she was assigned to Hong Kong.[43]

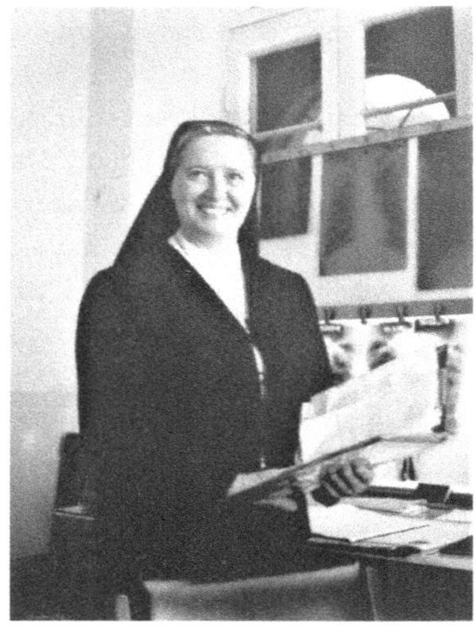

Figure 13.4 Sister Mary Aquinas
Source: Hong Kong Tuberculosis, Chest and Heart Diseases Association

Sister Aquinas arrived in Hong Kong on 17 January 1949 with a few nurses from Ireland, about one month prior to the opening of Ruttonjee Sanatorium. TB was prevalent before the war in Hong Kong, only to worsen after the war because of poverty and overcrowding. In 1948, TB accounted for 14.6% of all deaths. In 1952, Hong Kong had the highest notification rate of TB in its history, standing at 700/100,000.[44] Indeed, the South China Morning Post called TB "Public Enemy No. 1" in its report on the opening of Ruttonjee Sanatorium.[45] In the same report, it was noted that the idea of a sanatorium was proposed by Dr. Selwyn-Clarke before the war, and it took a generous donation from Mr. Ruttonjee to bring it to fruition.

Sister Aquinas became Medical Superintendent of the Sanatorium, leading her team to treat TB patients who required inpatient care. The government established Hong Kong Government Tuberculosis Service and organized a coordinated anti-tuberculosis treatment program in 1947, which provided extensive outpatient drug treatment for most of the patients with tuberculosis. The more serious cases were referred to hospitals such as Ruttonjee Sanatorium, Haven of Hope Sanatorium (built by Junk Bay Medical Relief Society), and Tung Wah Hospitals. Sister Aquinas soon discovered that the number of beds in the sanatorium was far fewer than the demand, because most of the time she had more than 800 patients on her waiting list for admission.[46] A new Jockey Club Wing was added in 1953, increasing the number of beds from 120 to 220.[47] Three years later, again with another donation from Mr. Ruttonjee, Freni Memorial Convalescent Home with 106 beds was built across the road from the sanatorium, further easing the bed shortage.[48]

The Government Tuberculosis Service carried out a case-finding program using contact tracing and annual chest X-ray examination of civil servants and teachers. Mobile miniature chest X-ray surveys were carried out for case finding in the 1950s and 1960s.[49] In addition, a BCG vaccination program for prevention of TB began in 1952. Three teams, each consisting of three vaccinators and one clerk, were provided by the Medical Department and trained by the WHO personnel to perform tuberculin testing and vaccination. The Hong Kong Anti-Tuberculosis Association, an NGO, recruited a fourth team at Ruttonjee Sanatorium to perform vaccinations for the general public.

In addition to inpatient service, the Hong Kong Anti-Tuberculosis Association ran its own follow-up clinic, public education program, and a tuberculosis insurance scheme for private companies. Tuberculosis rehabilitation service was provided by World Service of The Lutheran World Federation.

Sister Aquinas received a WHO scholarship to study TB at the University of Wales at Cardiff in 1952 and obtained a Tuberculosis Disease Diploma the following year. In 1955, she was elected Fellow of the American College of Chest Physicians. She went on postgraduate study again in London in 1958.[50] Her special research areas covered drug resistance, re-treatment, and adverse reactions to anti-tuberculosis drugs.[51] Her expertise in TB treatment was recognized in the 1960s, when she was invited to collaborate in clinical trials with the British Medical Research Council and the Hong Kong Government

Tuberculosis Service.[52] Though these studies were performed in Hong Kong, the findings were widely applicable to other parts of the world; for example, the studies on directly observed therapy (DOT) and short-course multiple antituberculosis drug treatment. The current standard treatment of TB of six months using four anti-TB drugs, preferably by DOT, stemmed from the results of these MRC trials.[53]

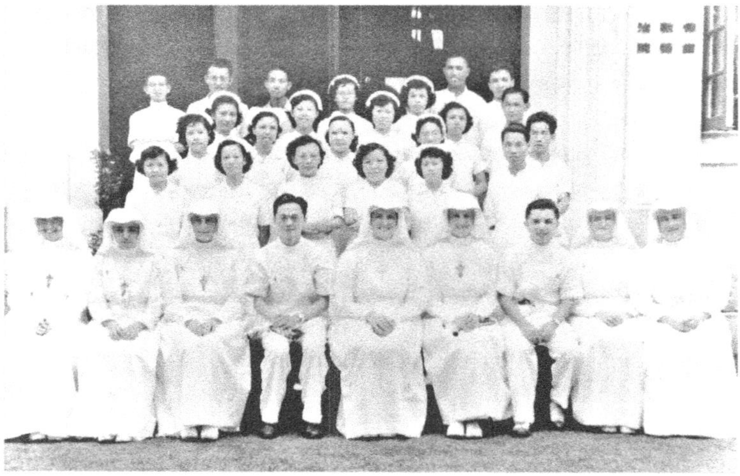

Figure 13.5 Sister Mary Aquinas (seated, center), Sister Mary Gabriel (next to Sister Aquinas) and staff of Ruttonjee Sanatorium, 1952
Source: Hong Kong Tuberculosis, Chest and Heart Diseases Association

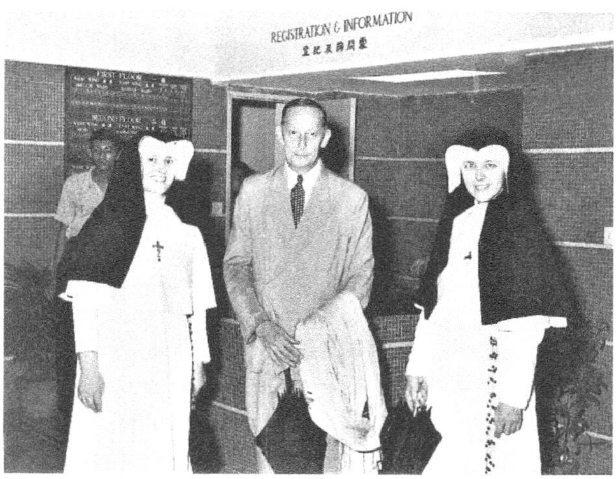

Figure 13.6 Sister Mary Aquinas (standing L) and Mr. Donovan Benson, Vice-Chairman of Anti-TB Association (1949–1962)
Source: HKMMS, reproduced with permission

Sister Aquinas had the honor to be the first woman to receive the Sir Robert Philip[54] Gold Medal in 1964. A citation appearing in Health, a publication of the British Chest and Heart Association, in June 1965 said: "A Chest Conference would hardly be the same without her. This medal is given every few years to an outstanding figure in the Commonwealth tuberculous campaign ... Her compassion, her skill, her patience and her dedication were beyond praise and left all of us who have known her, richer for her example and help."[55] Sister Aquinas's vast experience in TB control made her a much sought-after speaker, and she was happy to travel and share her expertise especially with developing countries in Asia and Africa. She received more honors in the 1970s: MRCP (Edinburgh, honorary, 1973) and FRCP (Edinburgh, honorary, 1977).[56] Being a religious woman, humility and dedication to the poor remained at her core despite increasing professional eminence. The Columban Sisters opened St Joseph's Caritas Clinic in 1966, to serve the rural community in Ta Kwu Ling, and Sister Aquinas attended the clinic every Saturday.[57]

By the end of the 1960s, mortality due to TB had dropped significantly, from 83.8/100,000 in 1958 to 37.8/100,000 in 1968. The decline in infant deaths from TB from 162 to three per year during the same decade was even more remarkable. There was no longer a lack of TB specialists and no lack of hospital beds, as patients could be admitted readily if needed.[58] As TB gradually came under control, Sister Aquinas turned her attention to the care of drug addicts, who were known to have a higher prevalence of TB.[59] No doubt many became patients under her care in the sanatorium. After the war, heroin had replaced opium as the dominant form of addiction in Hong Kong. It was estimated that the total number of drug addicts could be as high as 150,000 to 180,000 in the late 1950s.[60] As an active member of Society for the Aid and Rehabilitation of Drug Abusers (SARDA), which was formed in 1961, she had a lifelong interest in the welfare of drug addicts. She was a member of the Action Committee Against Narcotics, which was formed in 1965 to advise the government on policies and strategies about the control of drug abuse. She was Chair of SARDA from 1981 until her death. In her last hours, Sister Mary Greaney asked if she had any last words. She replied: "Keep an eye on SARDA."[61] SARDA named a center after her: Sister Aquinas Memorial Women's Treatment Center.

Sister Aquinas was also very active in the local medical community, contributing her expertise to many organizations. She had been President of the Hong Kong Branch of the British Medical Association and Vice-President of HKMA. She represented the British Medical Association on the Hong Kong Medical Council and Pharmacy and Poisons Board. She was also a member of the Hong Kong Medical Development Advisory Committee, which advised the government on healthcare policies. As a chest physician and a member of the Hong Kong and Macau Chapter of the American College of Chest Physicians (ACCP) before the formation of the Hong Kong Thoracic Society in 1986, Sister Aquinas played a leading role in the establishment of respiratory medicine as a specialty.[62] Sister Aquinas was a staunch supporter of the formation of the Hong Kong College of General Practitioners and was honorary secretary of the interim council, which was formed in 1975.[63] Dr. Zoltan Lett remembered that Sister Aquinas supported and attended the meetings of the Society of Anesthetists of Hong Kong in the 1950s. He recalled: "Her always cheerful, friendly, and unassuming nature … and even enthusiasm when matters such as ether or spinal anesthesia for tuberculous patients were discussed."[64] She was Chairman of the Society of Community Medicine in 1976. Her most enduring influence on the local medical community was her teaching of medical students on TB during her long association with the Medical Faculty, HKU, as an honorary teacher since 1952.

As a Catholic nun, it was natural that she was an executive member of the Catholic Marriage Advisory Council of Hong Kong and Chair of the medical subcommittee. She was active in the guilds of Catholic doctors and nurses and participated in other local communities such as being President (1979–1981) of Soroptimist International of Hong Kong, which had a mission to educate, empower, and enable women and girls. She was also Vice-chair of the Community Advice Bureau in 1983.[65] For her contributions to the control of TB and other community work in Hong Kong, she was awarded Doctor of Social Science, honoris causa, by HKU in 1978,[66] OBE in 1985, and was presented to Her Majesty Queen Elizabeth II at Buckingham Palace.[67]

Sister Aquinas died on 25 November 1985 in Ruttonjee Sanatorium after a brief illness. An obituary in the *British Medical Journal* noted that her life was characterized by selfless service to others and by extraordinary joy, graciousness, and good humor.[68] A Sister Mary Aquinas Museum was opened in 1991 on the first floor of the new Ruttonjee Hospital. It was relocated to the LG3 lobby of the Hospital in 2008 and renamed Ruttonjee Hospital Time Gallery. The Hong Kong Tuberculosis, Chest and Heart Diseases Association (previously Hong Kong Anti-Tuberculosis Association) also set up a scholarship (Sister Mary Aquinas and Purviz & Rusy Shroff Scholarship) in her memory, to be awarded to medical students with good performance at the TB Module of the Integrated Block.[69]

Sister Mary Gabriel O'Mahony
紀寶儀 (1921–2006)
MBE, FRCP

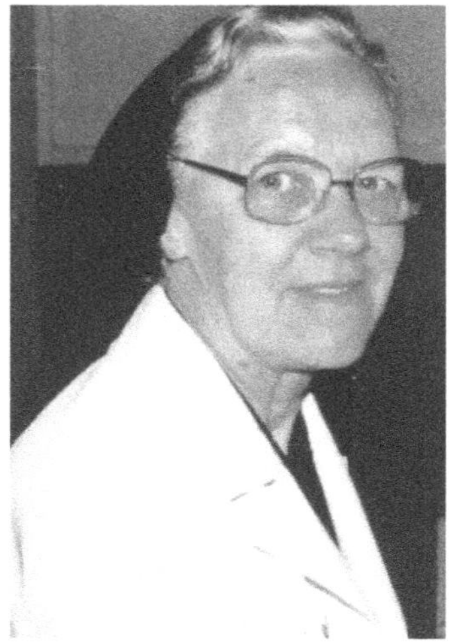

Figure 13.7 Sister Mary Gabriel

Source: Hong Kong Tuberculosis, Chest and Heart Diseases Association

Sister Mary Gabriel O'Mahony was born on 21 May 1921 in the County of Cork, Ireland. She was the third child of a Catholic family of eight. The O'Mahony family lived in the parish of Bishop Gavin, the cofounder of the Columban Fathers, who happened to be a classmate of Sister Gabriel's father. This might explain why four daughters in the family became nuns. Gabriel joined the Columban Sisters at the young age of 17, in 1938. She was sent to study medicine at University College Dublin together with Sister Aquinas. After graduation in 1947, she went for postgraduate studies of chest diseases in Boston, USA, and in London, England. She arrived in Hong Kong in 1950 and worked at Ruttonjee Sanatorium until 1988—all her professional life.[70]

In 1957, Sister Gabriel spent a year in the UK for further studies and obtained her MRCP.[71] Sister Gabriel was keen on research and widely published her findings. She was a collaborator of the MRC Working Party on Tuberculosis of the Spine and contributed to knowledge on children with TB spine.[72] When the Columban Sisters were invited to take over the operation of Sandy Bay Convalescent Home for disabled children in 1960, Sister Gabriel and Sister Aquinas were visiting consultant physicians.[73] Another area of special interest for Sister Gabriel was childhood tuberculosis, especially tuberculous meningitis. Before the widespread use of BCG, tuberculosis was prevalent in children and a major cause of mortality. Sister Gabriel had set aside a special hospital ward for TB meningitis patients and invited neurosurgeons to assist when necessary. She collaborated with a neurologist from CUHK, Dr. Robert Teoh, to study the various aspects of diagnosis and treatment of this dreaded condition. She also performed and published her research findings in relation to asthma and allergy.[74] Her dedication to her work was much appreciated by her colleagues, who noted: "It cost her many sleepless nights and harried days as she watched over children with TB meningitis, or tried a new drug regime on someone whose lungs were riddled with the bacillus."[75]

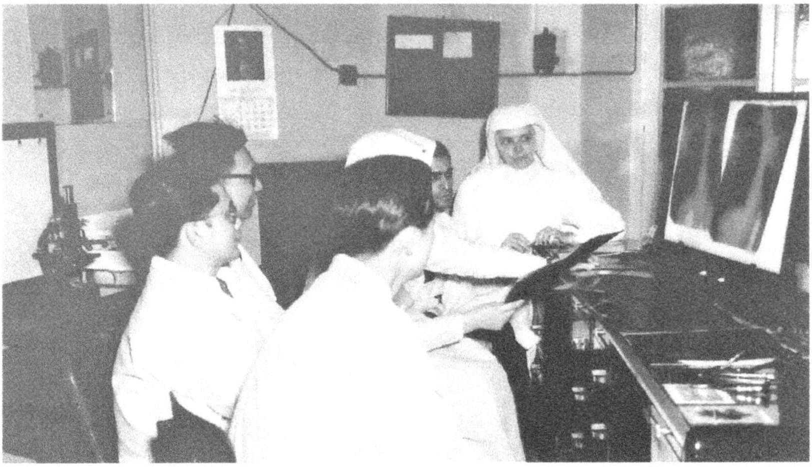

Figure 13.8 Sister Mary Gabriel with her students in Ruttonjee Sanatorium
Source: Hong Kong Tuberculosis, Chest and Heart Diseases Association

Like Sister Aquinas, she was often invited to attend conferences to share her expertise. In 1966, she was invited to deliver a lecture on TB in Hong Kong at Cambridge University. She attended MRC research meetings on TB of the bone and joints at Brompton Hospital, London.[76] Administrative duties finally fell on her shoulders when Sister Aquinas passed away in 1985. Since TB patients were declining in the 1970s, the Sanatorium Board decided in 1979 to transform the sanatorium into a general hospital.[77] With the change in the role of Ruttonjee Sanatorium, the future of the Columban Sisters was at a turning point. Sister Gabriel searched for a new ministry where the services of the sisters would be most needed and she found her answer in hospice care for cancer patients. As a clinician, she often observed that most cancer patients died in overcrowded public hospitals, screened off in a corner of a ward with no room for relatives to visit or stay. Doctors and nurses caring for these patients were often as distressed as the relatives were, because of their inability to cope with dying patients.[78] Although there was already a palliative care team at Our Lady of Maryknoll Hospital in 1982, hospice service had not taken root in Hong Kong.[79] In June 1985, Dr. Vincent Tse, oncologist of Queen Elizabeth Hospital, called for a meeting of people who were interested in hospice care. As a result, the Society for the Promotion of Hospice Care was formed later that year, Sister Gabriel as chairman with its headquarters in a small office at Ruttonjee Sanatorium. The founding members included Dr. Vincent Tse, Sister Mary Greaney, Lucy Chung (a nurse with hospice training from Maryknoll Hospital), and others.[80] A palliative care team was started in Ruttonjee in 1986 with two nurses (Sister Greaney and Sister Ryan), a physiotherapist, a social worker, two counsellors, and a doctor.[81] When Ruttonjee Sanatorium was finally turned into a general hospital in 1988, the Columban Sisters decided to withdraw and left the sanatorium. For Sister Gabriel and Sister Greaney, this would mean more time and effort available for the promotion of hospice care in Hong Kong. The Hospice Home Care Program was started at the end of 1988, with Sister Greaney as nurse and Sister Gabriel as part-time doctor. Sister Gabriel spared no effort to advocate for hospice care and find resources for a hospice facility.[82] As a result of her tireless efforts, Bradbury Hospice was opened in Shatin in 1992, a landmark achievement for the society.

Less well known, perhaps, were her contributions to pediatrics. Pediatrics used to be a unit in the Department of Medicine at HKU. In 1964, it became a separate department, two years after Professor Elaine Field was appointed the first Professor of Pediatrics. The earliest special service for children was probably the isolation and rehabilitation facilities for children with pulmonary TB and tuberculous meningitis at Ruttonjee Sanatorium. Dr. Yeung Chap-yung, retired Professor of Paediatrics at HKU, said, "Hong Kong had been lucky to have two highly devoted ladies, the late Sister Aquinas and Sister Gabriel who had demonstrated tremendous love and devotion to look after children with various tuberculosis diseases."[83] Last, but not least, was the influence on generations of medical students taught by her. Her teaching was invariably focused on patients, often humorous, and always inspiring. The tea and biscuits and informal discussion after the formal teaching were especially appreciated by students.[84]

Sister Gabriel no doubt made a very significant contribution in the control of TB in Hong Kong. She was also a pioneer in the introduction of hospice care and an important figure in the development of respiratory medicine in Hong Kong. She was a Fellow of the American College of Chest Physicians as early as 1956 and a founding council member of Hong Kong Thoracic Society when it was first established in 1986, as well as the first Honorary Fellow of the Hong Kong Academy of Medicine in 1996. In recognition of her significant contributions to respiratory medicine, she was conferred the first Life Honorary Membership of Hong Kong Thoracic Society in 1990.[85] She was also awarded MBE in 1990 for her care of the sick.

In 1997, her health failed after a heart attack, and she decided to return to Ireland. On her last evening in Hong Kong, which happened to be very cold, she did not forget to deliver food to street sleepers in Yau Ma Tei, showing her deep devotion to the less fortunate.[86] In retirement in Ireland, she relished the time she had for scripture and prayer and wrote a book on the story of the Columban Sisters in Hong Kong.[87] She passed away on 26 August 2006.

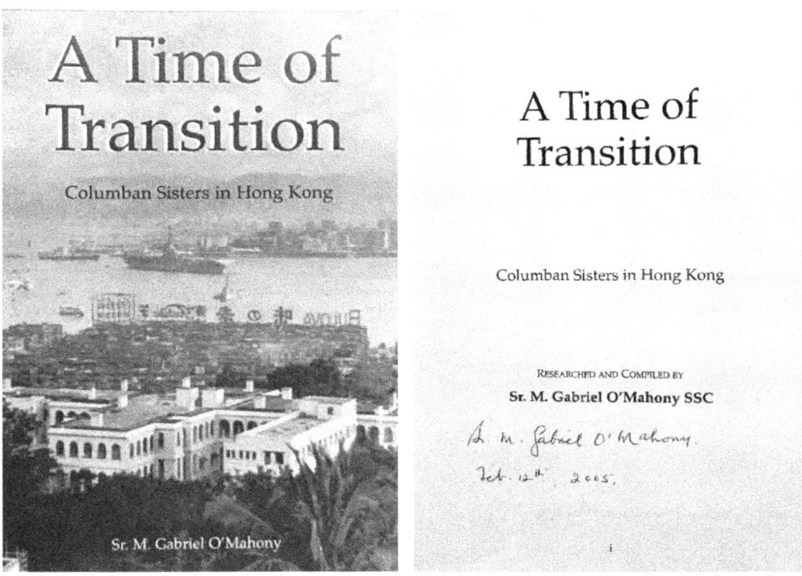

Figure 13.9a and b *A Time of Transition* by Sister M. Gabriel of the story of the Columban Sisters in Hong Kong

Source: Wong Tai-wai

The Congregation of the Missionary Sisters of St. Columban left Hong Kong in December 2015, ending their 67 years of service in Hong Kong. In 1949, when they began their work at Ruttonjee Sanatorium, Bishop Valtorta had this to say about them: "They were there by a special dispensation of Divine Providence. In their work they might not be able to instruct 'pagan' in the ordinary way, but they must bring people to Our Lord by showing them the 'Gospel in Action' by their gentleness, kindness and sympathy and by seeing Christ in them ..."[88] By providing dedicated, holistic care to their patients, the sisters had, indeed, delivered the "Gospel in Action."

Conclusion

This book is a collection of stories of the lives of many remarkable pioneers and leaders in the field of medicine who had shaped the medical and health services of Hong Kong today. The work of these exceptional individuals from diverse backgrounds over a period of 170 years formed the backbone of the medical development of Hong Kong.

Although Western medicine was introduced by the medical missionaries from the London Missionary Society as early as 1842 after Hong Kong was ceded to the British, it did not take root until they founded the Alice Memorial Hospital and the Hong Kong College of Medicine for Chinese in 1887. These two institutions together provided medical care and enabled Chinese young men to propagate Western medicine in Hong Kong. Other Catholic and Protestant missions also established hospitals and clinics and their presence contributed greatly to the medical services in Hong Kong especially in the early decades after World War II. The last medical missionary doctor from the LMS, Dr. E. Paterson, a visionary, built in 1973 the United Christian Hospital, which is "without walls" and has a number of community health programs to bring healthcare to the community. Their contributions were irreplaceable.

The early government medical officers played a vital role in the prevention of infectious diseases epidemics. Some of these medical officers were visionaries. For example, Dr. P. B. C. Ayres, the Colonial Surgeon (1873–1897), had the foresight to warn the government repeatedly over the years that the deplorable unhygienic condition of the Chinese quarters would lead to an epidemic of "unenviable renown" but all his words fell on deaf ears, resulting in the plague hitting Hong Kong in 1894 as he had anticipated. His successors had to work hard to improve the sanitation in Hong Kong and to build up the public medical and health system. Just before World War II, the public medical and health infrastructure was well-established, backed by public health laws to safeguard the health of Hong Kong's citizens. The progressive reduction in prevalent infectious diseases in the 1960s was the result of the incessant efforts of the officers of the Government Medical and Health Department. The shift of resources from preventive care to curative medicine after the 1970s allowed the government specialists to fulfil their vision of bringing up-to-date advances in technology to various special branches of medicine in Hong Kong.

Hong Kong has been blessed with many far-sighted and dedicated medical educators. When Dr. Patrick Manson advocated for the establishment of the Hong Kong College of Medicine in 1887, he envisaged introducing Western medicine not just to Hong Kong but also to China. When the Faculty of Medicine, the University of Hong Kong, was founded, the first few professors including Professors John Anderson and Herbert G. Earle had the same vision of spreading Western medicine to China in mind because they believed that Chinese medicine had no scientific basis. They, together with the Rockefeller Foundation professors, built a solid foundation for the Faculty of Medicine in the university. After World War II, despite limited resources, the university medical educators dedicated their efforts to rehabilitate the university and to train both undergraduates and specialists to satisfy the demands of a rapidly expanding population despite the lack of resources. In the end they not only fulfilled their role in education but also their mission in research which placed Hong Kong on the world map in each of their areas of interest. Before World War II, expatriate doctors dominated the medical scene as expected. At present, the vast majority of the doctors in both the public and the private sector, the academic staff, and the consultants of the public medical and health services are Chinese and graduates of the two universities in Hong Kong.[1] We are all beneficiaries of the early medical educators.

Primary care services in the community were mostly provided by doctors in the private sector. Hong Kong has been fortunate to have a number of public-minded private practitioners who devoted their spare time to charity work to improve the health of the underprivileged. A few even took up public office to effectively improve the medical services of Hong Kong and to ensure provision of social and medical services for the elderly and the disabled. Despite the wide wealth gap in Hong Kong, the impoverished in the city enjoyed the same public medical services as the rest of the society with their fees and medication cost waived by the social welfare service as needed.

While the medical and health development of a region is highly dependent on its economy, a healthy population is, in turn, crucial to its educational and social advancement, leading to its prosperity. By the 1990s, Hong Kong had public medical and health and education systems which helped to produce a healthy and well-educated population, a flourishing civil society, and a thriving economy that its citizens were proud of. By 2011, the men and women in Hong Kong led the world in longevity, and its medical and health system is on par with those in other advanced economies. These achievements would not be possible without these visionary and devoted pioneers and leaders in the medical profession, their professionalism and their selflessness. This group of notable doctors were endowed with different talents: some were brilliant clinicians who loved the contact with patients and helped them to restore health, some were imaginative and innovative researchers and scientists, some were passionate teachers, and others were interested in statistics and healthcare policies. Despite their varied interests and talents, their ultimate goal was not different—to heal and to improve the health of the people in Hong Kong. They were similar to their medical missionary colleagues who followed their motto "heal the bodies and save the souls," bringing the gospel to the people by their love in action.

We hope the spirit of service and dedication of this group of notable doctors would inspire future generations of young men and women in the medical profession to follow their footsteps, irrespective of the motivating factors to excel and the socio-economic environment of their time.

Appendix
Hong Kong Medical and Health Agencies and Principal Officers

Name of Government Medical and Health Agency

Year	Name
1843–1872	Colonial Surgeon's Office
1872–1958	Medical Department
1958–1989	Medical and Health Department
1989–present	Department of Health, and Hospital Authority

Name of Principal Officers of Hong Kong Medical and Health Agencies

Year	Name of Public Medical and Health Services
1843–1897	Colonial Surgeon
1897–1929	Principal Civil Medical Officer
1929–1936	Director of Medical and Sanitary Services
1936–1941, 1946–1950	Director of Medical Services
1950–1989	Director of Medical and Health Services
1989-present	Director of Health, and Chief Executive of Hospital Authority

Notes

Preface

1. Moira Chan-Yeung, *A Medical History of Hong Kong: 1842–1941* (The Chinese University of Hong Kong Press, 2018); *A Medical History of Hong Kong: 1942–2015* (The Chinese University of Hong Kong Press, 2019); *A Medical History of Hong Kong: The Development and Contributions of Outpatient Services* (The Chinese University of Hong Kong Press, 2021).
2. Hong Kong Museum of Medical Sciences Society, *Plague, SARS and the Story of Medicine in Hong Kong* (Hong Kong University Press, 2006).
3. "Why Hong Kong Has the Longest Life Expectancy in the World," CUHK eNews, January 2021, https://www.oal.cuhk.edu.hk/cuhkenews_202101_life_expectancy/; Hong Kong Has the Highest Life Expectancy in the World—What Is the Secret Behind It?" SCMP, 26 October 2019, https://www.scmp.com/magazines/post-magazine/long-reads/article/3034349/hong-kong-has-highest-life-expectancy-world-what?campaign=3034349&module=perpetual_scroll_0&pgtype=article.

Chapter 1

1. Robin Boyd, *The Witness of the Student Christian Movement* (London: Society of Promoting Christian Knowledge, 2007), 1.
2. G. H. Choa, *"Heal the Sick" Was Their Motto. The Protestant Medical Missionaries in China* (Hong Kong: The Chinese University of Hong Kong Press, 1990), 24–25.
3. William Lockhart, *The Medical Missionary in China: A Narrative of Twenty Years' Experience* (London: Hurst and Blackett, 1861).
4. "Obituary, Benjamin Hobson, MB, MRCP," *Brit Med J*, (29 March 1873): 355.
5. Choa, *"Heal the Sick" Was their Motto*, 26.
6. Ibid., 38–39.
7. Ibid., 50.
8. Marilyn Laura Bowman, *James Legge and the Confucian Classics: Brilliant Scot in the Turmoil of Colonial Hong Kong* (Vancouver: Simon Fraser University, 2015), 280.
9. Choa, *"Heal the Sick" Was their Motto*, 67–68.
10. Hobson, Benjamin, "Report of the Medical Missionary Society's Hospital at Hongkong," *Chinese Repository* 14 (1844): 380–381.

11. The Medical Missionary Society was first formed in 1838 in Guangzhou to support Dr. Peter Parker and the Eye Hospital. In 1845, some of the members of the Medical Missionary Society left for Hong Kong and established a branch in Hong Kong.
12. C. T. Smith, *A Sense of History: Studies in the Social and Urban History of Hong Kong* (Hong Kong: Hong Kong Educational Publishing Co., 1995), 299–302.
13. Chuang-Ye Hong, and Fu-Mei Wang. "Chinese Translation of English Textbooks on Internal Medicine from the 1850s to the 1940s," ScienceDirect, *Journal of the Chinese Medical Association* 77 (2014): 277–282.
14. S. M. Hillier, and J. A. Jewell, *Health Care and Traditional Medicine in China* (London: Routledge and Kegan Paul, 1983), 11.
15. T. M. K. Wong, "Local Voluntarism: The Medical Mission of the London Missionary Society in Hong Kong 1842–1923," in *Healing Bodies Saving Souls: Medical Mission in Asia and Africa*, ed. D. Hardiman (Amsterdam-New York, Rodopi, 2006), 91
16. Ibid., 92.

Chapter 2

1. Pottinger to Stanley, 17 July 1843, CO 129/2, 96–99.
2. Moira Chan-Yeung, *A Medical History of Hong Kong, 1842–1941* (Hong Kong: The Chinese University of Hong Kong Press, 2018), 18–22.
3. Treasury Chambers on Hong Kong Government Civil Hospital, 9 January 1849, CO 129/31, 69–74.
4. Hong Kong Blue Book, 1845
5. "Obituary, John Murray," *Brit Med J*, 8 August 1903, 339.
6. Lister to Colonial Secretary, 22 April 1869, Report on Tung Wa Hospital, 1896, VI–VII; MacDonnell to Granville, 9 April 1870, CO 129/138/726, 146.
7. *China Mail*, 14 February 1872.
8. UK Parliament, "1842 Report on the Sanitary Condition of the Laboring Population of Great Britain," 1842, accessed on 6 February 2023, https://www.parliament.uk/about/living-heritage/transformingsociety/livinglearning/coll-9-health1/health-02/#:~:text=1842%20Sanitary%20Report,Chadwick%20(1800%2D1890).
9. "Obituary, Philip Burnard Chenery Ayres. CMG, MRCS Eng. LRCP Edin, Late Colonial Surgeon and Inspector of Hospitals, Hong Kong," The Thames Database, taken from an obituary notice of 28 October 1899, printed in *the Lancet*, accessed on 6 February 2023, http://www.thamehistory.net/people/Ayres.htm.
10. Colonial Surgeon Annual Report for 1874 (Original) in Hong Kong Administrative Report (HKAR), 1879, 25–41.
11. Colonial Surgeon Report 1874, Tung Wa Hospital, Hong Kong Blue Book, 1874.
12. O. Chadwick, Report on the Sanitary Condition of Hong Kong, CO 882/4, Hong Kong Government, 1882, 1–59.
13. Chan-Yeung, *A Medical History of Hong Kong, 1842–1941*, 125–127.

14. Colonial Surgeon Annual Report for the year 1893, Hong Kong Sessional Papers (HKSP) 1894, 364.
15. Colonial Surgeon Annual Reports 1894–1929, HKSP, 1895 to 1930.
16. Medical Committee Report, HKSP 1895, 549 (i) and (ii).
17. Contagious Disease Ordinance 1867, Historical Laws of Hong Kong Online, accessed on 6 February 2023, https://oelawhk.lib.hku.hk/items/show/237.
18. Colonial Surgeon Annual Report 1878, The Lock Hospital, HKSP, 1879.
19. "Obituary, Philip B. C. Ayres, CMG, MRCS," *Br Med J*, 2 (1899): 1140.
20. Colonial Surgeon Annual Report for 1890, Government Civil Hospital, HKSP, 1891, No 27/91, 328.
21. H. W. Wylie, "Colonial Surgeon Extraordinary—The Era of Dr. P. B. C. Ayres, CMG," *The Bulletin-Journal of the Society of Medical Officer of Health Hong Kong,* 1 (1969): 9–19.
22. Minutes on Reorganization of the Medical Department and Sanitary Board, Colonial Office, 18 May 1895, CO 129/267/163, 407–416.
23. Robinson to Knutsford, Registration of Births and Deaths, 23 September 1892, Enclosed in Colonial Surgeon to Colonial Secretary, Public Dispensaries, 16 August 1892, CO 129/256/280, 212–215.
24. Colonial Surgeon Annual Reports for 1882 in Hong Kong Blue Book 1882 and 1887 to 1893 in HKSP 1888 to 1894.
25. H. W. Wylie, "Colonial Surgeon Extraordinary," 9–19.
26. Ibid.
27. "Obituary, Philip Burnard Chenery Ayres, CMG, MRCS Eng. LRCP Edin., Late Colonial Surgeon and Inspector of Hospitals, Hong Kong," The Thames Database, taken from an obituary notice of 28 October 1899, printed in *the Lancet*.
28. "Obituary, John Mitford Atkinson, M.B. (Lond.)," *Brit Med J*, 16 June 1917, 827.
29. "Atkinson, John Mitford (1887–1912)," *Biographic Dictionary of Medical Practitioners in Hong Kong: 1841–1941*, accessed on 6 February 2023, https://hkmd1841-1941.blogspot.com/2013/07/dr-john-mitford-atkinson-1887-1912.html.
30. "History of the Development of the ICD," accessed 6 February 2023, https://cdn.who.int/media/docs/default-source/classification/icd/historyoficd.pdf?sfvrsn=b9e617af_3.
31. J. M. Atkinson, "The Malarial Fevers of Hong Kong," *The Lancet*, 28 April 1894, 1054–1060.
32. "Imperial Gift. Medicos Handsomely Rewarded," *South China Morning Post*, 27 February 1905.
33. "Obituary. John Mitford Atkinson, M.B. (Lond.)," *Brit Med J*, 16 June 1917, 817.
34. Ibid.
35. "Cattle Disease in Hong Kong. The Recent Outbreak at the Dairy Farm," *South China Morning Post*, 22 April 1907.
36. "The Dairy Farm: Entirely Free from Infection," *South China Morning Post*, 3 July 1907.
37. Robinson to Chamberlain, Reorganization of the Sanitary Board, 5 March 1896. CO 129/271/53, 365–371.

38. C. P. Lucas, Minutes in Colonial Office, Sanitary Commissioners, 12 March 1903, CO 129/320, 439; Blake to Chamberlain, Sanitary Board Constitution, 28 August 1903, CO 129/318/413, 320–334.
39. Nathan to the Earl of Elgin, Irregularities in the Sanitary Department, 26 November 1906, CO 129/336, Confidential, 132.
40. May to Elgin, Commission to investigate the Sanitary Department, 29 May 1907, CO 129/340, 399–417. The Commissioners were: E. A. Hewitt, Fung Wa-chun, Lau Chu-pak, Henry Humphreys, and A. Shelton Hooper.
41. Nathan to Colonial Secretary, 10 April 1906, Enclosed in May to Elgin, 29 May 1907, CO 129/340, 418.
42. Atkinson's Response to the Report of the Sanitary Commission of 1907, Enclosed in May to Elgin, 29 May 1907. CO 129/340, Confidential, 420–432; "Sanitary Commission, Hon. Dr. Atkinson's Defense, Administration of Two Departments too Heavy for Him," *South China Morning Post*, 7 June 1907.
43. A. R. Wellington, Public Health in Hong Kong, The Need to Reorganize the Medical and Sanitary Services and for the Establishment of an Up-to-date System, 2 October 1931, CO 129/531/131, 17–45.
44. "Death of Dr. Atkinson, Former PCMO of Hong Kong," *South China Morning Post*, 2 June 1917.
45. Arnold Wright and H. A. Cartwright, *Twentieth Century Impressions of Hong Kong, Shanghai and Other Treaty Ports*, Volume 1 (London: Lloyds Greater Britain publishing Company, 1908), 265.
46. Report of the Commission to Enquire into the Existence of Insanitary Properties in the Colony, Hong Kong: printed by Noronha and Co, Government Printers, 1898.
47. E. G. Pryor, "A Historical Review of Housing Conditions in Hong Kong," *Journal of Hong Kong Branch of Royal Asiatic Society* 12 (1972): 89–129, accessed on 6 February 2023, https://www.jstor.org/stable/23881566.
48. Colonial Surgeon's Annual Report or Medical Officer of Health Annual report 1874–1938. Number of cases of enteric fever each year, HKSP or HKAR, 1874–1938.
49. Medical Officer of Health, Report to the Sanitary Board for 1896, HKSP 1897, 357.
50. Report of the Medical Officer of Health, Sanitary Report 1895, HKSP, 1896, 349.
51. Report of the Medical Officer of Health for 1900, HKSP, 1901, 401.
52. May to Lytton, 21 July 1904, CO 129/323/291, 241.
53. I. C. Petrie, "The Problem of Infant Mortality in Hong Kong 1886–1937," MA Thesis, The University of British Columbia, August 1996.
54. "Midwives Ordinance 1910, 2 September 1910," Historical Laws of Hong Kong Online, accessed on 6 February 2023, https://oelawhk.lib.hku.hk/items/show/1245.
55. F. Lugard to Lewis Harcourt, 25 July 1911, Nursing Institute, CO 129/378/267, 392–97.
56. Medical and Health Services Annual Report 1939, HKAR 1939, M18.
57. Daniel Ham, "Management of Malaria and Leprosy in Hong Kong and the International Settlement of Shanghai 1880s–1940s," PhD dissertation, Corpus Christi College, University of Cambridge, September 2012, 159–160.

58. "Notes and Comments. Francis Clark," *Caduceus* 7(4) (1928): 290.
59. *The Lancet*, 2 May 1908, 1314. Dr. Francis Clark, Medical Officer of Health in Hong Kong was elected the first general secretary–treasurer of the Far Eastern Association of Tropical Medicine.
60. Chan-Yeung, *A Medical History of Hong Kong, 1842–1941*, 221.
61. Medical and Sanitary Report for Year 1911, HKAR, 1911, L23.
62. D. Arnold, "British India and the 'Beriberi Problem' 1798–1942," *Med History* 54 (2010): 295–314.
63. "Notes and Comments," *Caduceus*, 7, 4 (1928): 290.
64. Frank Ching, *130 Years of Medicine in Hong Kong: From the College of Medicine for Chinese to Li Ka Shing Faculty of Medicine* (Singapore: Springer Nature, 2018), 59.
65. "Men's Insect Enemies: Dr. Clark's Lecture. Plague, Malaria and Typhoid," *South China Morning Post*, 9 May 1922.
66. "Malaria in Hong Kong," *South China Morning Post*, 22 December 1910.
67. Arnold Wright and H. A. Cartwright, Twentieth Century Impressions of Hong Kong, Shanghai and Other Treaty Ports, 265.
68. "Corinthian Yacht Club," *South China Morning Post*, 25 January 1906 and 21 November 1914.
69. Faith C. S. Ho, *Western Medicine for Chinese: How the Hong Kong College of Medicine Achieved a Breakthrough* (Hong Kong: Hong Kong University Press, 2017), 29–30.
70. Arnold Wright and H. A. Cartwright, *Twentieth Century Impressions of Hong Kong, Shanghai and Other Treaty Ports*, 265.
71. Blake to Chamberlain, on Bacteriologist, 12 June 1901, CO 129/305/221, 350.
72. William Hunter to Government House, Hong Kong, on Requirements for a Bacteriology Laboratory, 25 October 1901. Enclosed in CO 129/307/440, 300–304.
73. "Morgue/Public Mortuary (2nd generation), Hill Road," Gwulo, accessed on 26 April 2022, https://gwulo.com/node/30723.
74. William Hunter, Report of the Government Bacteriologist for the Year 1906, HKSP 1907, Annex L 474–482.
75. C. Y. Wang, "Infantile Tetanus (*Tetanus neonatorum*) in Hong Kong: Its Prevalence and Sources of Infection," *Caduceus* 6 (1927): 249.
76. William Hunter, Report of the Government Bacteriologist for the Year 1903, HKSP 1904, 263–264.
77. Ibid., 124–126.
78. William Hunter, Report of the Government Bacteriologist, 1905, HKSP 1906, 380. Enclosed in Lugard to Elgin, 12 October 1907, CO 129/341/258, 489–517.
79. William Hunter, Wilfred V. M. Koch, A Research into the Etiology of Beriberi. Report for the Year 1906. HKSP 1907, No 11/1906, 123–145.
80. University of Durham to the Colonial Office, 3 October 1907, CO 129/345, 640.
81. Secretary of Committee of Management, Colonial Office, 8 October 1907, CO 129/345, 643.
82. William Hunter to Sir Patrick Manson, 26 July 1906, CO 129/338, 650.
83. Governor Frederick Lugard to Colonial Office, Death of Hunter, 10 June 1909, CO 129/356, Telegram, 322.

84. "Obituary, A. R. Wellington, CMG, MRCS, LRCP, DPH, DTM&H," *Brit Med J*, 25, November 1961, 1439.
85. Sarawak became part of Malaya in 1963.
86. Robert E. Sniden, "Malaria, Mosquitoes and the Legacy of Ronald Ross," accessed on 6 February 2023, https://www.ncbi.nlm.nih.gov/pmc/articles/PMC2636258/.
87. A. R. Wellington, "Public Health in Hong Kong, The Need to Reorganize the Medical and Sanitary Services and for the Establishment of an Up-to-Date System," 2 October 1931, CO 129/531/131, 17–45.
88. A. R. Wellington, "Changes in the Public Health Organization of Hong Kong During the Period 1929–1937," *HKSP* 1937, no. 4/1937, 103–112.
89. A. R. Wellington, Medical and Sanitary Report for the Year 1935, HKAR, 1935, M11–13.
90. Report of the Railway Medical Officer for the Year 1906, HKSP 1907, Annex H, 457.
91. Medical and Sanitary Report for the Year 1934, HKAR 1934, Section X, M95.
92. Moira Chan-Yeung, *A Medical History of Hong Kong: The Development and Contributions of Outpatient Services* (Hong Kong: The Chinese University of Hong Kong Press, 2021), 75–83.
93. C. M. Fung, *A History of Queen Mary Hospital, Hong Kong 1937–1997* (Hong Kong: Queen Mary Hospital Hong Kong, 1997), 5
94. Extract from Report of the Technical Committee for the Reorganization and Improvement of Existing Official Hospitals and Clinical Facilities of the Colony of Hong Kong 1938–1939, Annual Medical Report for 1939, HKAR 1939, Appendix 2, M105–M110.
95. Medical and Sanitary Reports 1901–1938, HKSP or HKAR 1901–1938.
96. Hong Kong Government Gazette, 24 November 1900, HKGRO, 1700.
97. Daniel Ham, "Management of Malaria and Leprosy in Hong Kong and the International Settlement of Shanghai 1880s–1940s," 176–177.
98. "Malaria Lectures: Sanitary Board Decision to Reproduce," *China Mail*, 2 April 1940, 8. A. R. Wellington, "Malaria in Its Relation to Man and Mosquitoes," *Caduceus*, 8, 3 (1929): 117–129. "The Menace of Malaria. Its Relation to Men and Mosquitoes, History of the Parasite," *South China Morning Post*, 12 June 1929. "Life History of Mosquitoes, Man's Fight Against Malaria," *South China Morning Post*, 19 February 1930. "Life History of Mosquitoes, War against the Enemy of Man, a Scientific Problem," *South China Morning Post*, 22 February 1930. "Tuberculosis and Smallpox, The Vaccination Problem," *South China Morning Post*, 6 September 1930.
99. A. R. Wellington, "The Life History of Mosquitoes," *Caduceus* 9, 1, (1930): 15.
100. A. R. Wellington, Medical and Sanitary Report for the Year 1933, HKAR, 1933, M137 Appendix B.
101. Medical and Sanitary Report for Year 1936, HKAR, 1936, M126.
102. "Obituary, A. R. Wellington, CMG, MRCS, LRCP, DPH, DTM&H," *Brit Med J* 25, November 1961, 1439.
103. "Dr. Selwyn-Clarke Appointed as Successor to Dr. A. R. Wellington," *South China Morning Post*, 1 July 1937.

Chapter 3

1. Gerald H. Choa, *The Life and Times of Sir Kai Ho Kai* (Hong Kong, The Chinese University of Hong Kong Press, 1998), 57–59.
2. The Alice Memorial Hospital, Hong Kong, Historical Sketch, 1 September 1887, Hong Kong Printers at the China Mail Office, 3.
3. Edge (Missionary in Hong Kong) to Thompson (Foreign Secretary, London Missionary Society, LMS) 27 February 1882, LMS Box 9, 1882, no. 176.
4. Chalmers (Local Missionary) to Thompson, 18 November 1884 and 12 September 1884, LMS Box 10, 1884, no. 184.
5. J. Chalmers, 24 December 1884. LMS Box 10, 1884, no. 190; Report of the Alice Memorial and Nethersole Hospital for 1902 in Connection with the London Missionary Society for the year 1902, printed at the China Mail Office, 1903.
6. Thomson (Medical Superintendent of AMH) to Thompson, 20 May 1892, LMS Box 11, 1892, no. 208.
7. Thomson to Thompson, 11 September 1893, LMS Box 12, 1893, no. 214.
8. Gibson to Cousins. 15 May 1903, LMS Box 15, 1903, no. 274.
9. E. H. Paterson, *A Hospital for Hong Kong: Centenary History of Alice Ho Miu Ling Nethersole Hospital, Hong Kong, 1887–1987* (Hong Kong: Alice Ho Miu Ling Nethersole Hospital, 1987), 46–48.
10. Ibid., 89–90.
11. Ching, *130 Years of Medicine in Hong Kong: From the College of Medicine for Chinese to Li Ka Shing Faculty of Medicine*, 24.
12. Ibid., 25.
13. Peter Cunich, *A History of the University of Hong Kong, 1911–1945* (Hong Kong: Hong Kong University Press, 2012), 48.
14. Gerald H. Choa, *The Life and Times of Sir Kai Ho Kai*, 63–64. Li Hongzhang was Viceroy of Zhili and Huguang in 1887.
15. Dafydd Emrys Evans, *Constancy of Purpose: An Account of the Foundation and History of Hong Kong College of Medicine and the Faculty of Medicine of the University of Hong Kong 1887–1987* (Hong Kong: Hong Kong University Press, 1987), 37–38.
16. Ibid., 31.
17. Ibid., 39.
18. Cunich, *A History of the University of Hong Kong 1911–1945*, 72.
19. Faith C. S. Ho, *Western Medicine for Chinese: How the Hong Kong College of Medicine Achieved a Breakthrough*, 17.
20. Cunich, *A History of the University of Hong Kong 1911–1945*, 69–70.
21. Choa, *The Life and Times of Sir Kai Ho Kai*, 16–17.
22. Choa, *The Life and Times of Sir Kai Ho Kai*, 20–21.
23. May Holdsworth, and Christopher Munn, *Dictionary of Hong Kong Biography* (Hong Kong: Hong Kong University Press, 2011), 188–189.
24. Choa, *The Life and Times of Sir Kai Ho Kai*, 24–25.
25. Chalmers to Thompson, 18 November 1884 and 12 September 1884, LMS Box 10, 1884, no. 184.

26. Ching, *130 Years of Medicine in Hong Kong*, 25.
27. Choa, *The Life and Times of Sir Kai Ho Kai*, 77–78.
28. Report of the Medical Officer of Health for 1895–1910, HKSP, 1896–1911.
29. Proposal for a Hospital for Women and Children, Jubilee Celebration Enclosed in CO 129/275/96 468–69; Chater to Blake, Jubilee Hospital and Nursing Institute, 30 June 1899, Enclosed in Blake to Chamberlain 6 September 1899. CO 129/293/254, 340–345.
30. Gibson to Cousins, 15 May 1903, LMS Box 15, 1903, no. 274 (Opening of Alice Memorial Maternity Hospital).
31. Gibson to Cousins, 12 September 1902, LMS Box 15, 1902, no. 268–269.
32. Choa, *The Life and Times of Sir Kai Ho Kai*, 165–175.
33. Dr Ho Kai's Protest Against the 1887 Public Health Bill, Submitted to the Government by the Sanitary Board, and the Board's Rejoinder Thereto, HKSP 1887, no. 30/87, 403–407.
34. Chan-Yeung, *A Medical History of Hong Kong, 1842–1941*, 126–128.
35. Choa, *The Life and Times of Sir Kai Ho Kai, 131*.
36. A Freemasonry Lodge is a basic organization unit in Freemasonry.
37. Choa, *The Life and Times of Sir Kai Ho Kai*, 189.
38. "Sir Kai Ho Kai," *South China Morning Post*, 27 February 1914.
39. Choa, *The Life and Times of Sir Kai Ho Kai*, 192.
40. Ibid., 31.
41. "Sir Kai Ho Kai, Honored by Chinese Merchants," *South China Morning Post*, 30 April 1914. "Sir Kai Ho Kai," Honored by Influential Chinese," *South China Morning Post*, 8 June 1914.
42. "The Late Sir Kai Ho Kai. Tribute from the Bar," *South China Morning Post*, 23 July 1914.
43. Kelvin K. W. To and Kwok-Yung Yuen, "In memory of Patrick Manson, Founding Father of Tropical Medicine and the Discovery of Vector-borne Infections," *Emerging Microbes and Infections* 1:1, 1–7, DOI: 10.1038/emi.2012.32.
44. "Tercentenary Tribute to Sir P. Manson. His Great Work in Hong Kong and South China," *South China Morning Post*, 5 December 1960.
45. Kelvin K. W. To and Kwok-Yung Yuen, "In Memory of Patrick Manson."
46. Patrick Manson, "Remarks on an Operation for Abscesses of the Liver," *Brit Med J*, 1 (1892): 163–167.
47. Eli Chernin, "Sir Patrick Manson: An Annotated Bibliography and a Note on a Collected Set of His Writings," *Reviews of Infectious Diseases* 5 (2) (1983): 356–387.
48. Kelvin K. W. To and Kwok-Yung Yuen, "In Memory of Patrick Manson."
49. Philip Manson Bahr, "Sir Patrick Manson: The Founder of the Medical College of Hong Kong (October 1, 1887), and Its First Dean," *Elixir*, Spring (1956): 22–30.
50. B. F. Eldridge, "Patrick Manson and the Discovery Age of Vector Biology," memorial lecture, delivered at the 58th annual meeting of the American Mosquito Control Association, Corpus Christi, Texas, on 16 March 1992, 217.
51. Philip Manson Bahr, "Sir Patrick Manson," 22–30.
52. Kelvin K. W. To and Kwok-Yung Yuen, "In Memory of Patrick Manson."

53. "Tercentenary Tribute to Sir P. Manson: His Great Work in Hong Kong and South China," *South China Morning Post*, 5 December 1960.
54. Kelvin K. W. To and Kwok-Yung Yuen, "In Memory of Patrick Manson."
55. Philip Manson Bahr, "Sir Patrick Manson," 22–30.
56. Marsh to Secretary of State for the Colonies, Sanitary Board, Appointment of Unofficial Members, 11 August 1886, CO 129/228/259, 146.
57. Choa, *The Life and Times of Sir Kai Ho Kai*, 63.
58. Moira Chan-Yeung, *Lam Woo. Master Builder, Revolutionary and Philanthropist* (Hong Kong: The Chinese University of Hong Kong Press, 2017), 133–134; Purchase of IL47, Memorial 26094, HKRS 490-28-261, Hong Kong Public Records Office.
59. Kelvin K. W. To and Kwok-Yung Yuen, "In Memory of Patrick Manson."
60. Holdsworth and Munn, *Dictionary of Hong Kong Biography*, 307.
61. B. F. Eldridge, "Patrick Manson and the Discovery Age of Vector Biology,"218.
62. Kristin D. Hussey, "Sir Patrick Manson at Home: 21 Queen Anne Street as a Hybrid Space," *J R Coll Physicians Edin* 49 (2019): 84–91.
63. Ibid..
64. "Sir Patrick Manson. His Retirement," *South China Morning Post*, 15 August 1912.
65. "Overnight Cables. Death of Sir Patrick Manson: A Benefactor of Hong Kong. The Father of Dairy Farm," *South China Morning Post*, 11 April 1922.
66. Ching, *130 Years of Medicine in Hong Kong*, 250.
67. Mark Harrison, "Cantlie, Sir James," *Oxford Dictionary of National Biography*, accessed on 6 February 2023, https://www.oxforddnb.com/view/10.1093/ref:odnb/9780198614128.001.0001/odnb-9780198614128-e-50530.
68. Jean Cantlie Stewart, *The Quality of Mercy: The Lives of Sir James and Lady Cantlie* (New York: Unwin Hyman, First Edition 1983), 43.
69. Stewart, *The Quality of Mercy*, 86–95.
70. Cecily Liu, "Family Proud of Long, Strong Bond with China" *China Daily*, 3 January 2019, accessed on 6 February 2023, https://global.chinadaily.com.cn/a/201901/03/WS5c2ce352a310d91214053242.html.
71. Thomas S. N. Chen and Peter S. Y. Chen. "The Accomplishments of Sir James Cantlie," *J Med Biography* 7 (1999): 197–199.
72. Stewart, *The Quality of Mercy*, 51–52.
73. Ibid., 52.
74. Harry Y. J. Wu, "Triturator for Smallpox Vaccine Production," *Hong Kong Med J*, 25 (2019) 86–88.
75. Alexander Yersin discovered the plague bacillus, *Pasteurella pestis*, during the 1894 plague epidemic in Hong Kong.
76. Daniel Ham, "The Management of Leprosy and Malaria in Hong Kong and the International Settlement in Shanghai, 1880s–1940s," 37–41.
77. Stewart, *The Quality of Mercy*, 56.
78. Cunich, *A History of the University of Hong Kong*, 28.
79. Mark Harrison, "Cantlie, Sir James."
80. Ibid.

81. "Obituary, Sir James Cantlie, Venerable Hong Kong Doctor," *South China Morning Post*, 31 May 1926.
82. Mark Harrison, "Cantlie, Sir James."
83. "Obituary, Sir James Cantlie, Venerable Hong Kong Doctor," *South China Morning Post*, 31 May 1926.
84. "Statue of Dr Cantlie," *South China Morning Post*, 20 March 1947.
85. "A Man Overlooked: A Faded Memory of a Glorious Career," Armenians in India–Behind the Scenes Forgotten History, accessed on 6 February 2023, https://chater-genealogy.blogspot.com/2015/01/a-man-overlooked-faded-memory-of.html.
86. Ibid. Paul Chater was a highly successful businessman especially in land development. He was knighted in 1902 for his contributions in land reclamation in Hong Kong and serving in Executive Council for a number of years.
87. Katherine Mattock, *Hong Kong Practice: Drs. Anderson and Partners, The First 100 Years* (Hong Kong: Anderson and Partners, Link Print Ltd., 1984), 6–7.
88. Ibid., 14.
89. Ibid., 24.
90. "A Man Overlooked: A Faded Memory of a Glorious Career," Armenians in India—Behind the Scenes Forgotten History.
91. Mattock, *Hong Kong Practice*, 40.
92. Cunich, *A History of the University of Hong Kong*, Volume 1, 51–52.
93. "A Man Overlooked: A Faded Memory of a Glorious Career," Armenians in India—Behind the Scenes Forgotten History.
94. Mattock, *Hong Kong Practice*, 14.
95. "A Man Overlooked: A Faded Memory of a Glorious Career," Armenians in India—Behind the Scenes Forgotten History.
96. Historical Sketch of the Alice Memorial Hospital, 1 September 1887, The London Missionary Society, Hong Kong, Printed at the China Mail Office, 1887, 7.
97. E. H. Paterson, *A Hospital for Hong Kong*, 23–24.
98. Ibid., 24.
99. Ho, *Western Medicine for Chinese*, 34–36.
100. "Presentation to the Dr. J. C. Thomson," *South China Morning Post*, 11 December 1909.
101. Ching, *130 Years of Medicine in Hong Kong*, 56.
102. Ibid., 56, 58.
103. Cunich, *A History of the University of Hong Kong, 1911–1945*, 55.
104. Paterson, *A Hospital for Hong Kong*, 41.
105. Governor Robinson to Joseph Chamberlain (Secretary of State for the Colonies) Appointment of Dr. J. C. Thomson, CO 129/276/145, 172–173.
106. Ibid.
107. Ho, *Western Medicine for Chinese*, 36.
108. The Commission, Report on the Tung Wa Hospital, HKSP 1896.
109. Elizabeth Sinn, *Power and Charity: A Chinese Merchant Elite in Colonial Hong Kong* (Hong Kong: Hong Kong University Press, 2001), 82–120.

110. Commissioners' recommendations, Tung Wa Hospital Report, HKSP 1896, xxx–xxxii.
111. Annual Reports of Inspecting Medical Officers of Tung Wa Hospital from 1897 to 1903, HKSP 1898 to 1904.
112. Ibid.
113. Ibid.
114. Moira Chan-Yeung, *A Medical History of Hong Kong, 1842 to 1941*, 77.
115. Report of the Inspecting Medical Officer of the Tung Wa Hospital, HKAR, 1908.
116. Ho, *Western Medicine for Chinese*, 144.
117. Colonial Surgeon Annual Reports, 1885 and 1890. HKSP 1886 and HKSP 1891.
118. J. C. Thomson, Report regarding the Mosquitoes that Occur in the Colony of Hong Kong, Enclosed in Gascoigne to Chamberlain, 18 August 1902, CO 129/312/365, 224–226.
119. J. M. Green to C. P. Lucas 26 September 1902, CO 129/312/365, 219.
120. The Governor to the Earl of Crewe, Secretary of State for the Colonies, 13 September 1909, CO 129/357/265, 509–510.
121. "Presentation of Farewell Address to Dr. J. C. Thomson. Tung Wa Hospital Directors' Appreciation," *The China Mail*, 24 December 1909. "Tung Wa Hospital. Presentation to Dr Thomson," *South China Morning Post*, 24 December 1909.
122. Arnold Wright, *Twentieth Century Impressions of Hong Kong, Shanghai, and Other Treaty Ports of China* (London: Lloyd's Greater Britain Publishing Co., Ltd., 1908), 180.
123. Ho, *Western Medicine for Chinese*, 216.
124. A. Starling, F. Ho, L. Luke, S. C. Tso, and Edwin Yu, *Plague, SARS and the Story of Medicine in Hong Kong* (Hong Kong: Hong Kong University Press, 2006), 152.
125. "Hong Kong College of Medicine," *South China Morning Post*, 9 February 1909.
126. Arnold Wright, *Twentieth Century Impressions of Hong Kong*, 180; "Huashang renming lu" 華商人名錄, *Wah Kiu Yat Po*, 25 July 1910 documenting that he moved his office to Wellington Street. It seems that the licentiates could conduct private practice locally provided they only attended to Chinese patients despite the Medical Practitioner Registration Ordinance.
127. Ho Ko-tsun, *Chi shizihui chuji jijiu yaofa* 赤十字會初級急救要法 (Hong Kong: Juzhen shulou, 1908).
128. "Dr. Ho Ko-tsun Passed Away" 何高俊醫生逝世, *Wah Kiu Yat Po*, 7 June 1953.
129. Rudi Butt, *Biographical Dictionary of Medical Practitioners in Hong Kong: 1841–1941*, accessed on 6 February 2023, https://hkmd1841-1941.blogspot.com/2013/09/dr-ho-ko-tsun-1901.
130. Ho Ko-tsun, "Guangdongsheng zhengfu qudi yiwu zhi yuanyin" 廣東省政府取締醫務之原因, *Zhonghua Yibao* 中華醫報, 6(1913), 1–10.
131. "Canton News: Canton, January 19 Sanitary Board Notice," *South China Morning Post*, 23 January 1912, 11; "Plague in Canton: Measures for Prevention, Canton," *South China Morning Post*, 24 April 1913, 6.
132. Ho Ko-tsun, "Yu zhongguo kexue fada dang yi zhongguowen shouke bing yi kexue shubao yijianshu" 欲中國科學發達當以中國文授課並譯科學書報意見書, *Hsin Min Pao*, 4 (6) (1917): 38–40; 4 (7) (1917): 38–41.

133. "Reform in Canton: Many Official Changes. The Terrors of Martial Law," *South China Morning Post*, 24 September 1913, 7.
134. Chan-Yeung, *A Medical History of Hong Kong: The Development and Contributions of Outpatient Services*, 15–16.
135. Ibid., 31.
136. M. Chan-Yeung, "Eastern District (Wanchai) Dispensary and Plague Hospital," *Hong Kong Med J*, 25(6) (2019): 503–505.
137. "Wanchai Dispensary: Completion of a Modern Maternity Ward, a Gift to the Poor," *South China Morning Post*, 11 December 1931, 13.
138. "Kowloon Dispensary: New Recreation Ground Opened Tennis and Croquet," *South China Morning Post*, 16 September 1936, 10.
139. "Colourful Ceremony: Governor Presents Insignia to Twenty-Three H. K. Residents," *South China Morning Post*, 31 December 1949, 5.
140. W. C. Chau, and F. I. Tseung, "The Hong Kong Chinese Medical Association," *The Bulletin of the Hong Kong Chinese Medical Association*, 1(1) (1948): 8–12.
141. "Yeung Wo Hospital's New Building: Extension Formally Opened by Mrs. Kotewall," *South China Morning Post*, 19 May 1932, 9.
142. Secretary for Chinese Affairs to Accounts, 1 September 1949, Hong Kong Public Records Office, HKRS621-1-18.
143. "Dr. Ho Ko-tsun: Ashes Scattered at Sea, Launch Service," *South China Morning Post*, 12 June 1953, 8.

Chapter 4

1. Evans, *Constancy of Purpose*, 40.
2. Cunich, *A History of the University of Hong Kong*, 176.
3. Evans, *Constancy of Purpose*, 46.
4. L. Ride, "The Faculty of Medicine," in Brian Harrison, *The University of Hong Kong: The First 50 Years (1911–1961)* (Hong Kong: Hong Kong University Press, 1964), 104–107.
5. Cunich, *A History of the University of Hong Kong*, 224–226.
6. Evans, *Constancy of Purpose*, 56.
7. Ibid., 55–58.
8. Ibid., 59.
9. Julia Chan, and N. G. Patil, *Digby: A Remarkable Life* (Hong Kong: Hong Kong University Press, 2006), 3.
10. Ibid., 8.
11. Evans, *Constancy of Purpose*, 151
12. "Hong Kong University: The Rockefeller Gift," *South China Morning Post*, 11 July 1922, 6.
13. "Notes and Comments," *Caduceus*, 1(1) (1922): 5–6.
14. "University of Hong Kong: Medical Society," *South China Morning Post*, 11 October 1919, 3.

15. S. W. Phoon, "Kenelm Hutchinson Digby, O.B.E., F.R.C.S. An Appreciation," *Bulletin of the Hong Kong Chinese Medical Association*, 7 (1955): 26–28.
16. K. H. Digby, "Presidential Address on Clinical Research," *Caduceus*, 3(1) (1924): 31–36.
17. "Review: A Plea for The Tonsils," *British Medical Journal*, 2 (3070) (1919): 562.
18. Kenelm H. Digby, "What Is a 'Diseased' Tonsil"? *British Medical Journal*, 1 (3260) (1923): 1075.
19. A. G. M. Severn, and K. H. Digby, "Two Cases of Intrahepatic Stone Formation and Suppression of Bile," *Caduceus*, 3(3) (1924): 145–150; K. H. Digby, "Common-Duct Stones of Liver Origin," *The British Journal of Surgery*, 17 (1930): 578–591.
20. K. H. Digby, G. H. Thomas, and S. T. Hsiu, "Notes on Carcinoma of the Nasopharynx," *Caduceus*, 9 (2) (1930): 45–68.
21. K. H. Digby, "Nasopharyngeal Carcinoma," *The British Journal of Surgery*, 27 (1941): 517–537.
22. K. H. Digby, "A Suggestion for the Treatment of Early Phthisis by Upper Intercostals Nerve Block," *Caduceus*, 3(3) (1924): 111–112.
23. K. H. Digby, "A Few Observations on the Properties of Ivory as a Material for Use in Bone Surgery," *Caduceus*, 3(3) (1924): 103–110.
24. S. W. Phoon, "Kenelm Hutchinson Digby, O.B.E., F.R.C.S. An Appreciation," 26–28; A Department of Orthopedics was only formed after the war.
25. Louis Fu, "The Contributions of Kenelm Hutchinson Digby to Orthopedics in Hong Kong Part 1," *Journal of Orthopedics, Trauma and Rehabilitation*, 19 (2015): 66–71.
26. "Medals Awarded: Hongkong Recipients Representative Public Services," *South China Morning Post*, 15 May 1937, 9.
27. "The Birthday Honors," *British Medical Journal*, 1 (4093) (1939): 1247.
28. "Honorary Degrees: Hong Kong University Congregation Opening of New Building for the School of Surgery," *South China Morning Post*, 8 January 1935, 11
29. Evans, *Constancy of Purpose*, 200.
30. Emily Hahn, *China to Me* (London: Virago, 1987), 319.
31. Mabel Winifred Redwood, *It Was Like This...* (Oxford: Isis; large print edition, 2003), 204–205.
32. Chan and Patil, *Digby: A Remarkable Life*, 15.
33. Chan and Patil, *Digby: A Remarkable Life*, 25; K. H. Digby, and J. B. Enticknap, "The Immunization Function of the Rabbit Vermiform Appendix," Br J Exp Pathol, 35 (3) (1954): 294–298.
34. Chan and Patil, *Digby: A Remarkable Life*, 29.
35. S. W. Phoon, "Kenelm Hutchinson Digby, O.B.E., F.R.C.S. An Appreciation," 26–28.
36. "Kenelm Hutchison Digby," *Elixir*, May 1954: 67–69.
37. Chan and Patil, *Digby: A Remarkable Life*, 29–31.
38. Ibid., 16.
39. Osman was a student from Malaya who graduated from HKU in 1924. He was assistant to Professor of Pathology in HKU from 1925 to 1930. He returned to Malaya in 1930.

40. "Doctor Wedded: Marriage of Hongkong University Professor Osman-Kotwall," *South China Morning Post*, 9 November 1929, 10.
41. "Herbert Earle," Prabook, accessed on 6 February 2023, https://prabook.com/web/herbert.earle/2347211.
42. Evans, *Constancy of Purpose*, 46–48.
43. Ibid., 55–56.
44. Ching, *130 Years of Medicine in Hong Kong*, 127.
45. Henry Lester was an altruistic Englishman, a landowner, and philanthropist who left his estate to the welfare of Shanghai. His legacy included two institutes, for medical and technical research, as well as several hospitals and schools, institutes for the blind, the poor, and orphans. Professor Earle was the second person from HKU recruited by the institute to help develop the medical institute. Professor John Anderson was the first. See "Altruistic Englishman Who Invested in Welfare of Shanghai," Shine, accessed on 6 February 2023, https://www.shine.cn/feature/art-culture/1907047873/.
46. "Herbert Earle," Prabook, accessed on 28 January 2022, https://prabook.com/web/herbert.earle/2347211.
47. H. G. Earle, "Basal Metabolism," *Caduceus*, 1 (1922): 81–85.
48. "Herbert Gastineau Earle. Doctor of Laws *honoris causa*. Congregation 1936," The University of Hong Kong, accessed on 28 January 2022, https://www4.hku.hk/hongrads/citations/m-a-m-b-herbert-gastineau-earle.
49. "Dr. Herbert G. Earle: Former Hong Kong Resident Dies on Way Home," *South China Morning Post*, 21 June 1946.
50. Faith C. S. Ho, "Hong Kong's First Professor of Pathology and the Laboratory of the Royal College of Physicians of Edinburgh," *J R Coll Physicians Edin*, 41 (2011): 67–72.
51. *Wongs and Wangs Chronicle* (privately published, 2005), 173–174.
52. Li Shu-fan, *Hong Kong Surgeon* (New York: E. P. Dutton, 1964), 25.
53. Ibid., 30.
54. Wang was on a McGunn Research Scholarship, a Carnegie Research Fellowship, and a Freeland Barbour Fellowship of the Royal College of Physicians of Edinburgh. Faith C. S. Ho, "Hong Kong's First Professor of Pathology and the Laboratory of the Royal College of Physicians of Edinburgh," 67–72.
55. Faith C. S. Ho. "Hong Kong's First Professor of Pathology and the Laboratory of the Royal College of Physicians of Edinburgh," 67–72.
56. Correspondence between William Hornell, VC of HKU and Sir William Peel, Governor of HK and Chancellor of the University, the British Minister in Peking, Sir Miles Lampson, the Foreign Office, March–April 1931, CO 129/531/9, 24–28.
57. Ching, *130 Years of Medicine in Hong Kong*, 125.
58. C. Y. Wang, "Infantile Tetanus (Tetanus Neonatorum) in Hong Kong: Its Prevalence and Source of Infection," *Caduceus*, 6 (1927): 249–252
59. Ching, *130 Years of Medicine in Hong Kong*, 126
60. U. S. Khoo. "Handbook of Pathology," *Hong Kong Med J*, 24(5) (2018): 546–548.
61. Faith C. S. Ho, "Hong Kong's First Professor of Pathology and the Laboratory of the Royal College of Physicians of Edinburgh," 67–72.

62. *Caduceus*, 2(1) (1923).
63. Faith C. S. Ho, "Hong Kong's First Professor of Pathology and the Laboratory of the Royal College of Physicians of Edinburgh," 67–72.
64. Ching, *130 Years of Medicine in Hong Kong*, 133–134.
65. Faith C. S. Ho, "Hong Kong's First Professor of Pathology and the Laboratory of the Royal College of Physicians of Edinburgh," 71.
66. Philip Manson-Bahr, "Obituary. John Anderson MA, MD, BSc, MRCP, DTM and H," *Brit Med J*, April 11, 1931: 647–648.
67. N. T. Mackintosh to the Colonial Secretary Hong Kong, 23 June 1922, CO 129/478, 475–476.
68. Herbert Earle to the Board of Education, 14 July 1922, CO 129/478, 473.
69. R. T. Leiper to the Secretary, Board of Education, 13 December 1922, CO 129/478, 490–491.
70. The Board of Education to the Colonial Office, 18 December 1922, CO 129/478, 488–489.
71. Medical and Sanitary Report 1927, Hong Kong Administrative Reports, 1927, M [1] 12–13.
72. Faith C. S. Ho, "Dr. Tseung Fat Im's Notebook of Professor Anderson's Lectures, 1924," *Hong Kong Med J*, 22 (2016): 298–299.
73. Medical and Sanitary Report, 1927, Hong Kong Administrative Report, 1927, M(1)12.
74. Choa, *The Life and Times of Sir Kai Ho Kai*, 75.
75. Medical and Sanitary Report, 1922, Hong Kong Administrative Reports, M(1) 9, 10 and 18.
76. Medical and Sanitary Report, 1928, Hong Kong Administrative Reports 1928, M23.
77. "Hospital Work at the University Clinics," *Caduceus*, 3(1) (1924): 40–41.
78. *Caduceus*, 2(3) (1923): 158–159.
79. "Hospital Work at the University Clinics," *Caduceus*, 3(1) (1924): 40–41.
80. John Anderson, "The Present Position of Malaria in Hong Kong," *Caduceus*, 6(2) (1927): 105–115.
81. Philip Manson-Bahr, "Obituary: John Anderson MA, MD, BSc, MRCP, DTM and H," *Brit Med J*, April 11, 1931; 647–648.
82. "Late Dr. Anderson. Memorial Meeting Held at University. Tribute Paid," *South China Morning Post*, 2 April 1931.
83. Carol C. L .Tsang, "Out of the Dark: Women's Medicine and Women's Disease in Colonial Hong Kong," Dissertation for the Degree of Doctor of Philosophy, the University of Hong Kong, 2011, 87.
84. Evans, *Constancy of Purpose*, 59.
85. "The Medical Curriculum," *Caduceus*, 2(1) (1923): 8.
86. Tsang, "Out of the Dark," 80.
87. R. E. Tottenham, *A Surgeon's Journey*, 121–124. Quoted in Carol C. L. Tsang, "Knowing Chinese Women: Richard Tottenham and Colonial Medicine in Interwar Hong Kong," *JRASHKB*, 53 (2013): 167–181.

88. Ibid., 126–128. Quoted in Carol C. L. Tsang, "Knowing Chinese Women: Richard Tottenham and Colonial Medicine in Interwar Hong Kong," 167–179.
89. R. E. Tottenham, "Maternity Work in the Colony of Hong Kong," *Caduceus*, 5(2) (1926): 82–87.
90. Tsang, "Out of the Dark," 92–93.
91. "The History of the Rotunda Hospital Dublin," The Rotunda Hospital Dublin, accessed on 6 February 2023, https://rotunda.ie/history-of-rotunda-hospital/.
92. Gordon King, "The History of Tsan Yuk Hospital 1922–1955," *Bulletin of the Hong Kong Chinese Medical Association*, 8 (1956): 31–39.
93. Peel to Cunliffe-Lister, Tsan Yuk—A free gift to the Government, 4 May 1933, CO 129/544/1; Peel to Cunliffe-Lister, Tsan Yuk—A free gift to the Government, 7 May 1933, CO 129/549/6.
94. R. E. Tottenham, "Some Observations on the History and Treatment of Eclampsia," *Caduceus*, 7(1) (1928): 8–13.
95. R. E. Tottenham, "Strictures of the Vagina among the Chinese," *Caduceus*, 6(2) (1927): 150–154.
96. Tsang, "Out of the Dark," 98.
97. *Caduceus*, 1926 to 1936, in one of the issues of respective years. .
98. R. E. Tottenham, and E. C. Crichton, "Clinical Report of the Rotunda Hospital for One Year. November 1st, 1913, to October 31st, 1914," *Transactions of the Royal Academy of Medicine in Ireland*, 3 (1) (1915): 287–325.
99. Tsang, "Out of the Dark," 107.
100. "Dr. R. E. Tottenham. University Professor Leaving," *South China Morning Post*, 9 May 1935.

Chapter 5

1. Chan-Yeung, *A Medical History of Hong Kong: The Development and Contribution of Outpatient Services*, 14–16.
2. Li Shu-fan, *Hong Kong Surgeon* (New York: Dutton, 1964), 52.
3. Evans, *Constancy of Purpose*, 39.
4. Hong Kong Government Gazette, 1904, 1905 (5 May 1905, 636–367), 1915 (7 May 1915, 240–242), 1925 (8 May 1925, 167–173), 1935 (10 May 1945, 573–592), 1941 (9 May 1941, 704–733).
5. Hong Kong Government Gazette, 1904.
6. Hong Kong Government Gazette, 1941, 9 May 1941, 704–733.
7. Li Shu Pui, *Brit Med J*, 331 (7421) (2005): 908.
8. Cunich, *A History of the University of Hong Kong*, 239.
9. "Li Shu Fan, Doctor of Laws *honoris causa*. 55th Congregation (1961)," The University of Hong Kong, accessed on 6 February 2023, https://www4.hku.hk/hongrads/citations/mb-chb-frcs-shu-fan-li-li-shu-fan.
10. Li, *Hong Kong Surgeon*, 30.
11. Ching, *130 Years of Medicine in Hong Kong*, 80.

12. Li, *Hong Kong Surgeon*, 31.
13. Ibid., 49.
14. Li Shu Fan, "Reminiscence of 50 Years of Medical Work in Hong Kong and China," *Bull of the Hong Kong Chinese Medical Association*, 10 (1958): 161–173.
15. Li, *Hong Kong Surgeon*, 50.
16. Hong Kong College of Surgeons, *Healing with the Scalpel: From the First Colonial Surgeon to the College of Surgeons of Hong Kong* (Hong Kong: Hong Kong Academy of Medicine Press, 2010), 55.
17. Li, *Hong Kong Surgeon*, 52.
18. "Yeung Wo Hospital's New Building Extension Formally Opened by Mrs. Kotewall Yesterday," *South China Morning Post*, 19 May, 1932.
19. Li Shu Fan, "Reminiscence of 50 years of Medical Work in Hong Kong and China," *Bull of the Hong Kong Chinese Medical Association*, 10 (1958): 170. Thoracoplasty is a surgical procedure that was originally designed to permanently collapse the cavities of pulmonary tuberculosis by removing the ribs from the chest wall. It involved resection of multiple ribs, allowing the apposition of parietal to the visceral or mediastinal pleura.
20. S. F. Lee, "The Surgical Side of General Practice," *Caduceus*, 5(1) (1926): 14–19.
21. S. F. Li, "Recent Development and Observations on Spinal Anesthesia under Novocaine Caffeine Compound," *Caduceus*, 6(3) (1927): 326.
22. "Li Shu Fan, Doctor of Laws *honoris causa*, 55th Congregation (1961)," The University of Hong Kong, accessed on 6 February 2023, https://www4.hku.hk/hongrads/citations/mb-chb-frcs-shu-fan-li-li-shu-fan.
23. "Dr. Li's Questions. Nuisance and Flies in Kennedy Town," *South China Morning Post*, 20 July 1932; "Health in Schools. Questions regarding Medical Inspection," *South China Morning Post*, 27 February 1932; "Small Pox in Hong Kong. Replies to Li's Questions," *South China Morning Post*, 15 March 1933.
24. "New Councilors. Dr. Li Shu Fan and Mr. Leo d'Almada," *South China Morning Post*, 22 January 1937.
25. "A Valued Member. Dr Li Shu-fan's Service on Legislative Council. Retirement Regrets," *South China Morning Post*, 21 February 1941.
26. Li, *Hong Kong Surgeon*, 141.
27. Ibid., 145.
28. "Dr Li Shu Fan. Returning from America with Hospital Plans," *South China Morning Post*, 23 July 1948.
29. College of Surgeons of Hong Kong, *Healing with the Scalpel: From the First Colonial Surgeon to the College of Surgeons of Hong Kong*, 59.
30. Li, *Hong Kong Surgeon*, 57.
31. Ibid., 61.
32. "Himalayas Tiger Hunt," *South China Morning Post*, 3 August 1955; "Leopard Hunt. Dr. Li Shu Fan's Success in Safari," *South China Morning Post*, 28 May 1958; "Elephant Hunting. Dr. Li Shu Fan Tells Rotarians of His African Safari," *South China Morning Post*, 13 June 1958.
33. "Dr Li Shu Fan 'bags the big five'," *South China Morning Post*, 16 February 1958.
34. "Generous Land Gift Solves University's Major Problem," *South China Morning Post*, 25 January 1961.

35. "Donors Praised at Foundation Ceremony," *South China Morning Post*, 4 March 1963.
36. "Li Shu Fan, Doctor of Laws, *honoris causa*, 55th Congregation (1961)," The University of Hong Kong.
37. Li, *Hong Kong Surgeon*, 1964.
38. "Death of Dr. Li Shu-Fan," *South China Morning Post*, 25 November 1966.
39. Ho, *Western Medicine for Chinese*, 58.
40. Herbert K. Lau, "Dr Arthur W. Woo. Rejuvenated the Broken Hong Kong Rotary Club in 1945," accessed on 17 February, 2023, http://old.rotary3450.org/woo-a-w-dr/.
41. "Obituary Notices. A. W. Woo, OBE, MBBS, FRCS," *Br Med J*, 11 April 1964, accessed on 23 April 2022, https://www.bmj.com/content/bmj/1/5388/988.full.pdf.
42. Ibid.
43. "Woo Wai-tak, Arthur (1919–d.1964)," *Biographical Dictionary of Medical Practitioners in Hong Kong: 1841–1941*, accessed on 6 February 2023, https://hkmd1841-1941.blogspot.com/2013/09/woo-wai-tak-arthur-1919.html.
44. "Obituary Notices. A. W. Woo, OBE, MBBS, FRCS."
45. Holdsworth and Munn, *Dictionary of Hong Kong Biography*, 465.
46. "Woo Wai-tak, Arthur (1919–d.1964)," *Biographical Dictionary of Medical Practitioners in Hong Kong, 1841–1941*.
47. "Obituary Notices. A. W. Woo, OBE, MBBS, FRCS."
48. "Broadcast Appeal. Dr. Arthur Woo Addressed the Chinese, the Cost of Radium," *South China Morning Post*, 24 May 1934.
49. Hao Ran 浩然, "Hu Huide yisheng Xianggang haimian shiyi diyiren" 胡惠德醫生香港海面施醫第一人, *Christian Weekly*, no. 2461, 23 October 2011.
50. Holdsworth and Munn, *Dictionary of Hong Kong Biography*, 466.
51. Medical and Sanitary Report for the Year 1933, HKAR, 1933, M111–115.
52. "Rotary Club. Appointments of Officers for the Year," *South China Morning Post*, 27 June, 1941.
53. A region in Northeast China, specifically the three provinces of Heilongjiang, Jilin, and Liaoning, but broadly also including the eastern Inner Mongolian prefectures of Hulunbuir, Hinggan, Tongliao, and Chifeng, and sometimes Xilingol League.
54. The January 28 Incident or Shanghai Incident (28 January–3 March 1932) was a conflict between China and Japan that took place in the Shanghai International Settlement. Following the Japanese invasion of Manchuria, there were anti-Japanese demonstrations in the International Settlement. The Japanese Government sent a sect of militant ultranationalist Japanese Buddhist monks belonging to the Nichiren sect to Shanghai. The monks shouted anti-Chinese, pro-Japanese nationalist slogans in Shanghai, promoting Japanese rule over East Asia. In response, a Chinese mob formed, killing one monk and injuring two. The Japanese in Shanghai rioted and burned down a factory, killing two Chinese. Heavy fighting broke out, and China appealed with no success to the League of Nations. A truce was finally reached on 5 May, calling for Japanese military withdrawal and an end to Chinese boycotts of Japanese products.

55. Holdsworth and Munn, *Dictionary of Hong Kong Biography*, 466.
56. "Taipo Orphanage: Large Party Attends Yesterday's at Home," *South China Morning Post*, 25 April 1948.
57. Ho, *Western Medicine for Chinese*, 58.
58. "Rotary Conference. Prevailing Political Situation Responsible for Closures. Dr. Arthur Woo Elected Convenor," *South China Morning Post*, 28 May 1951.
59. Herbert K. Lau, "Dr Arthur W. Woo: Rejuvenated the Broken Hong Kong Rotary Club in 1945," accessed on 2 September 2022, http://old.rotary3450.org/woo-a-w-dr/.
60. "Personalities. Doctor Arthur Woo Returns from American Tour. Aid for Lingnan," *South China Morning Post*, 24 October 1947.
61. "Dr. Arthur Woo Honored by Hospital," *South China Morning Post*, 13 January 1956.
62. "Obituary Notices. A. W. Woo, OBE, MBBS, FRCS."
63. "Death of Dr. Arthur Wai-tak Woo," *South China Morning Post*, 4 March 1964.
64. "Obituary Notices. A. W. Woo, OBE, MBBS, FRCS."
65. "Prize Distribution, Queen's College," *South China Morning Post*, 27 January 1919.
66. Herbert K. Lau, "Hong Kong Rotarian Dr. Tseung Fat-im, Instrumental in Forming the United College and the Establishment of the Chinese University of Hong Kong," 1 September 2017, accessed on 2 September 2022, http://old.rotary3450.org/tseung-fat-im-hong-kong-dr/.
67. Faith C. S. Ho, "Dr. Tseung Fat-im's Notebook of Professor John Anderson's lectures, 1924," *Hong Kong Med J*, 22 (2016): 299–300.
68. Both notebooks were donated by Dr. Siu Yuk-tong to the Museum in 2001.
69. F. I. Tseung, "Diabetes Mellitus: The significance of Biochemical Tests in its Diagnosis and Treatment," *Caduceus*, 5(3) (1926): 197–226.
70. "Dr. Tseung Fat Im, M.B.B.S. (Hong Kong)," in *The Prominent Chinese in Hong Kong (1937)*, edited by Woo Sing-lim, 1937 (Hong Kong: Sunyata, 2019).
71. "Tseung Fat Im, Doctor of Laws *honoris causa*, 72nd Congregation, 1969," The University of Hong Kong, accessed on 5 February 2022, https://www4.hku.hk/hongrads/graduates/obe-mb-bs-jp-fat-im-tseung-tseung-fat-im.
72. The New Territories Medical Benevolent Society (MBS) had its financial foundation from H. & L. Kadoorie, E. M. Raymond, and J. E. Joseph, who were impressed by the number of diseases and amount of poverty in the New Territories after a tour. The MBS came into being on 25 May 1930. In the beginning, enthusiastic doctors and their nurses spent Sundays treating patients in various centers in the New Territories, such as Tsuen Wan, Tuen Mun, and Ping Shan. The society was responsible for the necessary medical supply and medications for the clinics. Later, it employed doctors to work part-time in these clinics three times a week rather than only on Sundays. Later still, permanent clinics were set up in the centers with a resident doctor, a nurse, and a dispenser.
73. Medical and Sanitary Report for the Year 1933, HKAR, 1933, M111–115.
74. Herbert K. Lau, "Hong Kong Rotarian Dr. Tseung Fat-im, Instrumental in Forming the United College, and the Establishment of the Chinese University of Hong Kong," accessed on 6 February 2023, http://old.rotary3450.org/tseung-fat-im-hong-kong-dr/.

75. Tseung Fat Im, "Dr. F. I. Tseung, C.St. J. New Commissioner of St. John Ambulance Brigade, Hong Kong," accessed on 6 February 2023, http://old.rotary3450.org/tseung-fat-im-hong-kong-dr/ .
76. "Dr. Tseung Fat-im, M.B.B.S. (Hong Kong)," in *The Prominent Chinese in Hong Kong (1937)*.
77. Social worker in a hospital.
78. "Hospital Report. Alice Memorial's Activities during Occupation. Tribute to the Staff," *South China Morning Post*, 18 December 1946.
79. Chan-Yeung, *A Medical History of Hong Kong: The Development and Contributions of Outpatient Services*, 39.
80. D. J. S. Crozier (Director of Education in Hong Kong) to Colonial Office, 26 May 1957, The Post-Secondary Colleges of Hong Kong, CO 1030/571, 286–289.
81. "History," United College, The Chinese University of Hong Kong, accessed on 28 February 2022, https://www.uc.cuhk.edu.hk/tc/about/history/.
82. D. J. S. Crozier to J. C. Burgh, Colonial Office, 7 November 1960, in CO 1030/1093.
83. Report of the Committee on Higher Education 1952, The Keswick Report, Hong Kong Government Printers, 1952.
84. A. N. H. Ng-Lun, *Quest for Excellence: A History of the Chinese University of Hong Kong* (Hong Kong: The Chinese University of Hong Kong Press, 1994), 1–34.
85. Tseung Fat-im, "Dr. F. I. Tseung, C.St. J. New Commissioner of St. John Ambulance Brigade, Hong Kong," accessed on 2 September 2022, http://old.rotary3450.org/tseung-fat-im-hong-kong-dr/.
86. "Tseung Fat Im, Doctor of Laws (*honoris causa*). 72nd Congregation 1969," The University of Hong Kong, accessed on 6 February 2023, https://www4.hku.hk/hongrads/graduates/obe-mb-bs-jp-fat-im-tseung-tseung-fat-im.

Chapter 6

1. Laura Jefferson, Karen Bloor, and Alan Maynard, "Women in Medicine: Historical Perspectives and Recent Trends," *British Medical Bulletin*, 114 (2015): 5–15.
2. Ibid.
3. "Editorial," *The Lancet* (1878, 17 August): 226–227.
4. Laura Jefferson, Karen Bloor, and Alan Maynard, "Women in Medicine: Historical Perspectives and Recent Trends," *British Medical Bulletin*, 114 (2015): 5–15.
5. "Chinese Medical Women," *British Medical Journal*, 15 April 1899: 927–928.
6. Sara Tucker, *The Canton Hospital and Medicine in Nineteenth Century China, 1835–1900* (Ann Arbor, MI: University Microfilms International, 1986), 201.
7. Ibid., 272.
8. J. George, "The Lady Doctor's 'Warm welcome,' Dr. Alice Sibree and the Early Years of Hong Kong's Maternity Service 1903–1909," *Journal of the Hong Kong Branch of the Royal Asiatic Society*, 33(1993): 81–109.
9. "Women Students: Bigger Hostel for Undergraduates Wanted. Appeal to the Public," *South China Morning Post*, 17 January 1927, 8.

10. "Notes and Comments," *Caduceus*, 7(4) (1928): 291.
11. Irene Cheng, *Intercultural Reminiscences* (Hong Kong: David C. Lam Institute for East-West Studies, Hong Kong Baptist University, 1997), 105.
12. "Notes and Comments," *Caduceus*, 1(1) (1922): 8.
13. Colonial Secretariat, *Report on Women' Salary Scales in Public Service* (Hong Kong: Government Printer 1962), 1
14. "Petition by Doctors: Approach to Mr. Sandys for Equal Treatment," South China Sunday Post, 17 March 1963.
15. Colonial Secretariat, *Report on Women' Salary Scales in Public Service* (Hong Kong: Government Printer 1962), 2.
16. Colonial Secretariat, *Report on Women's Salary Scales in the Public Service* (Hong Kong: Government Printer 1962), 5.
17. Colonial Secretariat, *Report on Women's Salary Scales in the Public Service* (Hong Kong: Government Printer 1962), 6, 9.
18. "Petition by Doctors: Approach to Mr. Sandys for Equal Treatment," South China Sunday Post, 17 March 1963; "Question about H. K. Women Doctors' Pay Raised in Lords: London," *South China Morning Post*, 9 April 1963, 10 April 1963.
19. "Equal Pay for Women in Civil Services Proposed by 1975," *South China Morning Post*, 29 February 1968.
20. "Married Women Doctors Disappointed with Improved Conditions," *South China Morning Post Special Report*, 27 October 1969, 6.
21. Second Report on Civil Service Pay, Hong Kong. Standing Commission on Civil Service Salaries and Conditions of Service. Hong Kong: The Commission 1980, 78 para 8.11.
22. Janet George, "The Lady Doctor's 'Warm Welcome': Dr. Alice Sibree and the Early Years of Hong Kong's Maternity Service 1903–1909," *JRASHKB*, 33 (1993): 87.
23. Medical Officer of Health, Report to the Sanitary Board, Hong Kong Sessional Papers, 1896 to 1907.
24. Anne W. M. Chow, "Root of Hong Kong Midwifery," *HKJGOM*, 1 (2000): 72–80.
25. May to Lyttelton, 21 July 1904, CO 129/323 #291, 240–243.
26. Janet George, "Moving with Chinese Opinion: Hong Kong's Maternity Service 1881–1941," PhD Thesis, University of Sydney, 1992, 116.
27. Anne W. M. Chow, "Root of Hong Kong Midwifery," *HKJGOM*, 1 (2000):72–80.
28. Report of the Principal Civil Medical Officer and Medical Officer of Health for 1907, HKSP, 1908, 409–410.
29. "Editorial," *The Lancet*, 17 August 1878: 226–227.
30. Janet George, "Moving with Chinese Opinion: Hong Kong's Maternity Service 1881–1941," PhD Thesis, University of Sydney, 1992, 116.
31. Minutes of HK District Committee Annual Meeting, 2 March 1909, London Missionary Society Box 18, 1909, no. 311.
32. Lugard to Harcourt, 27 July 1911, regarding Nursing Institute, CO 129/378/267, 391–398.
33. Hong Kong Government Gazette, 31 July 1914, 255.

34. "Dr. Alice Deborah Hickling, M.B.E.," *Caduceus*, 7(4) (1928): 292.
35. Hong Kong Blue Book 1918, Dr. Wilfred Pearce, Medical Officer of Health was away for 12 months in 1918–1919; Dr. Hickling was the one most qualified for the job and she was appointed Acting Medical Officer of Health for the duration.
36. "Obituary. Dr. Alice Deborah Hickling," *British Medical Journal*, 6 October 1928, 635.
37. Moira Chan-Yeung, "Eastern District (Wan Chai) Dispensary and Plague Hospital," *Hong Kong Med J*, 25 (2019): 503–505.
38. Severn to Colonial Office, Site for a Maternity Hospital, 30 April 1919, CO 129/454/139, 344; Registrar General's Report for 1919, Hong Kong Administrative Reports 1919, C10.
39. Gordon King, "The History of Tsan Yuk Hospital, 1922–1955," *Bulletin of the Hong Kong Chinese Medical Association*, 8 (1956):31–39.
40. Ibid.
41. Hong Kong Blue Book, 1923–1928.
42. Tsang, "Out of the Dark: Women's Medicine and Women's Disease in Colonial Hong Kong," 96–97.
43. Gordon King, "The History of the Tsan Yuk Hospital, 1922–1955," *Bulletin of the Hong Kong Chinese Medical Association*, 8 (1956):31–39.
44. Medical and Sanitary Reports for the Year 1932, HKAR 1932, M69–70.
45. "The Late Dr. Mrs. Hickling," *South China Morning Post*, December 1, 1929.
46. Gordon King, "The History of Tsan Yuk Hospital, 1922–1955," *Bulletin of the Hong Kong Chinese Medical Association*, 8 (1956): 31–39.
47. Sir Robert Ho Tung was a Eurasian but he regarded himself a Chinese.
48. Irene Cheng, *Intercultural Reminiscences* (Hong Kong: David C. Lam Institute for East-West Studies, Hong Kong Baptist University, 1997), 74–84.
49. Student Card of Eva Ho Tung, University Archives, University of Hong Kong.
50. "Notes and Comments," *Caduceus*, 6(1) (1927): 83.
51. "Varsity Degrees," *South China Morning Post*, 12 January 1927, 8.
52. "Notes and Comments," *Caduceus*, 7(2) (1928): 101.
53. "Notes and Comment," *Caduceus*, 7(3) (1928): 184.
54. "Notes and Comments," *Caduceus*, 8(1) (1929): 69.
55. Dr. Eva Ho Tung was present in a photograph in the farewell gathering of Prof. Tottenham in May 1935, *45th Anniversary Brochure, Obstetrical and Gynaecological Society* (1961–2006), 64.
56. *The Kung Sheung Daily News*, 28 April 1937.
57. "Clinical Report of the Department of Obstetrics and Gynecology of the University of Hong Kong 1937 and 1938," *Caduceus*, 18(2) (1939): 144.
58. Israel Epstein, *Woman in World History: Life and Times of Soong Ching Ling (Mme. Sun Yat-sen)* (Beijing, China: New World Press, distributed by China International Book Trading Co.,1995), 365.
59. Lindsay Ride, "The Test of War," in *Dispersal and Renewal: Hong Kong University During the War Years*, eds. Clifford Matthews and Oswald Cheung (Hong Kong: Hong Kong University Press, 1998), 12.

60. "Anti-epidemic War: Dr. Eva Ho Tung among Chungking Workers, Kweiyang Red Cross," *South China Morning Post*, 30 May 1939, 14.
61. Jean Gittins, *Stanley: Behind the Barbed Wire* (Hong Kong: Hong Kong University Press, 1982), 25.
62. *Kung Sheung Daily News*, 12 March 1946.
63. Cheng, *Intercultural Reminiscences*, 440.
64. Hong Kong Blue Book 1921
65. "Italian Convent School: Yesterday's Prize Distribution," *South China Morning Post*, 26 January 1922, 12.
66. Student Card of Lai Po Chuen. University Archives, University of Hong Kong.
67. Ibid.
68. "Notes and Comments," *Caduceus*, 7(3) (1928 Aug): 186.
69. Moira Chan-Yeung, "Dr Alice Hickling (1876–1928): the Doctor Who Changed the Paradigm of Maternal Care in Hong Kong," *Hong Kong Med J*, 27(5) (2021), 389–391.
70. Hong Kong Blue Book 1928.
71. Hong Kong Blue Book 1929.
72. S. K. Lam, and P. C. Lai, "Colonic Ether in Obstetrics and Gynecology," *Caduceus*, 7(4) (1928 Nov): 238–243.
73. Hong Kong Government Gazette May 1933 no. 317.
74. Hong Kong Government Gazette June 23 1939 no. 501–503.
75. Midwife Ordinance 1910, September 1910. Historical Laws of Hong Kong Online.
76. Report of the Medical Department for the Year 1937. HHAR 1937, M41.
77. School Hygiene Report. Medical Reports for the Year 1931. HKAR 1931, M46. Medical and Sanitary Report for the Year 1929, HKAR 1929, M37.
78. "Anti-TB Association: Standing Commission to Be Created Soon by Governor," *South China Morning Post*, 26 April 1941, 8.
79. "Ambulance Work in Hong Kong: Mr. E. Ralphs Guest of Honor at Dinner," *South China Morning Post*, 28 March 1930, 13.
80. "Ambulance Work: Vital Part Played in Colony's Defence. Report on Activities," *South China Morning Post & the Hongkong Telegraph*, 16 October 1945, 3.
81. "St. John Ambulance: List of Awards for Work During Hostilities. Question of Payments," *South China Morning Post*, 6 November 1946, 4.
82. Report Compiled by Direction of His Excellency Mr. F. C. Gimson, CMG, of Duties Performed by Dr. P. S. Selwyn-Clarke, Director of Medical Services, and Non-interned Staff and Volunteer Helpers, during the Occupation of Hong Kong by the Japanese Forces, CO129/592/1, 25.
83. "Anti-TB Association: Governor Elected Patron at Annual Meeting. Appeal for Support," *South China Morning Post*, 28 September 1946, 7.
84. "Medical Birthday Honors," *Brit Med J* (22 June 1946), 961.
85. The Hong Kong Civil Service List for 1949, Government Printers.
86. "New Baby Clinic at Wan Chai," *South China Morning Post*, 23 March 1932.

87. "Great Step Forward: Opening of the Violet Peel Health Center," *Hong Kong Daily Press*, 14 May 1935.
88. Medical and Sanitary Report for the Year 1935, HKAR 1935, M68.
89. The Hong Kong Civil Service List for 1949, Government Printers.
90. "Local Staff: More Chinese Civil Servants Promoted Government's New Policy Operates," *South China Morning Post*, 5 February 1947, 1.
91. *Family Health Service, Department of Health, 80th Anniversary Family Health Service 2012* (Hong Kong: The Government of Hong Kong SAR, 2012), 13.
92. *The Bulletin of Hong Kong Chinese Medical Association*, 21 (1969): 146.
93. Man-wui Richard Ho, *Tan xuexi yi mingshi* 談學習憶名師 (Hong Kong: The Commercial Press, 2017), 123.
94. The Hong Kong Civil Service List for 1949, Government Printers.
95. "High Post for HK Graduate: University Appoints Woman Professor," *South China Sunday Post-Herald*, 17 February 1957, 1.

Chapter 7

1. G. C. Emerson, *Hong Kong Internment 1942–1945: Life in Japanese Civilian Camp at Stanley* (Hong Kong: Hong Kong University Press, 2008), 36.
2. Report Compiled by Direction of His Excellency Mr. F. C. Gimson, CMG, of Duties Performed by Dr. P. S. Selwyn-Clarke, Director of Medical Services, and Non-interned Staff and Volunteer Helpers, during the Occupation of Hong Kong by the Japanese Forces, CO129/592/1, 20.
3. Edwin Ride, *BAAG: Hong Kong Resistance, 1942–1945* (Hong Kong: Oxford University Press, 1981), 165.
4. "Escape from Hong Kong: Lieut.-Col Gordon King Tells Exciting Tale of Journey into China," *South China Morning Post & the Hongkong Telegraph*, 27 February 1946, 5.
5. Holdsworth and Munn, *Dictionary of Hong Kong Biography*, 387.
6. Saw Swee-Hock, and Chiu Wing Kin, "Population Growth and Redistribution in Hong Kong, 1841–1975," *Southeast Asian Journal of Social Science*, Vol. 4, No. 1 (1975), 126.
7. Sir Geoffry Northcote, Governor, Hong Kong Hansard, 13 October 1938, 119–123.
8. P. S. Selwyn-Clark, Report of the Technical Committee for the Reorganization and Improvement of Existing Official Hospital and Clinical Facilities of the Colony of Hong Kong, 1938–1939, 10.
9. "Anti-TB Association: Standing Commission to be Created Soon by Governor," *South China Morning Post*, 26 April 1941, 8.
10. "Spitting in Public: Control Law Passed by Legislative Council," *South China Morning Post*, 26 April 1940, 10.
11. Percy Selwyn Selwyn-Clarke, *Footprints, the Memoirs of Selwyn Selwyn-Clarke* (United Kingdom: Sino-American Publishing Company, 1975), 61.
12. "Value of Soya Bean: Stressed by Director of Medical Services," *South China Morning Post*, 23 May 1941, 7.

13. "Under the Japanese: Hong Kong's Director of Medical Services Tells History that Exciting December...,"*South China Morning Post & the Hongkong Telegraph*, 7 February 1946, 9.
14. Selwyn-Clarke, *Footprints, the Memoirs of Selwyn Selwyn-Clarke*, 62.
15. Ibid., 68.
16. Report Compiled by Direction of His Excellency Mr. F. C. Gimson, CMG, of Duties Performed by Dr. P. S. Selwyn-Clarke, Director of Medical Services, and Non-interned Staff and Volunteer Helpers, during the Occupation of Hong Kong by the Japanese Forces, CO129/592/#1, 20.
17. P. D. Angus, Report on the Work Undertaken by Dr. P. S. Selwyn-Clarke, Following the Occupation of Hong Kong by the Japanese in December 1941, CO129/592/#1, 47–59.
18. Report Compiled by Direction of His Excellency Mr. F. C. Gimson, CMG, of Duties Performed by Dr. P. S. Selwyn-Clarke, Director of Medical Services, and Non-interned Staff and Volunteer Helpers, during the Occupation of Hong Kong by the Japanese Forces, CO129/592/#1, 25.
19. Ibid., 27.
20. N. C. Macleod, An Account by the Deputy Director of Health Services of the Organization of Health Services in Stanley Internment Camp, In Report on Medical and Health Conditions in Hong Kong for the Period, 1 January 1942 to 31 August 1945, His Majesty's Stationery Office, 1946, 33.
21. M. Horder, "The Hard-Boiled Saint: Selwyn-Clarke in Hong Kong," *Brit Med J*, 311 (1995): 492–495.
22. Selwyn-Clarke, Footprints, 107.
23. Ibid., 109.
24. "Dr Selwyn-Clarke: Tung Wah Hospitals' Officials Say Farewell. Good Deeds Recalled," *South China Morning Post*, 26 April 1947, 6.
25. "New Nurses' Quarters: Selwyn-Clarke Nurses' Home at Kwong Wah Hospital, Opening Ceremony," *South China Morning Post*, 5 January 1952, 8. After World War II, all government reports printed Tung Wa Hospital as Tung Wah Hospital. Kwong Wah Hospital has always been printed as Kwong Wah Hospital from its inception.
26. Holdsworth and Munn, *Dictionary of Hong Kong Biography*, 388–389.
27. "Memorial Service," *South China Morning Post*, 24 March 1976, 5.
28. J. R. Poynter, "Ride, Sir Lindsay Tasman (1898–1977)," Australian Dictionary of Biography, National Centre of Biography, Australian National University, https://adb.anu.edu.au/biography/ride-sir-lindsay-tasman-11524/text20557, published first in hardcopy in 2002, accessed online on 3 February 2024.
29. "Sir Lindsay Ride's Death Ends Close Links with Hongkong for Almost 50 Years," *South China Morning Post*, 19 October 1977, 6.
30. Lindsay Ride, K. D. Ling, E. Q. Lim, and S. F. Cheng. "Some Biochemical Aspects of Acute Cholera," *Caduceus*, 17(4) (1938): 175–201.
31. Gordon King, and L. T. Ride. "The Relation of Vitamin B1 Deficiency to the Pregnancy Anemias—A Study of 371 Cases of Beri-beri Complicating Pregnancy," *J Obstetrics Gynecology British Empire*, LII (2) (1945): 1–18.
32. Lindsay Ride, "Fifty Years of Medical Education in Hong Kong," *Caduceus*, 16(2) (1937): 61.

33. Ibid., 58.
34. Evans, *Constancy of Purpose*, 73–74.
35. Lindsay Ride, "Medical Education in Hong Kong," *Caduceus*, 15(4) (1936): 159–171.
36. "Sir Lindsay Ride C.B.E., Ed., M.A., D.M," *British Medical Journal*, 2 (6096) (1977): 1228.
37. Edwin Ride, *BAAG: Hong Kong Resistance, 1942–1945* (Hong Kong: Oxford University Press, 1981), 165.
38. Chan Sui-jeung, *East River Column: Hong Kong Guerillas in the Second World War and After*, Royal Asiatic Society Hong Kong Studies Series (Hong Kong: Hong Kong University Press, 2009), 49.
39. Alan Birch, "Decisive Role in Survival of War-Ravaged Colony," *South China Morning Post*, 13 October 1973, 2.
40. Bernard Mellor, *The University of Hong Kong—An Informal History* (Hong Kong: Hong Kong University Press, 1980), 143–144.
41. "The Sir Lindsay and Lady Ride Memorial Fund," Royal Asiatic Society Hong Kong, accessed on 8 February 2023, http://www.royalasiaticsociety.org.hk/sir.
42. W. C. W. Nixon. "J. Preston Maxwell, M.D., F.R.C.S., F.R.C.O.G," *British Medical Journal*, 2(5251) (1961): 590–591.
43. Holdsworth and Munn, *"Dictionary of Hong Kong Biography,"* 226.
44. "Great Hall Scenes: University Used as a Trial Hospital. Patients Moved In," *South China Morning Post*, 15 August 1940, 4.
45. "Escape from Hong Kong: Lieut.-Col Gordon King Tells Exciting Tale of Journey into China," *South China Morning Post* & the Hongkong Telegraph, 27 February 1946, 5.
46. Gordon King, "An Episode in the History of the University," in C. Matthews and O. Cheung, *Dispersal and Renewal: Hong Kong University During the War Years* (Hong Kong: Hong Kong University Press, 1998), 87–88.
47. Ibid., 88–92.
48. Ibid., 96–97.
49. Ibid., 98.
50. "Professor Honored: Gordon King Prize Created by Graduates," *South China Morning Post*, 25 May 1951, 3.
51. Frank Ching, *130 Years of Medicine in Hong Kong*, 189.
52. "The University: Progress Made since Reoccupation, Annual Report," *South China Morning Post*, 22 February 1948, 7.
53. "Faculty of Medicine: Projected Development at University Outlined by Prof. Gordon King," *South China Morning Post*, 18 November 1948, 5.
54. "New Hong Kong University Obstetric Department: New Maternity Hospital," *Brit Med J*, 1 (4929) (1955): 1527–1528.
55. "Birth Control Action: Eugenics League Reviews Position after Five Years Significant Birthrate Decline," *South China Morning Post*, 9 May 1941, 8.
56. "Family Planning Assn: An Essential Part of Colony's Social Welfare Machinery," *South China Morning Post*, 13 March 1952, 5.

57. Saw Swee-Hock, and Chiu Wing Kin, "Population Growth and Redistribution in Hong Kong, 1841–1975," *Southeast Asian Journal of Social Science*, 4 (1) (975), 128.
58. Malcolm Allbrook, "King, Gordon (1900–1991)," *Australian Dictionary of Biography*, Volume 1, 2021, 480–481.
59. "Hongkong FPA Gets Full-time Director," *South China Morning Post*, 12 January 1972, 7.

Chapter 8

1. Hong Kong Department of Medical and Health Services Annual Report 1946, Hong Kong Government, 4–5.
2. Ibid., 4–5.
3. Geoffrey Gilbert, "Valedictory: Dr. Isaac Newton Leaves Friday on Retirement," *South China Morning Post*, 2 July 1951.
4. Development of Medical Services in Hong Kong, Hong Kong Government, Government Printers, 1964.
5. "The Further Development of Medical and Health Services in Hong Kong," Hong Kong Government (Hong Kong: Hong Kong Government Printers, 1974).
6. Hong Kong Medical and Health Department Annual Reports 1953–1980.
7. "Global Strategy for Health for All by the Year 2000," World Health Organization, Geneva, 1981.
8. Dick Yeo, Excerpts from 'Glimpses of K. C.'s Life' which was read by Dick Yeo at the Memorial Service held in Mountfield Church on 18 June 2004, accessed on 14 February 2022, http://kcyeo.com/.
9. Hong Kong Blue Book 1939.
10. "Local Weddings: Miss Florence Ho Tung and Dr. K. C. Yeo," *South China Morning Post*, 25 March 1933.
11. Florence Yeo, *My Memories* (Pittsburgh, PA: Dorrance Publishing, 1994), 69–103.
12. Family Health Service, Department of Health, *80th Anniversary Family Health Service*, 2012 (Hong Kong: The Government of the Hong Kong SAR, 2012), 13.
13. S. H. Lee, *Prevention and Control of Communicable Diseases in Hong Kong* (Hong Kong: Government Printer, 1994), 43–45.
14. Hong Kong Medical and Health Department Annual Report, 1947, 11.
15. "Anti-Cholera Campaign," *South China Morning Post*, 20 July 1951; "Medical Department Report: Review by Director," *South China Morning Post*, 24 January 1953.
16. "Tuberculosis Control in Hong Kong," Hong Kong Government, accessed on 23 February 2022, https://www.info.gov.hk/tb_chest/doc/TBcon.pdf.
17. "New Director: Appointment for Dr. K. C. Yeo. Medical Services," *South China Morning Post*, 14 January 1952.
18. "Infectious Contacts. Government Measures for Control of Venereal Disease. Compulsory Treatment," *South China Morning Post*, 20 December 1951.
19. S. H. Lee, *Prevention and Control of Communicable Diseases in Hong Kong* (Hong Kong: Government Printer, 1994), 19–22.

20. Tuberculosis and Chest Service, Public Health Services Branch, Center for Health Protection, Department of Health, Government of the HKSAR Tuberculosis Manual, 2006, 105–111.
21. "Anti-TB Association. Mr. Ruttonjee's Appeal for Funds at Annual Meeting. Warning by Dr. K. C. Yeo," *South China Morning Post*, 28 February 1953. "Anti-TB Association. Plans for Additional Hospital Now Nearing Completion. Appeal for More Support," *South China Morning Post*, 26 February 1953.
22. "New T. B., Dental Clinic. To be Opened by Dr. the Hon K. C. Yeo at Kennedy Town Road Next Month," *South China Morning Post*, 19 March 1954.
23. Annual Report 2020, Tuberculosis and Chest Service of the Department of Health, Hong Kong SAR.
24. "Mission to Lepers. Flag Day Appeal Broadcast by Dr. The Hon K. C. Yeo. Work on Hay Ling Chau," *South China Morning Post*, 24 March 1956. Mimi Mo, "Biographic Notes. The Legacy of Dr. Kok Cheang Yeo, the first Chinese Director of Medical and Health Services of Hong Kong," *JRASHKB*, 54 (2014):181–194.
25. Moira Chan-Yeung, *A Medical History of Hong Kong: The Development and Contributions of Outpatient Clinics*, 92–93.
26. "Tung Wah Hospital. New Annex to Outpatient Department Opened," *South China Morning Post*, 30 March 1956.
27. "New Medical laboratory. Cardio-Respiratory Diagnosis. Opened by D.M.S.," *South China Morning Post*, 15 August, 1956.
28. Z Lett, "Obituary, Dr. Kok Cheang Yeo, CMG, MD, DPH, DTM& H," *Hong Kong College of Anesthesiologists, Newsletter*, September, 2004.
29. "Medical Registration. First Reading of Bill to Be Moved at Meeting Today. Council to Replace Board," *South China Morning Post*, 10 April 1957.
30. "Registration of Nurses. Bill to Amend Chapter of Ordinance," *South China Morning Post*, 6 October 1954.
31. Yeo, *My Memories*, 161–162.
32. "A Tribute to K. C. Yeo, 1 April 1903–24 May 2004," accessed on 15 February 2022, http://kcyeo.com/.
33. "Medical Department. Presentation Made to Dr. the Hon K. C. Yeo. Brilliant Administrator," *South China Morning Post*, 27 June 1957.
34. Patricia Lim, *Forgotten Souls: A Social History of the Hong Kong Cemetery* (Hong Kong: Hong Kong University Press, 2011), 509–510.
35. David Todd, "Gerald Hugh Choa (b.21 March 1921 d.3 December 2001)," *The Royal College of Physicians*, accessed on 7 February 2023, https://history.rcplondon.ac.uk/inspiring-physicians/gerald-hugh-choa.
36. Yu Y. L., abridged version of the talk given by Prof. Sir David Todd at the inauguration of the Medical History Interest Group held at the Hong Kong Museum of Medical Sciences on 17 January 2009. "Reminiscence of Three Former Teachers: Prof. AJS McFadzean, Dr. Stephan Chang and Prof. Gerald Choa," *Hong Kong Med J*, 15(4) (2009) 315–319.
37. Ibid.
38. Arthur van Langenberg, *From Scalpel to Spade: Surgeon's Road to Ithaka* (Hong Kong: The Chinese University of Hong Kong Press, 2021), 23.

39. "Dr. Choa Takes Over July 2, "*South China Morning Post*, 2 June 1970.
40. "History of the Hong Kong Doctors Union," Hong Kong Doctors Union, accessed on 7 February 2023, https://www.hkdu.org/en/about-us/history-hong-kong-doctors-union.
41. "Big Progress in Health of the People," *South China Morning Post*, 14 November 1974.
42. Hong Kong Medical and Health Department Annual Report for the Year 1974/75, 4.
43. "The Problem of Narcotic Drugs in Hong Kong," a White Paper laid before Legislative Council Hong Kong, 11 November 1959, 13–14. (Treatment of addiction)
44. Hong Kong Medical and Health Department Report for the Year 1959, 3.
45. Stuart Heaver, "Shek Kwu Chau, Hong Kong's Drug Rehabilitation Island—Changing Times at the Remote Haven," *South China Morning Post*, 30 October 2017, accessed on 7 February 2023, https://www.scmp.com/lifestyle/article/2117559/shek-kwu-chau-hong-kongs-drug-rehabilitation-island-changing-times-remote.
46. "Physical Rehabilitation, Methadone Maintenance," *South China Morning Post*, 8 July 1974.
47. "Employers Urged to Hire Cured Ex-addicts," *South China Morning Post*, 26 November 1970.
48. "Increase in Mental Illness," *South China Morning Post*, 15 May 1974.
49. "Don't Reject Mentally Sick," *South China Morning Post*, 25 May 1975.
50. "A Sharp Indictment of Our Hospitals," *South China Morning Post*, 15 November 1974.
51. "Development of Medical Services in Hong Kong," Hong Kong Government (Hong Kong: Hong Kong Government Printers, 1964).
52. "The Further Development of Medical and Health Services in Hong Kong," Hong Kong Government (Hong Kong: Hong Kong Government Printers, 1974).
53. "Steps to Relieve Overcrowding in Our Major Hospitals," *South China Morning Post*, 15 November 1974.
54. "Aim of Hospital Fee Rise," *South China Morning Post*, 1 May 1973.
55. Although the White Paper did not think that community nursing was possible in the foreseeable future, the United Christian Hospital program demonstrated the possibility. In 1979, the government began its own community nursing program.
56. "The Further Development of Medical and Health Services in Hong Kong," Hong Kong Government (Hong Kong: Hong Kong Government Printers, 1974).
57. "Rude Hospital Staff Will Be Disciplined," *South China Morning Post*, 8 June 1972.
58. "Dr. Choa to Retire Soon," *South China Morning Post*, 16 November 1976.
59. David Todd, "Gerald Hugh Choa (b.21 March 1921 d.3 December 2001)," *The Royal College of Physicians*, accessed on 7 February 2023, https://history.rcplondon.ac.uk/inspiring-physicians/gerald-hugh-choa.
60. Ibid.
61. A. R. Starling, *The Chance of a Lifetime: The Birth of a New Medical School in Hong Kong* (Hong Kong: The Chinese University of Hong Kong Press, 1988), 65–69.

62. Ibid., 72–73.
63. "Prof. Gerald CHOA, Our Founding Dean," Faculty of Medicine, CUHK, accessed on 18 February 2022, https://geraldchoa.med.cuhk.edu.hk/our_founding_dean.
64. G. H. Choa, *"Heal the Sick" Was Their Motto: The Protestant Medical Missionaries in China* (Hong Kong: The Chinese University of Hong Kong Press, 1990).
65. G. H. Choa, *The Life and Times of Sir Kai Ho Kai* (Hong Kong: The Chinese University of Hong Kong Press, 2000).
66. David Todd, "Gerald Hugh Choa (b.21 March 1921 d.3 December 2001)," *The Royal College of Physicians*, accessed on 7 February 2023, https://history.rcplondon.ac.uk/inspiring-physicians/gerald-hugh-choa.
67. Constance Chan, "Shiu-hung Lee, b.6 June 1933 d.9 January 2014," *The Royal College of Physicians*, accessed on 7 February 2023, https://history.rcplondon.ac.uk/inspiring-physicians/shiu-hung-lee.
68. Honorary Fellow. A Citation. Professor Lee Shiu Hung, SBS, ISO, MBBS, MD, DPH, DIH, FRCP (Lon), FFPH (UK), FAFOM (Aust), FFOK (UK). FRACMA (Aust), FHKAM (CM), Hon. Fellow (HKCCM), JP, accessed on 25 February 2024, https://honfellow.cuhk.edu.hk/Citation/en/8_leeshiuhung.pdf.
69. Hong Kong Medical and Health Department Annual Report 1962–1963, 3.
70. Constance Chan, "Shiu-hung Lee, b.6 June 1933 d.9 January 2014," *The Royal College of Physicians*, accessed on 7 February 2023, https://history.rcplondon.ac.uk/inspiring-physicians/shiu-hung-lee.
71. "Lee Tipped for New Role," *South China Morning Post*, 21 October 1988.
72. "Health for All, the Way Forward: Report of the Working Party on Primary Health Care," Hong Kong Government (Hong Kong: Hong Kong Government Printer, 1990).
73. R. Gauld and D. Gould, *The Hong Kong Health Sector* (Hong Kong: The Chinese University of Hong Kong Press, 2002), 83–84.
74. G. Leung and J. Bacon-Shone, *Hong Kong's Health System: Reflections, Perspectives and Visions* (Hong Kong: Hong Kong University Press, 2006), 146.
75. Honorary Fellow, A Citation, Professor Lee Shiu Hung, SBS, ISO, MBBS, MD, DPH, DIH, FRCP (Lon), FFPH (UK), FAFOM (Aust), FFOK (UK). FRACMA (Aust), FHKAM (CM), Hon. Fellow (HKCCM), JP, accessed on 25 February 2024, https://honfellow.cuhk.edu.hk/Citation/en/8_leeshiuhung.pdf.
76. "Milestone," The Jockey Club School of Public Health and Primary Care website, accessed on 7 February 2023, https://www.sphpc.cuhk.edu.hk/milestones.
77. Honorary Fellow, A Citation, Professor Lee Shiu Hung, SBS, ISO, MBBS, MD, DPH, DIH, FRCP (Lon), FFPH (UK), FAFOM (Aust), FFOK (UK). FRACMA (Aust), FHKAM (CM), Hon. Fellow (HKCCM), JP, accessed on 25 February 2024, https://honfellow.cuhk.edu.hk/Citation/en/8_leeshiuhung.pdf.
78. Colin Binns, Andy Lee, and Wah Yun Low, "Obituary, Professor Shiu-Hung Lee," *Asia-Pacific Journal of Public Health*, 26(2) (2014): 215–216.
79. "Building Healthy Cities. Guidelines for Implementing a healthy City Project in Hong Kong," Department of Health, 2007.
80. Honorary Fellow, A Citation, Professor Lee Shiu Hung, SBS, ISO, MBBS, MD, DPH, DIH, FRCP (Lon), FFPH (UK), FAFOM (Aust), FFOK (UK). FRACMA (Aust), FHKAM (CM), Hon. Fellow (HKCCM), JP.

81. "Director of Health Deeply Saddened by Death of Professor Lee Shiu-hung," Department of Health, The Government of the Hong Kong SAR, accessed on 7 February 2023, https://www.dh.gov.hk/english/press/2014/140109.html.
82. "Shiu-hung Lee, b.6 June 1933 d.9 January 2014," *The Royal College of Physicians*, accessed on 7 February 2023, https://history.rcplondon.ac.uk/inspiring-physicians/shiu-hung-lee.
83. Jacob W. T. Ng, and John Y. H. Ho, "An Addendum to 'Doctor for Society'—Professor Lee Shiu Hung: 'Pass on Benevolence, Pass on the Legend'," *Hong Kong Med J*, 20 (2) (2014): 169.

Chapter 9

1. Medical and Sanitary Report 1927, Hong Kong Administrative Reports, 1927, M [1] 12–13.
2. Gordon King, "The History of Tsan Yuk Hospital 1922–1955," *Bulletin of the Hong Kong Chinese Medical Association*, 8 (1956): 31–39.
3. Cunich, *A History of the University of Hong Kong*, 319–320.
4. C. M. Fung, *A History of Queen Mary Hospital, Hong Kong* (Hong Kong: Queen Mary Hospital, 1997), 17.
5. "Hay Ling Chau," International Leprosy Association—History of Leprosy, accessed on 8 February 2023, https://leprosyhistory.org/database/archive308.
6. Fung, *A History of Queen Mary Hospital*, Hong Kong, 25.
7. Vernon Ram, *Emperor Extraordinaire: The Life and Work of John HC Ho* (Hong Kong: Scientific Communications (HK) Ltd, 2003), 6–8.
8. Ibid., 10.
9. Ibid., 10–11.
10. Ibid., 29.
11. Ibid., 12–13.
12. Jane Parry, "Obituary: John HC Ho," *Brit Med J*, 331 (2005): 578.
13. A. W. M. Lee. "A Tribute to the Emperor Extraordinaire: The Legend of Professor John HC Ho," *J HK Coll Radiol*, 8 (2005): 117–120.
14. Ram, *Emperor Extraordinaire: The Life and Work of John HC Ho*, 21–25.
15. A. W. M. Lee. "A Tribute to the Emperor Extraordinaire: The Legend of Professor John HC Ho," *J HK Coll Radiol*, 8 (2005): 117–120.
16. Ram, *Emperor Extraordinaire: The Life and Work of John HC Ho*, 44.
17. Ibid., 45–46.
18. Nam Long Hospital was also a hospice and for the Chinese is a hospital for the "dying" and the hospital fell into disfavor.
19. L. Y. Fong, J. H. Ho, and D. P. Huang, "Preserved Foods as Possible Cancer Hazards: WA Rats Fed Salted Fish Have Mutagenic Urine," *Int J Cancer*, 23 (1979): 542–546.
20. John H. C. Ho. "An Epidemiologic and Clinical Study of Nasopharyngeal Carcinoma," *Int. I Radiation Oncology, Biology, Physics*, 4(3–4) (1978): 193–198.

21. A. W. M. Lee, "A Tribute to the Emperor Extraordinaire: The Legend of Professor John HC Ho," *J HK Coll Radiol*, 8 (2005): 117–120.
22. Ram, Emperor Extraordinaire: The Life and Work of John HC Ho, 50.
23. A. W. M. Lee, "A Tribute to the Emperor Extraordinaire: The Legend of Professor John HC Ho," *J HK Coll Radiol*, 8 (2005): 117–120.
24. Ibid.
25. 粒粒皆辛苦. This is a quotation from poet Li Shen 李紳 in the Tang Dynasty—《憫農》:「鋤禾日當午，汗滴禾下土。誰知盤中飧，粒粒皆辛苦？」(*Min Nong*: The farmers are working hard in the fields under the midday sun, with drops of their sweat falling onto the earth. Who understands that each and every grain in our bowl of rice has come from such strenuous labor?) (translation taken from Rey Chow, "Thinking with Food, Writing Off Center: Notes on Two Hong Kong Authors," in *Global Chinese Literature: Critical Essays*, eds. by Jing Tsu and David Der-wei Wang, Vol. 3 (Leiden: Koninklijke Brill NV, 2010), 135.
26. A. W. M. Lee, "A Tribute to the Emperor Extraordinaire: the Legend of Professor John HC Ho," *J HK Coll Radiol*, 8 (2005): 117–120.
27. "Founding Father of Mental Care," *South China Morning Post*, 21 August 1978.
28. The Victoria Institution is a memorial school, partly funded by public subscription intended for the erection of a permanent memorial to commemorate the Golden Jubilee of Queen Victoria in 1887, and partly supported by contributions from the Sultan and subscriptions from the prominent residents and the public.
29. T. W. Fan, "The Life and Works of Professor Pow-meng Yap", *Hong Kong Journal of Mental Health*, 28 (1999):16–20.
30. Report of the Acting Principal Civil Medical Officer for the Year 1900, HKSP 1901, 252. Dr. John Kerr, an American medical missionary, after retiring from the Canton Hospital in 1899, devoted all his time to caring for people with mental illness. Between 1876 and 1880, Kerr campaigned for the necessary and just treatment of patients in mental hospitals, but the city government did not want to build a mental hospital. Kerr used his own money to purchase 17 acres of land in Fangcun, as a building site for the hospital. With donors' assistance, two buildings were erected in 1898 as a hospital.
31. "Mental Illness: Talk by Dr. Yap," *South China Morning Post*, 29 May 1953.
32. "Mental Abnormality: Talk by Dr. Yap," *South China Morning Post*, 11 December 1953.
33. "Mental Hygiene: HK School Child's Problems, Guidance Clinic Need," *South China Morning Post*, 6 November 1951.
34. T. N. Foo, "The Mental Health Association of Hong Kong: A Brief History," in *Aspects of Mental Health Care: Hong Kong 1981*, ed. T. P. Khoo (Hong Kong: Mental Health Association of Hong Kong, 1981), 85–103.
35. W. H. Lo, "Development of Legislation for the Mentally Ill in Hong Kong," *J Hong Kong Psychiatr Assoc*, 8 (1988), 6–9.
36. Medical and Health Department Annual Report, 1965/1966, 29.
37. Edward L. Margetts, "Pow Meng Yap (1921–1971)," *Canad Psychiat Ass J*, 17 (1972): 253–254.
38. "Community Attitude to Mental Health Needs to Be Changed," *South China Morning Post*, 18 March 1988.

39. S. Liu, "The New Life and I," in *New Life Psychiatric Rehabilitation Association Annual Report 1990*, 49–51.

40. Ibid.; "Milestones," New Life Psychiatric Rehabilitation Association, accessed on 8 February 2023, https://www.nlpra.org.hk/55year/en/milestone.

41. Hong Kong Medical and Health Department Report for the Year 1966/1967, 28.

42. Hong Kong Medical and Health Department Report for the Year 1968/1969, 29.

43. Hong Kong Hospital Authority Statistical Report (2013a) for 2011/2012.

44. "Reasons for Suicide: Poverty, Illness, Unemployment Most Important Causes Here. Men and Women Ratios," *South China Morning Post*, 25 April 1956.

45. P. M. Yap, "Suicide in Hong Kong," *Journal of Mental Science*, 194 (1958): 261–301.

46. P. M. Yap, "Koro—A Culture-bound Depersonalization Syndrome," *British Journal of Psychiatry*, 111 (1965): 43–50.

47. P. M. Yap, "The Latah Reaction: Its Pathodynamics and Nosological Position," *Journal of Mental Science*, 98 (1952): 515–564.

48. Helen F. K. Chiu, "Professor Pow-Meng Yap: A Giant in Psychiatry from Hong Kong," *Asia-Pacific Psychiatry*, 4(2012): 84–86.

49. Edward L. Margetts, "Pow Meng Yap (1921–1971)," *Canad Psychiat Ass J*, 17 (1972): 253–254.

50. "Psychiatric Department for HKU," *South China Morning Post*, 8 May 1971.

51. Edward L. Margetts, "Pow Meng Yap (1921–1971)," *Canad Psychiat Ass J*, 17 (1972); 253–254.

52. Ronald Lo, "Obituary—Dr. Zoltan (Lefty) Lett," Royal College of Anesthetists, accessed on 8 February 2023, https://rcoa.ac.uk/obituary-dr-zoltan-lefty-lett.

53. Patrick P. Sim, "A Measure of Gold, Hong Kong Anesthesia at 50," *Anesthesiology*, 107(1) (2007): 153.

54. Ronald Lo, "Dr. Zoltan Lett, MD, DA, FRCA, FFARCS, FANZCA, FHKCA, FHKAM (Anes) on the Conferment of Honorary Fellowship of the Hong Kong College of Anesthesiologists at the 25th Congregation of the College," accessed on 8 February 2023, https://www.hkca.edu.hk/archives/HKCAbulletin/E-news/doc/Citation-Zoltan_Lett.pdf.

55. Patrick P. Sim, "A Measure of Gold, Hong Kong Anesthesia at 50," *Anesthesiology*, 107(1) (2007): 154.

56. "Colony's First Anesthetists Society Formed," *South China Morning Post*, 18 June 1954.

57. Roland Lo, "Dr. Zoltan Lett, MD, DA, FRCA, FFARCS, FANZCA, FHKCA, FHKAM (Anes) on the Conferment of Honorary Fellowship of the Hong Kong College of Anesthesiologists at the 25th Congregation of the College."

58. Ibid.

59. Ibid.

60. Patrick P. Sim, "A Measure of Gold, Hong Kong Anesthesia at 50," *Anesthesiology*, 107(1) (2007): 156.

61. Fiona E. Kelly , Kevin Fong, Nicholas Hirsch, and Jerry P. Nolan, "Intensive Care Medicine Is 60 years Old: The History and Future of the Intensive Care Unit," *Clin Med (Lond)*, 14(4) (2014): 376–379.

62. J. E. Calvin, K. Habet, and J. E. Parrillo, "Critical Care in the United States. Who Are We and How Did We Get Here?" *Crit Care Clin*, 13 (2) (1997): 363–376.
63. Z. Lett, *Anesthesia* (Hong Kong: Hong Kong University Press, 1983); Z. Lett, *History of Anesthesia in Hong Kong* (Hong Kong: Centre for Asian Studies, Hong Kong University, 1987); Z. Lett, and Ronald Lo, "Anesthesia and Intensive Care in Hong Kong: Evolution and Present Position," Centre for Asian Studies, Hong Kong University 1997; "Doctor Relates a Pathfinder Role," *South China Morning Post*, 20 June 1982.
64. "High Standards as the Gas Man Cometh," *South China Morning Post*, 28 March 1984.
65. Roland Lo, "Dr. Zoltan Lett, MD, DA, FRCA, FFARCS, FANZCA, FHKCA, FHKAM (Anes) on the Conferment of Honorary Fellowship of the Hong Kong College of Anesthesiologists at the 25th Congregation of the College."

Chapter 10

1. J. Duffin, *History of Medicine* (Toronto: University of Toronto Press, 1999), 344–345.
2. Cunich, *A History of the University of Hong Kong*, 362–363.
3. Colonial Office, Note on Present Position regarding Hong Kong University, 20 December 1947, CO 129/610/1.
4. Moira Chan-Yeung, *A Medical History of Hong Kong 1942–2015* (Hong Kong: The Chinese University of Hong Kong Press, 2019) 195–196.
5. Medical and Health Department Annual Reports 1953–1980.
6. "The Further Development of Medical and Health Services in Hong Kong," Hong Kong Government (Hong Kong: Hong Kong Government Printers, 1974).
7. David Todd, "Recent Developments in Medical Education in Hong Kong," in Hong Kong Museum of Medical Sciences Society, *Plague, SARS and the Story of Medicine in Hong Kong* (Hong Kong: Hong Kong University Press, 2006), 288–289.
8. Hong Kong Academy of Medicine, *In Pursuit of Excellence, The First 10 years 1993–2003* (Hong Kong: Hong Kong Academy of Medicine, 2003), 15–16.
9. Lau Chi-pang, and Liu Shuyong, *Hou baozhang jiazu shi* 侯寶璋家族史 (Hong Kong: Peace Book Co. Ltd., 2012), 12–14.
10. Citation: Hou Pao Chang, Doctor of Science *honoris causa*, 54th Congregation (1961), The University of Hong Kong, accessed on 7 February 2024, https://www4.hku.hk/hongrads/citations/md-pao-chang-hou-hou-pao-chang.
11. "Obituaries. Professor Hou Pao Chang," *Nature* 214, (1967): 539.
12. "HK University. Recent Appointments Made by the Council. Six Professors," *South China Morning Post*, 28 August 1948.
13. Lau Chi-pang, and Liu Shuyong, *Hou Baozhang jiazu shi*, 23–24.
14. Evans, *Constancy of Purpose*, 89–90.
15. Suyin Han, *My House Has Two Doors* (New York: Putnam Pub Group, 1980), 36.
16. "University Loses Two Professors," *South China Morning Post*, 1 June 1960.
17. "University Celebrates Golden Anniversary. Honorary Degrees Conferred at Special Congregation," *South China Morning Post*, 10 January 1961.

18. Fan Ka-wai, "Hou Pao-chang, (1893–1967): Pathologist and Historian of Chinese Medicine," *Journal of Medical Biography*, 14(2) (2006), accessed on 11 February 2022, https://journals.sagepub.com/doi/abs/10.1177/096777200601400407.
19. "Former HKU Professor Dies," *South China Morning Post*, 21 March 1967.
20. Lau Chi-pang, and Liu Shuyong, *Hou Baozhang jiazu shi*, 17, 24–26.
21. Roy Cameron, *Hou Pao Chang. Biliary Cirrhosis* (Edinburgh: Oliver and Boyd, 1962), quoted in Fan Ka-wai, "Hou Pao-chang, (1893–1967): Pathologist and Historian of Chinese Medicine.".
22. C. T. Huang, "Prof. Hou Pao-Chang," *Elixir*, 1, (1967), 15.
23. Pao-Chang Hou, "A History of Anatomy in China," *Yixue shi yu baojian zuzhi* (History of Medicine and Hygiene Organization 醫學史與保健組織), 1 (1) (1957): 64–73; quoted in Fan Ka-wai, "Hou Pao-chang, (1893–1967): Pathologist and Historian of Chinese Medicine.".
24. Pao-Chang Hou, "Malaria in Tang Poetry," *Present Day Chinese Medical Journal*, 9 (1961): 815–916, quoted in Fan Ka-wai, "Hou Pao-chang, (1893–1967): Pathologist and Historian of Chinese Medicine."
25. Joseph Needham, *Science and Civilization in China: Vol 1* (Cambridge: Cambridge University Press, 1954), 12, quoted in Fan Ka-wai, "Pao-chang Hou, (1893–1967): Pathologist and Historian of Chinese Medicine."
26. Lau Chi-pang, and Liu Shuyong, *Hou Baozhang jiazu shi*, 55–56.
27. Information from Centre for Research Collections, Edinburgh University Library.
28. Citation: James Blackburn Gibson, Doctor of Science, *honoris causa*, 118th Congregation (1983), The Hong Kong University.
29. James Blackburn Gibson, "The Hepatic Veins in Health and Disease," MD thesis, The Faculty of Medicine, University of Edinburgh, October 1958, accessed on 8 February 2024, https://era.ed.ac.uk/handle/1842/32270.
30. Citation: James Blackburn Gibson, Doctor of Science, *honoris causa*, 118th Congregation (1983), The Hong Kong University.
31. "History," Department of Pathology, School of Clinical Medicine, HKU, accessed on 6 February 2023, https://www.patho.hku.hk/en/About-Us/History.
32. Clarence C. K. Lam, "Journey through Quantitative Hematology," *Hong Kong Med J*, 26 (6) (2020): 556–558.
33. Ibid.
34. Ching, *130 Years of Medicine in Hong Kong*, 326–338
35. Citation: James Blackburn Gibson, Doctor of Science, *honoris causa*, 118th Congregation, 1983, The Hong Kong University.
36. Ching, *130 Years of Medicine in Hong Kong*, 346.
37. Rayson Huang, "Eulogy: Professor James Blackburn Gibson," Hong Kong University Digital Repository at HKUL, Interflow no. 71, March 1994.
38. "History," Department of Pathology, School of Clinical Medicine, The University of Hong Kong, accessed on 6 February 2023, https://www.patho.hku.hk/en/About-Us/History.
39. Citation: James Blackburn Gibson, Doctor of Science, *honoris causa*, 118th Congregation (1983), The Hong Kong University.
40. Rayson Huang, "Eulogy: Professor James Blackburn Gibson," Hong Kong University Digital Repository at HKUL, Interflow no. 71, March 1994.

41. Citation: James Blackburn Gibson, Doctor of Science, *honoris causa*, 118th Congregation (1983), The Hong Kong University.
42. "Obituary. A. J. S. McFadzean, OBE, DSc, MD, FRCP, FRCP Ed, FACP," *Brit Med J*, 6 (1974): 723.
43. "The Great Expansion—The McFadzean Era (1948–1974)," in *HKU Department of Medicine, 1995–2019, Impact Inspirations* (Hong Kong: The University of Hong Kong, 2021), 38–59.
44. Fung, *A History of Queen Mary Hospital Hong Kong*, 68.
45. Ibid., 101.
46. Y. L. Yu, abridged version of the talk given by Prof. Sir David Todd at the Inauguration of the Medical History Interest Group held at the Hong Kong Museum of Medical Sciences on 17 January 2009. "Reminiscence of Three Former Teachers: Prof. AJS McFadzean, Dr. Stephen Chang and Prof Gerald Choa," *Hong Kong Med J*, 15(4) (2009), 315–319.
47. Hong Kong Medical and Health Department Annual Reports, 1951 to 1971.
48. "The Great Expansion—The McFadzean Era (1948–1974)," in *HKU Department of Medicine, 1995–2019, Impact Inspirations* (Hong Kong: The University of Hong Kong, 2021), 50–51.
49. Ibid., 52.
50. "Hau-Cheong Kwaan," in *Centenary Tribute to Professor AJS McFadzean. A Legacy for Medicine in Hong Kong* (Hong Kong: Hong Kong Academy of Medicine, 2015), 34.
51. R. T. T. Young, "Vision and Mission. A History of the Department of Medicine," in *Achievements in Medicine, 1989–1995, Department of Medicine, HKU* (Hong Kong: ColorPrint Production Co., 1995), 1–13.
52. "T. K. Chan," in *Centenary Tribute to Professor AJS McFadzean*, 19.
53. Arthur Van Langenberg, *From Scalpel to Spade: A Surgeon's Road to Ithaka* (Hong Kong: The Chinese University of Hong Kong Press, 2021), 16.
54. "Donald Yu," in *Centenary Tribute to Professor AJS McFadzean*, 65.
55. David Todd, "Professor A. J. S. McFadzean—An Appreciation," *Caduceus*, Special issue, the McFadzean Memorial Issue, 1, 1975, 121–123.
56. David Todd, "Tribute," in *Centenary Tribute to Professor AJS McFadzean*, 8–9.
57. R. T. T. Young, "Vision and Mission. A History of the Department of Medicine," 2.
58. Y. L. Yu, abridged version of the talk given by Prof. Sir David Todd at the Inauguration of the Medical History Interest Group held at the Hong Kong Museum of Medical Sciences on 17 January 2009. "Reminiscence of Three Former Teachers: Prof. AJS McFadzean, Dr. Stephen Chang and Prof Gerald Choa," *Hong Kong Med J*, 15(4) (2009) 315–319.
59. "Sum-ping Lee," in *Centenary Tribute to Professor AJS McFadzean*, 42.
60. Y. L. Yu, abridged version of the talk given by Prof Sir David Todd at the Inauguration of the Medical History Interest Group held at the Hong Kong Museum of Medical Sciences on 17 January 2009. "Reminiscence of Three Former Teachers: Prof. AJS McFadzean, Dr. Stephen Chang and Prof Gerald Choa," *Hong Kong Med J*, 15(4) (2009) 315–319.
61. Richard Yu, "Preface," in *Centenary Tribute to Professor AJS McFadzean*, 7.
62. David Todd, "Professor A. J. S. McFadzean—An Appreciation," *Caduceus*, Special issue, the McFadzean Memorial Issue, 1, 1975, 121–123.

63. T. K. Chan, "Tribute and Biography: David Todd," in *Achievements in Medicine 1974–1989. Department of Medicine, Univerity of Hong Kong* (Hong Kong: Hong Kong Univerity Press), 1989, 1.
64. Interview of Professor Sir David Todd by DBS carried out on 1 December 2015, Steps (DBS School Magazine, Chinese section), 2016, 11–16.
65. T. K. Chan, "Tribute and Biography. David Todd," in *Achievements in Medicine 1974–1989, Department of Medicine, Univerity of Hong Kong*, 1.
66. Rosie Young, "Eulogy," In Memoriam: Professor Sir David Todd 1928–2017, accessed on 6 February 2023, https://www.med.hku.hk/remembertodd/Eulogy.pdf.
67. T. K. Chan, "Tribute and Biography. David Todd," in Achievements in Medicine 1974–1989. Department of Medicine, University of Hong, 1–2.
68. S. K. Lam, and W. M. Hui, "Achievements in Gastroenterology/Hepatology," in Achievements in Medicine 1974–1985, Department of Medicine, University of Hong Kong, 45–54.
69. K. L. Cheung, "Achievements in Cardiology," in Achievements in Medicine 1974–1989, Department of Medicine, University of Hong Kong, 28–32.
70. R. T. T. Young, C. Wang, K. S. L. Lam, K. K. Pun, and A. W. C. Kung, "Achievements in Endocrinology," in Achievements in Medicine 1974–1985, Department of Medicine, Univerity of Hong Kong, 37–44.
71. T. K. Chan, "Achievements in Haematology," in *Achievements in Medicine 1974–1989, Department of Medicine, Univerity of Hong Kong*, 64.
72. "Urgent Need for Medical Specialists," *South China Morning Post*, 29 August 1991.
73. Cindy L. K. Lam, "Obituary: Professor Sir David Todd, 1928–2017, Honorary Fellow, Hong Kong College of Family Physicians," accessed on 6 February 2023, https://www.hkcfp.org.hk/Upload/Commemorative/Obituary_and_Remembrances/obituary-Prof.%20DavidTodd.pdf.
74. R. T. T. Young, "Vision and Mission. A History of the Department of Medicine," in *Achievements in Medicine, 1985–1995, Department of Medicine, Univerity of Hong Kong*, 3.
75. R & D Funding, Hong Kong Annual Digest of Statistics, 2014.
76. "Research and Development Statistics," OECD, accessed on 17 March 2022, http://www.oecd.org/innovation/inno/researchanddevelopmentstatisticsrds.htm.
77. Citation: David Todd, Doctor of Science *honoris causa*, 143rd Congregation (1992), The University of Hong Kong, accessed on 6 February 2023, http://www4.hku.hk/hongrads/index.php/archive/graduate_detail/214.
78. T. K. Chan, "Tribute and Biography, David Todd," *Achievements in Medicine 1974–1989, Department of Medicine, Univerity of Hong Kong*, 2.
79. R. T. T. Young, "Visions and Missions. A History of the Department," *Achievements in Medicine 1989–1995, Department of Medicine, University of Hong Kong*, 3.
80. Hong Kong Academy of Medicine, *In Pursuit of Excellence*, 11–13.
81. "Medical Body to be approved," *South China Morning Post*, 20 July 1992.
82. Hong Kong Academy of Medicine, *In Pursuit of Excellence*, 15–16.
83. Ibid., 58–60.

84. "AIDS Groups Back Funding Advisers," *South China Morning Post*, 17 April 1993.
85. "Team Set to Act on Whitehead Report," *South China Morning Post*, 11 June 1994.
86. C. S. Lau, "Professor Sir David Todd," *Hong Kong Med J*, 23(2017): 541.
87. "A Knight Hospitaler," *South China Morning Post*, 2 July 1995.
88. T. K. Chan, "Tribute and Biography," in *Achievements in Medicine 1974–1989, Department of Medicine, Univerity of Hong Kong*, 2.
89. "In Memoriam: Professor Sir David Todd, 1928–2017," an online condolences book by LKS Faculty of Medicine, The University of Hong Kong, accessed on 6 February 2023, https://www.med.hku.hk/remembertodd/book.html.
90. Ching, *130 Years of Medicine in Hong Kong*, 260.
91. Ibid., 262–263.
92. Ibid., 270.
93. "Our History," School of Clinical Medicine, Department of Orthopaedics and Traumatology, HKU Med, accessed on 6 February 2023, https://www.ortho.hku.hk/about-us/history/.
94. Ibid.
95. "A Controlled Trial of Anterior Spinal Fusion and Debridement in the Surgical Management of Tuberculosis of the Spine in Patients on Standard Chemotherapy: A Study in Hong Kong," *The British Journal of Surgery*, 61 (1974): 853–866.
96. "Convalescent Home for Children. Relief for the Disabled. Lady Grantham Performed Opening Ceremony," *South China Morning Post*, 15 November 1956.
97. Ching, *130 Years of Medicine in Hong Kong*, 267–268.
98. Ibid., 275–279.
99. Alpaslan Senkoylu, "Arthur Ralph Hodgson," *The Journal of Turkish Spinal Surgery*, 23(3) 2012, 253–257.
100. Ching, *130 Years of Medicine in Hong Kong*, 280.
101. Lain Macintyre, and Lain MacLaren, *Surgeons' Lives: Royal College of Surgeons of Edinburgh: An Anthology of College Fellows Over 500 Years* (Edinburgh: Royal College of Surgeons of Edinburgh, 2005): 291–292. In the Middle Ages, soldiers who required surgery during and after battles were operated on by barber surgeons, who had razors and possessed good manual dexterity. In 1540, The Company of Barber Surgeons was formed as the specialist college for surgeons in the UK.
102. "Ong, Guan Bee (1921–2004)," Plarr's Lives of the Fellows, The Royal College of Surgeons of England, accessed on 6 February 2023, https://livesonline.rcseng.ac.uk/client/en_GB/lives/search/detailnonmodal/ent:$002f$002fSD_ASSET$002f0$002fSD_ASSET:372574/one?qu=Ong+Guan+B&te=ASSEThttps://livesonline.rcseng.ac.uk/client/en_GB/lives/search/results?qu=Ong+G.+B.&te=ASSET.
103. "First Chinese Professor of Surgery," *South China Morning Post*, 1 April 1964.
104. The Royal College of Surgeons of England, "Obituary: Guan Bee Ong," *BMJ*, 328 (2004): 771.
105. The College of Surgeons of Hong Kong, *Healing with a Scalpel, From the First Colonial Surgeon to the College of Surgeons of Hong Kong* (Hong Kong: Hong Kong Academy of Medicine Press, 2010), 97.

106. Raj M. Nambiar, "Obituary, Professor Tan Sri Guan Bee Ong, PSM, OBE, MD, DS, FAMS (Hon) (1921–10 January 2004"), *Annals Academy of Medicine*, May 2004, accessed on 6 February 2023, https://annals.edu.sg/pdf200405/V33N3p398.pdf.
107. "HKU Mourns the Death of Professor G. B. Ong, 12 Jan 2004," The University of Hong Kong, accessed on 28 February 2022, https://www.hku.hk/press/news_detail_4946.html.
108. Raj M. Nambiar, "Obituary, Professor Tan Sri Guan Bee Ong PSM, OBE, MD, DS, FAMS (Hon) (1921, 10 January 2004)," *Annals Academy of Medicine*, May 2004.
109. Ibid.
110. "HKU Mourns the Death of Professor G. B. Ong, 12 Jan 2004."
111. "Ong, Guan Bee (1921–2004)," Plarr's Lives of the Fellows, The Royal College of Surgeons of England.
112. Ibid.
113. The College of Surgeons of Hong Kong, *Healing with a Scalpel, From the First Colonial Surgeon to the College of Surgeons of Hong Kong*, 98.
114. Arthur Van Langenberg, From Scalpel to Spade, 50.
115. In Chinese: 玉不琢不成器, 嚴師出高徒.
116. Gabriel Leung, "Shizhiminggui de dayi—Wangyuanmei" 實至名歸的大醫——王源美, in *Dayi jingcheng: Xianggang yixue fazhan yibai sanshi nian* 大醫精誠：香港醫學發展一百三十年 (Hong Kong: Joint Publishing (HK) Co. Ltd., 2017) 106–109.
117. "A Silent Game of Patients…," *South China Morning Post*, 25 May, 1975.
118. "Nurses Must Heed This Plea," *South China Morning Post*, 4 January 1979.
119. "Doctor's Bitter Dose," *South China Morning Post*, 17 January 1979.
120. Leung, "Shizhiminggui de dayi," 106–109.
121. "HKU Mourns the Death of Professor G. B. Ong, 12 Jan 2004."

Chapter 11

1. Hong Kong Government, Hong Kong Annual Digest of Statistics 1954 to 2015.
2. Development of Medical Services in Hong Kong, Hong Kong Government, Government Printers, 1964.
3. Working Party on Primary Health Care Report 1990, 8.
4. G. Leung, and J. Bacon-Shone, *Hong Kong's Health System: Reflections, Perspectives and Visions* (Hong Kong: Hong Kong University Press, 2006), 145.
5. Albert Rodrigues, "A Hong Kong Doctor in War and Peace," in *Dispersal and Renewal, Hong Kong University During the War Years*, eds., Clifford Matthews and Oswald Cheung (Hong Kong: Hong Kong University Press, 1998), 203–205. Personal communication from Dr. Albert Edward Rodrigues, son of Sir Albert, about the musical instrument he played.
6. Charles Roland, "Sir Alert Rodrigues, M. D., POW Experiences as a MO in Hong Kong 1941–1945," interviewed in Hong Kong, China by Charles Roland 8 September 1987, Oral History Archives. Hannah Chair for the *History of Medicine*, McMaster University. Interview no. HCM 8–87.
7. Albert Rodrigues, "A Hong Kong Doctor in War and Peace," 206–207.

8. Holdsworth and Munn, *Dictionary of Hong Kong Biography*, 374.
9. Louis E. Keloon Ha, Wai Lun Tam, and Patrick Taveirne, eds., *The History of St. Paul's Hospital: Caring and Serving for 120 Years* (Hong Kong: Centre for Catholic Studies, The Chinese University of Hong Kong, 2018), 68.
10. Holdsworth and Munn, *Dictionary of Hong Kong Biography*, 374.
11. Personal information from Dr. A. E. Rodrigues.
12. Ibid.
13. The calculation was based on the census data of 1961, the average salary of the population, and the cost of various medical procedures.
14. Report of the Medical Development Advisory Committee 1973, Hong Kong Government Printer, Hong Kong, 2.
15. "The Problem of Narcotic Drugs in Hong Kong," a White Paper laid before Legislative Council, Hong Kong, 11 November 1959, 3.
16. Ibid., 13–14.
17. "Drug Addicts. Rehabilitation More Difficult Than Cure," *South China Morning Post*, 25 July 1968.
18. The Society for the Aid and Rehabilitation of Drug Abusers (SARDA), accessed on 7 February 2023, https://www.sarda.org.hk/eng/index.html.
19. "Shek Kwu Chau, Hong Kong's Drug Rehabilitation Island—Changing Times at the Remote Haven," *South China Morning Post*, 30 October 2017, accessed on 14 February 2020, https://www.scmp.com/lifestyle/article/2117559/shek-kwu-chau-hong-kongs-drug-rehabilitation-island-changing-times-remote.
20. "Shek Kwu Chau Plans Hospital, Reservoir," *South China Morning Post*, 16 December 1966.
21. Hong Kong Medical and Health Department Report for the Year 1967/1968, 29.
22. G. Choa, "An Odyssey to a Land of Woes," *Hong Kong Journal of Mental Health*, 28 (1999), 63.
23. "Philanthropist Knighted. Queen's Recognition for Twenty-two Residents. New Year Honors," *South China Morning Post*, 1 January 1964.
24. "School Medical service," *South China Morning Post*, 15 May 1962.
25. After the war, the School Health Program was reestablished for government schools initially and grant schools later. The program consisted of two parts: 1) school inspection of school premises to ensure the environment was fit for schooling; 2) medical examination of the students as they entered the program, and repeated at the ages of 5, 7, 10, 12, 15, and 18. Those found to have abnormalities would be referred to general or special outpatient services such as dental, eye, and ENT. Participants in the scheme only made an annual payment of HK$15 and enjoyed free medical, dental, and ophthalmologic attention. Children requiring hospitalization were admitted to government hospitals and only paid a nominal fee of HK$5. In 1953, the school population was around 200,000, and the number of participants in the School Health Program around 46,051 (less than 25%). The program required a large number of medical staff and a huge budget and yet only serving less than 25% of the school children. As a result, the medical and curative portion of the work was taken over by the establishment of the School Medical Service, separated from the rest of the School Health Service.

26. "Schools Skipping Medical Scheme: The LegCo meets," *South China Morning Post*, 19 October 1972.
27. "School Medical Service Still Disappointing," *South China Morning Post*, 5 October 1970.
28. "School Medical Plan Off to a New Start," *South China Morning Post*, 9 October 1988.
29. "President Says: Good Year for Badminton," *South China Morning Post*, 12 September 1968.
30. Hong Kong Sports Institute, accessed on 7 August 2023, https://www.hksi.org.hk.
31. "Rodrigues Award—Celebration of Sports Achievements," Development and Alumni Affairs Office, The University of Hong Kong, accessed on 7 February 2023, https://www.giving.hku.hk/rodrigues-award-celebration-of-sports-achievements; personal communication from Dr. Albert Edward Rodrigues.
32. "Dr. Rodrigues Honored by HK University: Honorary Degree at City Hall Graduation Ceremony," *South China Morning Post*, 15 November 1962.
33. "Chairman of University Council," *South China Morning Post*, 8 November 1967.
34. "Personalities. Wide Acclaim for New Hong Kong University Appointment," *South China Morning Post*, 17 January 1968.
35. Holdsworth and Munn, *Dictionary of Hong Kong Biography*, 375.
36. Citation, Harry Fang Sin Yang, Doctor of Laws *honoris causa*, 96th (1977) congregation, The University of Hong Kong, accessed on 7 February 2023, https://www4.hku.hk/hongrads/citations/obe-mb-bs-mchorth-frcse-facs-fracs-jp-harry-sin-yang-fang-harry-fang-sin-yang.
37. Harry S. Y. Fang, *Rehabilitation—A Life's Work* (Hong Kong: Hong Kong University Press, 2002), 18.
38. York Y. N. Chow, "Prof. Sir Harry S. Y. Fang," Repair, Reconstruct and Rehabilitate: Half a Century of Orthopedics in Hong Kong (Hong Kong: Hong Kong Academy of Medicine Press 2004), 174–176.
39. Fang discovered that the Sino-British Fellowship Trust originated from a fund collected by Bishop Ronald Hall, the Anglican Church of Hong Kong, in England, after the fall of Hong Kong in 1942, by preaching in a different church every week. At the end he would ask each parishioner to donate £1 to help the people of China. Soon he collected £3 million. A committee was formed to oversee the management and distribution of funds, to send money to China for medicine and education. At the end of the war, the residual money formed the Sino-British Fellowship Trust. Quoted from: Harry S. Y. Fang, *Rehabilitation—A Life's Work*, 34–35.
40. Harry S. Y. Fang, *Rehabilitation—A Life's Work*, 42.
41. York Y. N. Chow, "Obituary. Harry S. Y. Fang," *Journal of Orthopedic Surgery*, 17(3) (2009): 259–260.
42. The College of Surgeons of Hong Kong, *Healing with a Scalpel, From the First Colonial Surgeon to the College of Surgeons of Hong Kong* (Hong Kong: Hong Kong Academy of Medicine Press, 2020), 75.
43. "Professor Sir Harry Fang Sin-yang: Honorary Fellow of HKCOS 2005," The Hong Kong College of Orthopaedic Surgeons, accessed on 7 February 2023, https://www.hkcos.org.hk/aboutus_doc/Y2005_Sir%20Harry%20Fang.pdf.

44. Fang, *Rehabilitation—A Life's Work*, 72–73.
45. York Y. N. Chow, "Obituary. Harry S. Y. Fang," *Journal of Orthopedic Surgery*, 17(3) (2009): 259–260.
46. Fang, *Rehabilitation—A Life's Work*, 94.
47. York Y. N. Chow, "Obituary. Harry S. Y. Fang," *Journal of Orthopedic Surgery*, 17(3) (2009): 259–260.
48. Fang, *Rehabilitation—A Life's Work*, 91
49. "Integrating the Disabled into the Community: A United Effort," Hong Kong Government (Hong Kong: Hong Kong Government Printers, October 1977).
50. "White Paper on Rehabilitation. Equal Opportunities and Full Participation: A Better Tomorrow for All," May 1995, Hong Kong Government, accessed on 7 February 2023, https://www.lwb.gov.hk/tc/highlights/rpp/Report%20on%20Scoping%20Stage.pdf.
51. Herbert K. Lau, "Father of Rehabilitation in Asia, Sir Harry S. Y. Fang, M.B.B.S., M.Sc., J.P., Hon L.L.D. (HKU), D.S.Sc. D.Sc, Kt, G.B.M., C.B.E.," 10 August 2017, accessed on 7 February 2023, http://old.rotary3450.org/fang-harry-s-y/.
52. Fang, *Rehabilitation—A Life's Work*, 93.
53. "Fang Calls for Action on Unlicensed Doctors," *South China Morning Post*, 24 October 1975.
54. "Better Salaries. Answer to Chronic Doctor Shortage," *South China Morning Post*, 31 March 1977.
55. "Support for a Dental School," *South China Morning Post*, 31 October 1975.
56. "Disabled to Get Senior School in 1981," *South China Morning Post*, 10 May 1979.
57. "Home Ownership Worth Encouraging," *South China Morning Post*, 28 October 1975.
58. David Fang, "Harry S. Y. Fang—the Legend Lives On," *Hong Kong Med J*, 16 (5) (2009): 402.
59. Ibid.
60. "Sir Harry Sin-Yang Fang. Alumna, Surgery. Honorary Graduate, Doctor of Medicine, 1996. Orthopaedic Surgeon, Rehabilitation and Disability Champion," University of Liverpool, accessed on 7 February 2023, https://www.liverpool.ac.uk/hr/diversityandequality/events/bhm/honorarygraduates/harry,sin-yang,fang/.
61. David Fang, "Harry S. Y. Fang—The Legend Lives On," *Hong Kong Med J*, 16 (5) (2009): 402.
62. After the death of their father, Simon Lee, Peter's brother, took over the business and restructured it and expanded the business and greatly contributed to Hong Kong's development into a major shipping center and a transportation hub between China and the world.
63. Citation: Peter Chung Yin Lee, Doctor of Laws *honoris causa*, 96th Congregation (1977), the Hong Kong University, accessed on 11 February 2024, https://www4.hku.hk/hongrads/citations/mb-bs-jp-peter-chung-yin-lee-peter-lee-chung-yin.
64. "Government Loans to Students Urged," *South China Morning Post*, 14 May 1969.
65. "Department of Music for HKU Proposed," *South China Morning Post*, 14 January 1965.

66. Citation: Peter Chung Yin Lee, Doctor of Laws *honoris causa*, 96th Congregation, (1977), the Hong Kong University.
67. Hong Kong Civic Association was one of the two semi-political parties to participate in the Urban Council elections since the 1950s, alongside Reform Club of Hong Kong. It was established in 1954 by a group of teachers, professionals, and entrepreneurs.
68. The Reform Club was founded by expatriate barrister Brook Bernacchi in 1949, in the midst of the debate over the Young Plan, a plan for wide constitutional reform in Hong Kong. The immediate target of the club was to campaign for direct elections to the Legislative Council of Hong Kong.
69. Hong Kong University, *Growing with Hong Kong: The University and Its Graduates: The First 90 Years* (Hong Kong University Press, 2002), 273
70. "Civic Association Criticizes Government on Land Policy," *South China Morning Post*, 23 December 1964.
71. "Private Sector Could Help in Doctor Shortage," *South China Morning Post*, 26 September 1974.
72. "Control These Laboratories," *South China Morning Post*, 8 July 1975.
73. World Medical Association, accessed on 7 February 2023, https://www.wma.net/who-we-are/about-us/.
74. Peter C. Y. Lee "Keynote Address," in *15th Anniversary Celebration Commemorative* (Hong Kong: Hong Kong College of General Practitioner, 1993), 2.
75. Causes of deaths in 1970, 1990, 2010, Hong Kong Medical and Health Department Annual Reports, 1970, 1990 and 2010.
76. Stephen Foo, "In Memory of Dr. Peter CY Lee," Messages from Past Presidents, Council Members and Friends, The Obituary of Dr. Peter C. Y. Lee, Hong Kong College of Family Physicians, 2013, 14, accessed on 7 February 2023, https://www.hkcfp.org.hk/Upload/Commemorative/Obituary_and_Remembrances/obituary_Dr.PeterLee.pdf.
77. Peter C. Y. Lee, "Contributions and Influence of the Hong Kong College in the Development of Family Medicine in Hong Kong and around the World during the Past Quarter Century (1977–2002) as Seen Through the Eyes of Its Founding President," compiled and edited by Dr. Peter C. Y. Lee, March 2003, in *25th Anniversary Commemorative brochure* (Hong Kong: Hong Kong College of Family Physicians, 2003), 9.
78. Peter C. Y. Lee, "Keynote Address," in *15th Anniversary Celebration Commemorative* (Hong Kong: Hong Kong College of General Practitioner, 1993), 3.
79. Peter C. Y. Lee, "Keynote Address," in *15th Anniversary Celebration Commemorative* (Hong Kong: Hong Kong College of General Practitioner, 1993), 5.
80. *World Health Organization*, "Global Strategy for Health for All by the Year 2000," World Health Organization, Geneva, 1981.
81. "Health for All, the Way Ahead: Report of the Working Party on Primary Health Care," Hong Kong Government (Hong Kong: Hong Kong Government Printer, 1990).
82. Peter Lee, "Message from the Founding President," *The First 30 Years of the Hong Kong College of Family Physicians*, 20–21.
83. Stephen Foo, "In Memory of Dr. Peter C. Y. Lee," 14–15.

84. Peter Lee, "Introduction of General Practice/Family Medicine into China, The Role of HKCGP/HKCFP in the Early Years," Part 3, *The First 30 Years of the Hong Kong College of Family Physicians*, 155–156.

Chapter 12

1. Hung-kay Luk, *A History of Education in Hong Kong* (Hong Kong: Lord Wilson Heritage Trust, 2000), 73, 91.
2. Grace C. L. Mak, "Women and Education," in *Women and Girls in Hong Kong: Current Situation and Future Challenges*, ed. Susanne Y. P. Choi and Fanny M. Cheung (Hong Kong: Hong Kong Institute of Asia-Pacific Studies, The Chinese University of Hong Kong, 2012), 24.
3. "Gender and Educational Summary Grid for A Level Sociology," ReviseSociology, accessed on 2 February 2023, https://revisesociology.com/2017/04/19/gender-and-education-summary-grid-for-a-level-sociology/.
4. "Information Paper—Curriculum Development Institute," Panel on Education Paper, 17 October 1997, Legislative Council, HKSAR, accessed on 8 February 2023, https://www.legco.gov.hk/yr97-98/english/panels/ed/papers/ed1710-6.htm.
5. The University of Hong Kong Annual Report 2021, accessed on 8 February 2023, https://www4.hku.hk/pubunit/annualreport/ebook_AR2021/48-49/.
6. May Holdsworth and Christopher Munn, *Dictionary of Hong Kong Biography* (Hong Kong: Hong Kong University Press, 2011), 100.
7. "High Post for HK Graduate. University Appoints Woman Professor," *South China Morning Post*, 17 February 1957.
8. "Maternity Hospital Praised as One of World's Best," *South China Morning Post*, 26 May 1972.
9. Han Suyin, *My House Has Two Doors* (New York: Putnam Pub Group (T), 1980), 19.
10. Daphne Chun, "History of Cesarean Section," *Elixir*, Summer 1957, 16–24.
11. Moira Chan-Yeung, *A Medical History of Hong Kong—The Development of Outpatient Services* (Hong Kong: The Chinese University of Hong Kong Press, 2021), 136–137.
12. "Appointed to the Midwives Board," *South China Morning Post*, 14 January 1961.
13. Hong Kong Medical and Health Department Annual Reports 1949 to 1980; Hong Kong Annual Digest of Statistics, 1981 to 2000.
14. Citation, Daphne Chun Wai Chan, Doctor of Social Sciences *honoris causa*, 81st Congregation (1972), The University of Hong Kong, accessed on 16 February 2024, https://www4.hku.hk/hongrads/citations/o-b-e-m-b-b-s-h-k-f-r-c-s-e-f-r-c-o-g-daphne-wai-chan-chun-daphne-chun-wai-chan.
15. Holdsworth and Munn, *Dictionary of Hong Kong Biography*, 100.
16. "Radio and Television: Today Radio Hong Kong," *South China Morning Post*, 12 April 1963.
17. "Family Planning Can Save People from Misery," *South China Morning Post*, 30 August 1963.
18. "Safety of Birth Control," *South China Morning Post*, 27 August 1966.

19. "Family Planning Association: Urgent Appeal for Public Support Made. More Clinics and More Workers," *South China Morning Post*, 25 April 1957.
20. Hong Kong Medical and Health Department Annual Report 1958/1959, 1972/73.
21. "Government Urged to Shoulder Family Planning Task," *South China Morning Post*, 17 September 1965.
22. Hong Kong Medical and Health Department Annual Report, 1974/1975, 4.
23. Hong Kong Medical and Health Department Annual Report, 2003/2004.
24. "HK Requires 'Drastic' Population Program," *South China Morning Post*, 19 April 1974.
25. "The Planned Population," *South China Morning Post*, 23 May 1975.
26. "Birthday Honors: CBE Awards to Two Residents," *South China Morning Post*, 13 June 1959.
27. Citation, Daphne Chun Wai Chan, Doctor of Social Sciences, *honoris causa*, 81st congregation (1972), The University of Hong Kong.
28. Holdsworth and Munn, *Dictionary of Hong Kong Biography*, 100.
29. "Appointments in University of Hong Kong," *South China Morning Post*, 25 January 1962.
30. "Pediatrics in the Early Years," Department of Pediatrics, HKU, accessed on 8 February 2023, http://paed.hku.hk/menu/staff.html.
31. University of Hong Kong. *Department of Pediatrics. Silver Jubilee 25*, 1962–1987 (Hong Kong: Department of Pediatrics, HKU, 1987), 6–7.
32. Ibid.
33. "Pediatrics in the Early Years," Department of Pediatrics, HKU, accessed on 8 February 2023, http://paed.hku.hk/menu/staff.html.
34. "Pediatrics in the Early Years," Department of Pediatrics, HKU, accessed on 8 February 2023, http://paed.hku.hk/menu/staff.html.
35. "HK Pediatric Society Annual Meeting," *South China Morning Post*, 22 March 1963.
36. Flora Baber, "The Role of the Pediatrician in the Community of Hong Kong. Reflection on a Longitudinal Study 1967–1976," The Fourth Elaine Field Lecture delivered on 3 February 1977, Excelsior Hotel, Causeway Bay, Hong Kong, in *C. Elaine Field Lectures, 1974–1993*, (Hong Kong: Hong Kong Pediatric Society, 1994), 34–42.
37. Elaine Field School, accessed on 3 March 2023, https://www.sahk1963.org.hk/en_service.php?id=17.
38. "British Aid for Child Study Here," *South China Morning Post*, 13 October 1966.
39. Flora Baber, "The Role of the Pediatrician in the Community of Hong Kong. Reflection on a Longitudinal Study 1967–1976."
40. "Breaking into the World of Silence," *South China Morning Post*, 11 April 1971.

Chapter 13

1. Dr. F. R. Ashton, *Alice Ho Miu Ling Nethersole Hospital, Hong Kong, 1887–1967* (Hong Kong: Alice Ho Miu Ling Nethersole Hospital, 1967), 2–4.

2. Ibid., 23.
3. Sergio Ticozzi, *Historical Documents of the Hong Kong Catholic Church* (Hong Kong: Hong Kong Catholic Diocesan Archives, 1997), 36–37.
4. Ida Sala, *History of Our Canossian Missions: The First Fifty Years* (Hong Kong: Daughters of Charity of Canossa, 1997–2012), Volume 1, 28.
5. Center for Catholic Studies, *Caring and Serving for 120 Years: The history of St. Paul's Hospital* (Hong Kong: The Chinese University of Hong Kong, 2018), 12–13.
6. Ibid., 29–31.
7. Cindy Chu, *The Chinese Sisters of the Precious Blood and the Evolution of the Catholic Church* (Singapore: Palgrave Macmillan, 2016), 80, 112.
8. Sister M. Gabriel O'Mahony, *A Time of Transition: Columban Sisters in Hong Kong* (Magheramore, Wicklow: Columban Sisters, 2005, private circulation), 4–5.
9. Ibid., 6.
10. Ibid., 8.
11. Hospital ships were ships used to take care of the sick and injured before the Royal Navy Hospital was established. The hospital ship, *HMS Melville*, in service at that time, was found to be inadequate for the job; thus, the navy was eager to find a shore-based hospital (M. Humphries, *Ruttonjee Sanatorium: Life and Time* [Hong Kong: The Sanatorium, 1996], 17).
12. M. Humphries, Ruttonjee Sanatorium: Life and Time, 11–20.
13. Sister M. Gabriel O'Mahony, *A Time of Transition: Columban Sisters in Hong Kong*, 24.
14. Ibid., 16.
15. Andrew Paterson, "Edward Hamilton Paterson," *Brit Med J*, 348 (2014): 1250; Citation by Professor Francis Moore on the conferment to Dr. E. H. Paterson of Doctor of Social Sciences *honoris causa*, 124th Congregation (1985), by the University of Hong Kong, accessed on 16 February 2024, https://www4.hku.hk/hongrads/citations/o-b-e-m-b-b-s-f-r-c-s-edward-hamilton-paterson.
16. E. H. Paterson, *A Hospital for Hong Kong* (Hong Kong: Alice Ho Miu Ling Nethersole Hospital, 1987), 87–88.
17. E. H. Paterson, "Cleft Lips and Palates in Hong Kong," *Hong Kong Nursing Journal*, 22 (1977): 45–50.
18. "Operations Can Overcome Lip Deformity," *South China Morning Post*, 24 October 1976, 5.
19. Bilateral cleft lip is a severe deformity involving both sides of the upper lip, which is difficult to repair. Paterson fashioned the defect into a heptagon shape to facilitate its closure. A picture can be found in E. H. Paterson, "Cleft Lip Surgery," *Bulletin of the Hong Kong Chinese Medical Association*, 11 (1960): 77–81.
20. "Paterson, Edward Hamilton (1920–2013)," Plarr's Lives of the Fellows, Royal College of Surgeons of England, accessed on 6 February 2023, https://livesonline.rcseng.ac.uk/biogs/E005167b.htm.
21. E. H. Paterson, *Dreams and a Hospital* (Hong Kong: United Christian Medical Service, 2000), 2.
22. F. R. Ashton, *Alice Ho Miu Ling Nethersole Hospital, Hong Kong, 1887–1967* (Hong Kong: Alice Ho Miu Ling Nethersole Hospital, 1967), 24.

23. *Development of Medical Services in Hong Kong* (Hong Kong: Government Printer, 1964), 18.
24. E. H. Paterson, *Dreams and a Hospital*, 8
25. Ibid., 11.
26. E. H. Paterson, "The Kwun Tong Community Health Project," *Trop Doct*, 8 (1978): 85–89.
27. Paterson, *Dreams and a Hospital*, 20.
28. *Development of Medical Services in Hong Kong* (Hong Kong: Government Printer, 1964), 18.
29. Paterson, *Dreams and a Hospital*, 21–27.
30. "Health: Don't Rely on 'Pros'," *South China Morning Post*, 1 April 1976, 8.
31. E. H. Paterson, "The Kwun Tong Community Health Project," *Trop Doct*, 8 (1978): 85–89; E. H. Paterson, "Outside Europe. An Urban Community Health Project," *Brit Med J*, 280 (1980): 29–31.
32. M. J. Carter, *Community Nursing in Hong Kong: A Report on Behalf of the Community Nursing Committee* (Hong Kong: Hong Kong Council of Social Service, 1976).
33. "Hospitals Do Not Raise Standards," *South China Morning Post*, 9 October 1975, 7.
34. "The Further Development of Medical and Health Services in Hong Kong," Hong Kong Government (Hong Kong: Hong Kong Government Printers, 1974).
35. World Health Organization, "Report of the International Conference on Primary Health Care, Alma-Ata, USSR, 6–12 September 1978," accessed on 16 February 2024, https://www.unicef.org/media/85611/file/Alma-Ata-conference-1978-report.pdf.
36. *Health for All, The Way Ahead: Report of the Working Party on Primary Health Care* (Hong Kong: Government Printer, 1990), 224.
37. Paterson, *Dreams and a Hospital*, 61.
38. Paterson, *Dreams and a Hospital*, 84–91.
39. Citation by Professor Francis Moore on the conferment to Dr. E. H. Paterson of Doctor of Social Sciences *honoris causa*, 124th Congregation (1985), by the University of Hong Kong.
40. Paterson, *Dreams and a Hospital*, 80–81.
41. This is from a pamphlet for The Thanksgiving Service for the lives of Dr. and Mrs. E. H. Paterson on 26 Feb 2013 at Hop Yat Church, 11.
42. Andrew Paterson, "Edward Hamilton Paterson," *Brit Med J*, 348(2014): 1250.
43. Linde Lunney, "Monaghan, Cathleen (Sister Mary Aquinas)," in James McGuire and James Quinn, eds., *Dictionary of Irish Biography* (Cambridge: Cambridge University Press, 2009) 572–573.
44. Tuberculosis and Chest Service Annual Report, Department of Health, HKSAR, 2020.
45. "Public Enemy No. 1," *South China Morning Post*, 26 February 1949, 8.
46. "Ruttonjee Sanatorium: Preference Given to Residents of Colony, States Report Many on Waiting List," *South China Morning Post*, 23 February 1951, 8.
47. "Ruttonjee Sanatorium: Sir Arthur Morse Opens New Jockey Club Wing," *South China Morning Post*, 7 March 1953, 4.

48. "The Freni Memorial: Convalescent Home for Tuberculosis Patients. Big Gathering at Opening,"*South China Morning Post*, 3 August 1956, 6.
49. A. S. Moodie, "Tuberculosis in Hong Kong," *Tubercle, Lond.*, 44(1963): 334–345.
50. O'Mahony, *A Time of Transition: Columban Sisters in Hong Kong*, 16, 21.
51. M Humphries, *Ruttonjee Sanatorium: Life and Time*, 37.
52. Ibid., 23.
53. S. H. Lee. "The 60-Year Battle against Tuberculosis in Hong Kong—A Review of the Past and a Projection into the 21st Century," *Respirology*, 13 (Suppl. 3) (2008): S49–S55.
54. Sir Robert William Philip (1857–1939), a physician from Edinburgh, was the founder of TB dispensaries. He was knighted for his extensive work on TB in 1913.
55. O'Mahony, *A Time of Transition: Columban Sisters in Hong Kong*, 26–27.
56. Lunney, "Monaghan, Cathleen (Sister Mary Aquinas)," 572–573.
57. O'Mahony, *A Time of Transition: Columban Sisters in Hong Kong*, 37.
58. "Drop in TB Deaths Dramatic," *South China Morning Post*, 15 April 1969, 5.
59. A. S. Moodie. "Tuberculosis in Hong Kong," *Tubercle, Lond.*, 44 (1963): 334–345.
60. "The Problem of Narcotic Drugs in Hong Kong," A White Paper laid before Legislative Council, Hong Kong 11 November 1959, 3, 17.
61. O'Mahony, *A Time of Transition: Columban Sisters in Hong Kong*, 52.
62. David Hui, K. S. Chan, and H. S. Chan, "Introduction and History," joint website of the Hong Kong Thoracic Society and the Chest Delegation Hong Kong and Macau, accessed on 6 February 2023, https://hkts.hk/index/about/about-hong-kong-thoracic-society/introduction-and-history.
63. Henry F. K. Li, "Report from the Chairman," in HKCGP Inauguration Ceremony Commemorative Brochure 1979.
64. Z. Lett, "Obituary," *Brit Med J* (Clin Res Ed), 292 (1986): 208.
65. Lunney, "Monaghan, Cathleen (Sister Mary Aquinas)," 572–573.
66. Professor Peter Bernard Harris, Citation: Sister Mary Aquinas, Doctor of Social Sciences, *honoris causa*, 100th Congregation (1978), The University of Hong Kong.
67. M. Humphries, *Ruttonjee Sanatorium: Life and Time*, 37.
68. TAC, "Obituary, Sister Mary Aquinas, OBE, FRCPED," *Brit Med J* (Clin Res Ed), 292 (1986): 208.
69. Hong Kong Tuberculosis, Chest and Heart Diseases Association, 70th Anniversary Commemorative Album.
70. Holdsworth and Munn, *Dictionary of Hong Kong Biography* (Hong Kong: Hong Kong University Press, 2012), 156. And Redempta Twomey, "Homily at Funeral Mass of Sister Gabriel O'Mahony on August 29, 2006," accessed on 6 February 2023, http://www.columbansisters.org/rip/gabriel/gabriel_rip_homily.htm.
71. Holdsworth and Munn, *Dictionary of Hong Kong Biography*, 21.
72. H. Bailey, M. Gabriel, A. R. Hodgson, and J. S. Shin, "Tuberculosis of the Spine in Children. Operative Findings and Results in One Hundred Consecutive Patients Treated by Removal of the Lesion and Anterior Grafting," *J Bone & Joint Surg (Am)*,

54 (1972): 1633–1657; "Fourth Report of the Medical Research Council Working Party on Tuberculosis of the Spine. A Controlled Trial of Anterior Spinal Fusion and Debridement in the Surgical Management of Tuberculosis of the Spine in Patients on Standard Chemotherapy: A Study in Hong Kong," *Brit J Surg*, 61 (1974): 853–866.

73. O'Mahony, *A Time of Transition: Columban Sisters in Hong Kong*, 29–30.
74. Humphries, *Ruttonjee Sanatorium: Life and Time*, 41.
75. Redempta Twomey, "Homily at Funeral Mass of Sister Gabriel O'Mahony on August 29, 2006," accessed on 6 February 2023, http://www.columbansisters.org/rip/gabriel/gabriel_rip_homily.htm.
76. O'Mahony, *A Time of Transition: Columban Sisters in Hong Kong*, 27–28.
77. Ibid., 49.
78. Ibid., 70–71.
79. W. K. Yu, "Palliative Care in Practice," *The Hong Kong Practitioner*, 9(6) (1987): 2531–2544.
80. O'Mahony, *A Time of Transition: Columban Sisters in Hong Kong*, 71.
81. Sister M. Gabriel, "Doctor at Large-Hospice Care," *The Hong Kong Practitioner*, 10 (2) (1988): 3024–3027.
82. "Poor Cancer Funding Forces Search Elsewhere," *South China Morning Post*, 23 September 1987, 3;Helen Signy, "Commitment for Hospices 'Inadequate'," *South China Morning Post*, 14 November 1990, 7.
83. C. Y. Yeung, "Evolution of Child Health Care in Hong Kong," *HK J Paediatr* (New Series), 6 (2001): 66–71.
84. M. Humphries, "Obituary: Sister Mary Gabriel O'Mahoney," *Hong Kong Med J*, 12(5) (2006): 402.
85. Thomas Mok, Loretta Yam, and P. C. Wong, "Obituary. Sister Mary Gabriel O'Mahoney," joint website of the Hong Kong Thoracic Society and the Chest Delegation Hong Kong and Macau, accessed on 6 February 2023, https://hkts.hk/index/specials-events/obituary-and-condolences?detail=1&aid=250.
86. M. Humphries, "Obituary: Sister Mary Gabriel O'Mahoney," *Hong Kong Med J*, 12(5) (2006): 402.
87. Redempta Twomey, "Homily at Funeral Mass of Sister Gabriel O'Mahony on 29 August 2006," accessed on 27 September 2006, http://www.columbansisters.org/rip/gabriel/gabriel_rip_homily.htm.
88. O'Mahony, *A Time of Transition: Columban Sisters in Hong Kong*, 10.

Conclusion

1. The Faculty of Medicine of the second university in Hong Kong, The Chinese University of Hong Kong, was founded in 1981.

Glossary

Alberto Maria Rodrigues	羅理基
Au Tak	區德
Basic Red Cross First Aid	赤十字會初級急救要法
Bau Tsu-zung	鮑志成
Cheeloo University	齊魯大學
Chinese Nationalist Party	國民黨
Chiu Hin-yeung	趙顯揚
Chiu Bek-to	周默道
Chun Wai-chan, Daphne	秦惠珍
Chung Boon-chor, also Chung King-ue	鍾本初(鍾景儒)
Chusan	舟山
David Todd	達安輝
Edward Hamilton Paterson	巴治安
Fang Sin-yang, Harry	方心讓
First Lines of Practice of Surgery in the West	西醫略論
Fung Wa-chun	馮華川
G. H. Thomas	譚嘉士
Gerald Hugh Choa	蔡永業
Gordon King	王國棟
Guan Maocai	管茂材
Hanyang	漢陽
Ho Chung-chung	何中中
Ho Fuk-tong	何福堂
Ho Hung-chiu, John	何鴻超
Ho Kai	何啟

Ho Ko-tsun	何高俊
Ho Miu-ling	何妙齡
Ho Nai-hop	何乃合
Hong Kong Chinese Swimming Association	香港華人游泳會
Hou Pao-chang	侯寶璋
Huguang	湖廣
Jeu Hawk	趙學
Kam-li-fau	金利埠
Koloshan (Geleshan)	歌樂山
Kwan King-leung	關景良
Kung Yee Medical College	公醫醫學院
Lai Po-chuen, Pauline	賴寶川
Lai Po-kan	賴寶勤
Lao She	老舍
Lau Chu-pak	劉鑄伯
Lee Chung-yin, Peter	李仲賢
Lee Shiu-hung	李紹鴻
Leung Sheung-chi	梁尚志
Li Hongzhang	李鴻章
Li Shu-fan	李樹芬
Li Tsoo-yiu	李祖佑
Li Yuanhong	黎元洪
Lindsay Tasman Ride	賴廉士
Lo Man-kam	羅文錦
Long Jiguang	龍濟光
Ma Luk	馬祿
Mengzi	蒙自
Missionary Society of the Chinese Christian Council	華人基督教聯會
National Southwestern Associated University (Lianda)	國立西南聯合大學（聯大）
Natural Philosophy and Natural History	博物新編
Ng Choy, also Wu Ting-fang	伍才（伍廷芳）
Ong Guan Bee	王源美

Outline of Anatomy and Physiology	全體新知
Percy Selwyn Selwyn-Clarke	司徒永覺
Phoon Sek-wah	潘錫華
Practice of Medicine and Materia Medica	內科新說
Shibasaburo Kitasato	北里柴三郎
Sister Mary Aquinas Monaghan	亞規納 / 區貴雅
Sister Mary Gabriel O'Mahony	紀寶儀
Ta Kwu Ling	打鼓嶺
Tai Yuk Primary School	體育學校
To Chai Church	道濟會堂
Tong Meng Hui	同盟會
Treatise on Midwifery and Diseases of Children	婦嬰新說
Tsan Yuk Hospital	贊育醫院
Tsao Yen-chow	曹延洲
Tseung Fat-im	蔣法賢
Tso Lai-ki	曹麗姬
Tso Seen-wan	曹善允
Tso Shuk-kei	曹淑姬
Vice-Minister of Ministry of Health	衛生司副司長
Wan Man-kai	尹文楷
wan po	穩婆
Wang Chung-yik	王寵益
Wang Yuk-cho	王煜初
Woo Wai-tak, Arthur	胡惠德
Wu Tin-po	吳天保
Xing Zhong Hui	興中會
Yap Pow-meng	葉寶明
Yeo Kok-cheang	楊國璋
Zhili	直隸

Bibliography

Primary Sources

Archives

CO 129. Colonial Office, Hong Kong: Original Correspondence, 1838–1946

Council for World Mission Archives, South China. London Missionary Society (LMS) Box 9–19: 1882–1891

Elizabeth Ride Archive

University Archives, the University of Hong Kong

Hong Kong Government Reports Printed or Online

Hong Kong Administrative Report (HKAR) 1879–1883 and 1908–1939 from Hong Kong Government Reports online

Hong Kong Blue Book (HKBB) hard copies of 1845 to 1870 from Hong Kong University Library Special Collection and soft copies of 1871 to 1940 from Hong Kong Government Reports online

Hong Kong Sessional Papers (HKSP) 1884–1940 from Hong Kong Government Reports online

Hong Kong Government Gazette (HKGG) 1842–1848, 1853–1941 from Hong Kong Government Reports online

Hong Kong Civil Service List, Government Printers

Hong Kong Medical and Health Department Annual Reports, 1946–2000

Special Hong Kong Government Publications, Printed or Online

Chadwick, O. Report on the Sanitary Condition of Hong Kong. Hong Kong Government, 1882, 1–59.

Medical Committee Report. Hong Kong Government, HKSP 1895.

The Commission. Report on the Tung Wa Hospital, HKSP 1896.

Report of the Commission to Enquire into the Existence of Insanitary Properties in the Colony. Hong Kong: Noronha and Co, Government Printers, 1898.

Hunter, William. Report of the Government Bacteriologist for the Year 1906, HKSP 1907, Annex L 474–482.

Wellington, A. R. Changes in the Public Health Organization of Hong Kong During the Period 1929–1937, HKSP 1937, no 4/1937.

Selwyn-Clark, P. S. Report of the Technical Committee for the Reorganization and Improvement of Existing Official Hospital and Clinical Facilities of the Colony of Hong Kong, 1938–1939.

Report of the Committee on Higher Education 1952, The Keswick Report, Hong Kong Government Printers, 1952.

The Problem of Narcotic Drugs in Hong Kong. A White Paper laid before Legislative Council Hong Kong, 11 November 1959.

Colonial Secretariat. Report on Women's Salary Scales in Public Service. Government Printer, 1962.

Development of Medical Services in Hong Kong. Hong Kong Government, Government Printers, 1964.

Report of Advisory Committee on Clinics. Hong Kong Government, Hong Kong Government Printers, 1966.

Report of the Medical Development Advisory Committee, Hong Kong Government, Hong Kong Government Printer, 1973.

The Further Development of Medical and Health Services in Hong Kong. Hong Kong Government, Hong Kong Government Printers, 1974.

Integrating the Disabled into the Community: A United Effort. Hong Kong Government, Hong Kong Government Printers, October 1977.

Second Report on Civil Service Pay, Hong Kong. Standing Commission on Civil Service Salaries and Conditions of Service. Hong Kong: The Commission, 1980.

Health for All, the Way Forward: Report of the Working Party on Primary Health Care. Hong Kong: Government Printer, 1990.

Lee, S. H. Prevention and Control of Communicable Diseases in Hong Kong. Hong Kong Government Printers, 1994.

White Paper on Rehabilitation. Equal Opportunities and Full Participation: A Better Tomorrow for All. Hong Kong: Government Printer, 1995.

The Harvard Team, Improving Hong Kong's Healthcare System: Why and for Whom?, 1999. http://www.fhb.gov.hk/en/press_and_publications/consultation/HCS.HTM.

Tuberculosis Manual. Tuberculosis and Chest Service, Public Health Services Branch, Center for Health Protection, Department of Health, Government of the HKSAR, 2006.

Building Healthy Cities. Guidelines for Implementing a Healthy City Project in Hong Kong. Department of Health, The Government of the Hong Kong SAR, 2007.

Family Health Service, Department of Health. 80th Anniversary Family Health Service, 2012. The Government of the Hong Kong SAR, 2012.

Special Reports from Other Organizations

British Parliament. 1842 Report on the Sanitary Condition of the Laboring Population of Great Britain. https://www.parliament.uk/about/living-heritage/transformingsociety/livinglearning/coll-9-health1/health-02/#:~:text=1842%20Sanitary%20Report,Chadwick%20(1800%2D1890).

Macleod, N. C. "An Account by the Deputy Director of Health Services of the Organization of Health Services in Stanley Internment Camp." In Report on Medical and Health Conditions in Hong Kong for the Period, 1 January 1942 to 31 August 1945, His Majesty's Stationery Office, 1946.

Carter, M. J. Community Nursing in Hong Kong: A Report on Behalf of the Community Nursing Committee. Hong Kong Council of Social Service, 1976.

World Health Organization. Report of the International Conference on Primary Health Care, Alma-Ata, 1978.

World Health Organization. Global Strategy for Health for All by the Year 2000. Geneva, 1981.

Newspapers

South China Morning Post

China Mail

Hong Kong Telegraph

Hong Kong Daily Press

Kung Sheung Yat Po

Wah Kiu Yat Po

Books

Ashton, F. R. *Alice Ho Miu Ling Nethersole Hospital, Hong Kong, 1887–1967*. Hong Kong: Alice Ho Miu Ling Nethersole Hospital, 1967.

Bowman, Marilyn Laura. *James Legge and the Confucian Classics. Brilliant Scot in the Turmoil of Colonial Hong Kong.* Vancouver: Simon Fraser University, 2015.

Boyd, Robin. *The Witness of the Student Christian Movement*. London: Society of Promoting Christian Knowledge, 2007.

Chan, Julia, and N. G. Patil. *Digby: A Remarkable Life*. Hong Kong: Hong Kong University Press, 2006.

Chan, Sui-jeung. *East River Column: Hong Kong Guerillas in the Second World War and After*. Royal Asiatic Society Hong Kong Studies Series. Hong Kong: Hong Kong University Press, 2009.

Chan-Yeung, M. *A Medical History of Hong Kong, 1842–1941*. Hong Kong: The Chinese University of Hong Kong Press, 2018.

———. *A Medical History of Hong Kong: The Development and Contributions of Outpatient Services*. Hong Kong: The Chinese University of Hong Kong Press, 2021.

———. *Lam Woo. Master Builder, Revolutionary, and Philanthropist*. Hong Kong: The Chinese University of Hong Kong Press, 2017.

Cheng, Irene. *Intercultural Reminiscences*. Hong Kong: David C. Lam Institute for East-West Studies, Hong Kong Baptist University, 1997.

Ching, Frank. *130 Years of Medicine in Hong Kong. From the College of Medicine for Chinese to Li Ka Shing Faculty of Medicine*. Singapore: Springer Nature, 2018.

Choa G. H. *The Life and Times of Sir Kai Ho Kai.* 2nd Edition. Hong Kong: The Chinese University of Hong Kong Press, 2000.

———. *"Heal the Sick" Was Their Motto: The Protestant Medical Missionaries in China.* Hong Kong: The Chinese University of Hong Kong Press, 1990.

Chu, Cindy. *The Chinese Sisters of the Precious Blood and the Evolution of the Catholic Church.* Singapore: Palgrave Macmillan, 2016.

Cunich P. *A History of the University of Hong Kong.* Hong Kong: Hong Kong University Press, 2012.

Department of Medicine. *Achievements in Medicine 1974–1989. Department of Medicine, University of Hong Kong.* Hong Kong: Hong Kong University Press, 1989.

———. *Achievements in Medicine, 1989–1995. Department of Medicine, University of Hong Kong.* Hong Kong: ColorPrint Production Co., 1995.

———. *Centenary Tribute to Professor AJS McFadzean. A Legacy for Medicine in Hong Kong.* Hong Kong: Hong Kong Academy of Medicine Press, 2015.

———. *HKU Department of Medicine, 1995–2019, Impact Inspirations.* Hong Kong: Hong Kong University, 2021.

Department of Paediatrics. *Silver Jubilee 25, 1962–1987.* Department of Paediatrics, University of Hong Kong, 1987.

Duffin, J. *History of Medicine.* Toronto: University of Toronto Press, 1999.

Emerson, G. C. *Hong Kong Internment 1942–1945. Life in Japanese Civilian Camp at Stanley.* Hong Kong: Hong Kong University Press, 2008.

Epstein, Israel. *Woman in World History: Life and Times of Soong Ching Ling.* Beijing, China: New World Press, 1995.

Evans, D. E. *Constancy of Purpose. An Account of the Foundation and History of the Hong Kong College of Medicine and the Faculty of Medicine of the University of Hong Kong (1887–1987).* Hong Kong: Hong Kong University Press, 1987.

Fang, Harry S. Y. *Rehabilitation—A Life's Work.* Hong Kong: Hong Kong University Press, 2002.

Fung, Chi-Ming. *A History of Queen Mary Hospital 1937–1997.* Hong Kong: Queen Mary Hospital, 1997.

Gauld, R., and D. Gould. *The Hong Kong Health Sector.* Hong Kong: The Chinese University of Hong Kong Press, 2002.

Gittins, Jean. *Stanley: Behind the Barbed Wire.* Hong Kong: Hong Kong University Press, 1982.

Ha, Louis E. Keloon, Wai Lun Tam, and Patrick Taveirne, eds. *The History of St. Paul's Hospital: Caring and Serving for 120 Years.* Catholic Studies Publication Research Series (11), Centre for Catholic Studies, The Chinese University of Hong Kong. Hong Kong: Chinese University of Hong Kong Press, 2018.

Hahn, Emily. *China to Me.* London: Virago, 1987.

Han, Suyin. *My House Has Two Doors.* New York: Putnam Pub Group, 1980.

He, Gaojun. *Chishizi hui chuji jijiu yao fa* [Basic Red Cross First Aid]. Hong Kong: Juzhen Shu Lou, 1908.

Hillier, S. M., and J. A. Jewell. *Health Care and Traditional Medicine in China*. London: Routledge and Kegan Paul, 1983.

Ho, Faith C. S. *Western Medicine for Chinese: How the Hong Kong College of Medicine Achieved a Breakthrough*. Hong Kong: Hong Kong University Press, 2017.

Ho, Man-wui Richard. *Tan xuexi, yi mingshi*. [About studying and my teachers]. Hong Kong: The Commercial Press (H.K.) Ltd., 2017.

Ho, Michael. *When Science and Compassion Meet—A Turning Point in the History of Medicine in Hong Kong*. Hong Kong: Hong Kong Museum of Medical Sciences Society, 1997.

Holdsworth, May, and Christopher Munn. *Dictionary of Hong Kong Biography*. Hong Kong: Hong Kong University Press, 2011.

Hong Kong Academy of Medicine. *In Pursuit of Excellence, The first 10 Years 1993–2003*. Hong Kong: Hong Kong Academy of Medicine Press, 2003.

Hong Kong College of Surgeons. *Healing with the Scalpel: From the First Colonial Surgeon to the College of Surgeons of Hong Kong*. Hong Kong: Hong Kong Academy of Medicine Press, 2010.

Hong Kong Tuberculosis, Chest and Heart Diseases Association. *70th Anniversary Commemorative Album*. 2018.

Hong Kong University. *Growing with Hong Kong: The University and Its Graduates: The First 90 Years*. Hong Kong: Hong Kong University Press, 2002.

Humphries, M. *Ruttonjee Sanatorium: Life and Time*. Hong Kong: The Sanatorium, 1996.

Lett, Z. *Anesthesia*. Hong Kong: Hong Kong University Press, 1983.

———. *History of Anesthesia in Hong Kong*. Hong Kong: Centre for Asian Studies, Hong Kong University, 1987.

Lett, Z., and Ronald Lo. *Anesthesia and Intensive Care in Hong Kong: Evolution and Present Position*. Hong Kong: Centre for Asian Studies, Hong Kong University, 1997.

Leung, G., and J. Bacon-Shone. *Hong Kong's Health System: Reflections, Perspectives and Visions*. Hong Kong: Hong Kong University Press, 2006.

Li, S. F. *Hong Kong Surgeon*. New York: E. P. Dutton, 1964.

Lau, Chipang, and Liu Shuyong. *Hou Baozhang jiazu shi* [Family History of Hou Pao-chang]. Hong Kong: Peace Book Co. Ltd., 2012.

Lockhart, W. *The Medical Missionary in China: A Narrative of Twenty Years' Experience*. London: Hurst and Blackett Publishers, 1861.

Luk, Hung-kay. *A History of Education in Hong Kong*. Hong Kong: Lord Wilson Heritage Trust, 2000.

Mattock, K. *Hong Kong Practice. Drs. Anderson and Partners. The First Hundred Years*. Hong Kong: Dr. Anderson and Partners, Linkprint Ltd, 1984.

Mellor, Bernard. *The University of Hong Kong—An Informal History*. Hong Kong: Hong Kong University Press, 1980.

Needham, Joseph. *Science and Civilization in China: Vol 1*. Cambridge: Cambridge University Press, 1954.

Ng-Lun, A. N. H. *Quest for Excellence: A History of the Chinese University of Hong Kong*. Hong Kong: Chinese University of Hong Kong Press, 1994.

O'Mahony, M. Gabriel. *A Time of Transition: Columban Sisters in Hong Kong*. Magheramore, Wicklow: Columban Sisters, 2005, Private Circulation.

Paterson, E. H. *A Hospital for Hong Kong. Centenary History of Alice Ho Miu Ling Nethersole Hospital, Hong Kong, 1887–1987*. Hong Kong: Alice Ho Miu Ling Nethersole Hospital, 1987.

———. *Dreams and a Hospital*. Hong Kong: United Christian Medical Service, 2000.

Ram, Vernon. *Emperor Extraordinaire: The Life and Work of John HC Ho*. Hong Kong: Scientific Communications (HK) Ltd, 2003.

Redwood, M. W. *It Was Like This ...* Oxford: Isis; large print edition, 2003.

Ride, Edwin. *BAAG: Hong Kong Resistance, 1942–1945*. Hong Kong: Oxford University Press, 1981.

Sala, Ida. *History of Our Canossian Missions: The First Fifty Years, Hong Kong, 1860–1910*. Hong Kong: Daughters of Charity of Canossa, 1997.

Selwyn-Clarke, P. Selwyn. *Footprints: The Memoirs of Sir Selwyn Selwyn-Clarke*. Hong Kong: Sino-American Publishing, 1975

Sinn, E. *Power and Charity: A Chinese Merchant Elite in Colonial Hong Kong*. Hong Kong: Hong Kong University Press, 2003.

Smith, C. T. *A Sense of History: Studies of the Social and Urban History of Hong Kong*. Hong Kong: Hong Kong Educational Publishing Co. 1995.

Starling, A. R. *The Chance of a Life Time: The Birth of a New Medical School in Hong Kong*. Hong Kong: The Chinese University of Hong Kong Press, 1988.

Starling, A., F. Ho, L. Luke, S. C. Tso, and Edwin Yu. *Plague, SARS and the Story of Medicine in Hong Kong*. Hong Kong: Hong Kong University Press, 2006.

Stewart J. C. *The Quality of Mercy: The Lives of Sir James and Lady Cantlie*. New York: Unwin Hyman, first edition 1983.

Ticozzi, Sergio. *Historical Documents of the Hong Kong Catholic Church*. Hong Kong: Hong Kong Catholic Diocesan Archives, 1997.

Tucker, Sara. *The Canton Hospital and Medicine in Nineteenth Century China, 1835–1900*. Ann Arbor, MI: University Microfilms International, 1986.

van Langenberg, Arthur. *From Scalpel to Spade: A Surgeon's Road to Ithaka*. Hong Kong: The Chinese University of Hong Kong Press, 2021.

Wang Family. *Wongs and Wangs Chronicle*, privately published, 2005.

Wright, Arnold, and H. A. Cartwright. *Twentieth Century Impressions of Hong Kong, Shanghai and Other Treaty Ports*, Volume 1. London: Lloyds Greater Britain publishing Company, 1908.

Yeo, Florence. *My Memories*. Pittsburgh, PA: Dorrance Publishing, 1994.

Book Chapters

Allbrook, Malcolm. "King, Gordon (1900–1991)." In *Australian Dictionary of Biography*, Volume 19. Australia: ANU Press, 2021, 480–481.

Baber, Flora. "The Role of the Pediatrician in the Community of Hong Kong. Reflection on a Longitudinal Study 1967–76." In *C. Elaine Field Lectures, 1974–1993*. Hong Kong: Hong Kong Paediatric Society 1994, 34–42.

Chan, T. K. "Achievements in Haematology." In *Achievements in Medicine 1974–1989, Department of Medicine, University of Hong Kong*. Hong Kong: Hong Kong University Press, 1989, 64.

Chan, T. K. "Tribute and Biography: David Todd." In *Achievements in Medicine 1974–1989, Department of Medicine, University of Hong Kong*. Hong Kong: Hong Kong University Press, 1989, 1.

Cheung, K. L. "Achievements in Cardiology." In *Achievements in Medicine 1974–1989, Department of Medicine, University of Hong Kong*. Hong Kong: Hong Kong University Press, 1989, 28–32.

Chow, York Y. N. "Prof. Sir Harry S. Y. Fang." In Hong Kong College of Orthopedic Surgeons and the Hong Kong Orthopedic Association, *Repair, Reconstruct and Rehabilitate. Half a Century of Orthopedics in Hong Kong*. Hong Kong: Hong Kong Academy of Medicine Press, 2004, 174–176.

Foo, T. N. "The Mental Health Association of Hong Kong: A Brief History." In T. P. Khoo ed., *Aspects of Mental Health Care: Hong Kong 1981*. Hong Kong: Mental Health Association of Hong Kong, 1981, 85–103.

King, Gordon. "An Episode in the History of the University." In Clifford Matthews and Oswald Cheung eds., *Dispersal and Renewal: Hong Kong University During the War Years*. Hong Kong: Hong Kong University Press, 1998, 85–104.

Lee, Peter C. Y. "Keynote Address." In *15th Anniversary Celebration Commemorative*. Hong Kong: Hong Kong College of General Practitioner, 1993, 2.

———. "Contributions and Influence of the Hong Kong College in the Development of Family Medicine in Hong Kong and around the World during the Past Quarter Century (1977–2002) as Seen Through the Eyes of Its Founding President," March 2003. In *25th Anniversary Commemorative Brochure*. Hong Kong: Hong Kong College of Family Physicians, 2003, 9.

———. "Message from the Founding President." In *The First 30 Years of the Hong Kong College of Family Physicians*. Hong Kong: The Hong Kong College of Family Physicians, 2007, 20–21.

———. "Introduction of General Practice/Family Medicine into China, The Role of HKCGP/HKCFP in the Early Years." In *The First 30 Years of the Hong Kong College of Family Physicians*. Hong Kong: The Hong Kong College of Family Physicians, 2007, 155–56.

Leung, Gabriel. "Shizhiminggui de dayi—Wangyuanmei" [GB Ong—A Great Doctor]. In *Dayi jingcheng: Xianggang yixue fazhan yibai sanshi nian* [The Great Doctors: The Medical Development of Hong Kong in Its 130 Years]. Hong Kong: Joint publishing (HK) Co. Ltd., 2017, 106–109.

Li, Henry F. K. "Report from the Chairman." in HKCGP Inauguration Ceremony Commemorative Brochure 1979, 3.

Lunney, Linde. "Monaghan, Cathleen (Sister Mary Aquinas)." In James McGuire and James Quin, eds., *Dictionary of Irish Biography*. Cambridge: Cambridge University Press, 2009, 572–573.

Mak, Grace C. L. "Women and Education." In Susanne Y. P. Choi and Fanny M. Cheung, eds., *Women and Girls in Hong Kong: Current Situation and Future Challenges*. Hong Kong: Hong Kong Institute of Asia-Pacific Studies, The Chinese University of Hong Kong, 2012, 24.

Lam, S. K., and W. M. Hui, "Achievements in Gastroenterology/Hepatology." In *Achievements in Medicine 1974–1985, Department of Medicine, University of Hong Kong*. Hong Kong: Hong Kong University Press, 45–54.

Ride, L. "The Faculty of Medicine." In Brian Harrison, *The University of Hong Kong: The First 50 Years (1911–1961)*. Hong Kong: Hong Kong University Press, 1964, 104–107.

Ride, Lindsay. "The Test of War (Part 1)." In Clifford Matthews and Oswald Cheung, eds., *Dispersal and Renewal: Hong Kong University during the War Years*. Hong Kong: Hong Kong University Press, 1998, 9–24.

Rodrigues, Albert. "A Hong Kong Doctor in War and Peace." In *Dispersal and Renewal, Hong Kong University during the War Years*. Hong Kong: Hong Kong University Press, 1998, 203–205.

Todd, David. "Recent Developments in Medical Education in Hong Kong." In *Plague, SARS and the Story of Medicine in Hong Kong*, Hong Kong Museum of Medical Sciences Society. Hong Kong: Hong Kong University Press, 2006, 288–289.

Wong, T. M. K. "Local Voluntarism: The Medical Mission of the London Missionary Society in Hong Kong 1842–1923." In D. Hardiman, ed., *Healing Bodies Saving Souls: Medical Mission in Asia and Africa*. Amsterdam-New York, Rodopi, 2006.

Young, R. T. T. "Vision and Mission. A History of the Department of Medicine." In *Achievements in Medicine, 1989–1995, Department of Medicine, University of Hong Kong*. Hong Kong: ColorPrint Production Co., 1995, 1–13.

Young, R. T. T, C. Wang, K. S. L. Lam, K. K. Pun, and A. W. C. Kung. "Achievements in Endocrinology." In *Achievements in Medicine 1974–1989, Department of Medicine, University of Hong Kong*. Hong Kong: Hong Kong University Press, 1989, 37–44.

Thesis

George, Janet. "Moving with Chinese Opinion: Hong Kong's Maternity Service 1881–1941," PhD thesis, University of Sydney, 1992.

Ham, Daniel. "The Management of Malaria and Leprosy in Hong Kong and the International Settlement of Shanghai 1880s–1940s," PhD thesis, Corpus Christi College, Cambridge, England, 2013.

Petrie, I. C. "The Problem of Infant Mortality in Hong Kong 1886–1937," MA Thesis, The University of British Columbia, August 1996.

Tsang, Carol C. L. "Out of the Dark: Women's Medicine and Women's Disease in Colonial Hong Kong," PhD thesis, the University of Hong Kong, 2011.

Journal Articles, and Online Articles

Anderson, John. "The Present Position of Malaria in Hong Kong." *Caduceus*, 6(2) (1927): 105–115.

Anon. "Chinese Medical Women." *British Medical Journal*, 15 April 1899: 927–928.

Anon. "Notes and Comments." *Caduceus*, 1(1) (1922): 5–6.

Anon. "Notes and Comments." *Caduceus*, 1(1) (1922): 8.

Anon. "The Medical Curriculum." *Caduceus*, 2(1) (1923): 8.

Anon. "Hospital Work at the University Clinics." *Caduceus*, 3(1) (1924): 40–41

Anon. "Notes and Comments." *Caduceus*, 6(1) (1927): 83.

Anon. "Notes and Comments." *Caduceus*, 7(2) (1928): 101.

Anon. "Notes and Comment." *Caduceus* 7(3) (1928): 184.

Anon. "Notes and Comments." *Caduceus* 7(3) (1928): 186.

Anon. "Notes and Comments. Francis Clark," *Caduceus*, 7(4) (1928): 290.

Anon. "Notes and Comments." *Caduceus*, 7(4) (1928): 291.

Anon. "Dr. Alice Deborah Hickling, M.B.E." *Caduceus*, 7(4) (1928): 292.

Anon. "Notes and Comments." *Caduceus*, 8(1) (1929): 69.

Anon. "The Birthday Honors." *British Medical Journal*, 1 (4093) (1939): 1247.

Anon. "Medical Birthday Honors." *Brit Med J* (22 June 1946), 961.

Anon. "Kenelm Hutchinson Digby." *Elixir*, May 1954: 67–69.

Anon. "New Hong Kong University Obstetric Department: New Maternity Hospital." *Brit Med J*, 1 (4929) (1955): 1527–1528.

Anon. Interview of Professor Sir David Todd by DBS carried out on 1 December 2015. *Steps* (DBS School Magazine, Chinese section), 2016, 11–16.

Arnold, D. "British India and the 'Beriberi Problem' 1798–1942." *Med History*, 54 (2010): 295–314.

Bailey, H, M. Gabriel, A. R. Hodgson, and J. S. Shin. "Tuberculosis of the Spine in Children. Operative Findings and Results in One Hundred Consecutive Patients Treated by Removal of the Lesion and Anterior Grafting." *J Bone & Joint Surg* (Am), 54 (1972): 1633–1657.

Binns, Colin, Andy Lee, and Wah Yun Low. "Obituary, Professor Shiu-Hung Lee." *Asia-Pacific Journal of Public Health*, 26(2) (2014): 215–216.

Butt, Rudi. "Woo Wai-tak, Arthur (1919–1964)." Biographical Dictionary of Medical Practitioners in Hong Kong, 1841–1941. Accessed on 23 April 2022, https://hkmd1841-1941.blogspot.com/2013/09/woo-wai-tak-arthur-1919.html.

Chan-Yeung, M. "Eastern District (Wanchai) Dispensary and Plague Hospital." *Hong Kong Med J*, 25(6) (2019): 503–505.

Chan-Yeung, M. "Dr Alice Hickling (1876–1928): The Doctor Who Changed the Paradigm of Maternal Care in Hong Kong." *Hong Kong Med J*, 27(5) (2021), 389.

Chau, W. C., and F. I. Tseung, "The Hong Kong Chinese Medical Association." *The Bulletin of the Hong Kong Chinese Medical Association*, 1(1) (1948): 8–12.

Che, Thomas S. N., and Peter S. Y. Chen. "The Accomplishments of Sir James Cantlie." *J Med Biography*, 7 (1999): 197–199.

Chernin, Eli. "Sir Patrick Manson: An Annotated Bibliography and a Note on a Collected Set of His Writings." *Reviews of Infectious Diseases*, 5 (2) (1983):356–387.

Chiu, Helen F. K. "Professor Pow-Meng Yap: A Giant in Psychiatry from Hong Kong." *Asia-Pacific Psychiatry*, 4(2012): 84–86.

Choa, G. "An Odyssey to a Land of Woes." *Hong Kong Journal of Mental Health*, 28 (1999), 63.

Chow, Anne W. M. "Root of Hong Kong Midwifery." *HKJGOM*, 1 (2000): 72–80.

Chow, York Y. N. "Obituary. Harry S. Y. Fang." *Journal of Orthopedic Surgery*, 17(3) (2009): 259–260.

Chun, Daphne. "History of Cesarean Section." *Elixir*, Summer 1957, 16–24.

DeVine, Charles Leslie. "A Man Overlooked: A Faded Memory of a Glorious Career." Armenians in India—Behind the Scenes Forgotten History. Accessed on 11 January 2022, http://chater-genealogy.blogspot.com/2015/01/a-man-overlooked-faded-memory-of.html.

Digby, K. H. "Review: A Plea for the Tonsils." *British Medical Journal*, 2 (3070) (1919): 562.

———. "What Is a 'Diseased' Tonsil"? *British Medical Journal*, 1 (3260) (1923): 1075.

———. "A Suggestion for the Treatment of Early Phthisis by Upper Intercostals Nerve Block." *Caduceus*, 3(3) (1924): 111–112.

———. "A Few Observations on the Properties of Ivory as a Material for Use in Bone Surgery." *Caduceus*, 3(3) (1924): 103–110.

———. "Presidential Address on Clinical Research." *Caduceus*, 3(1) (1924): 31–36.

———. "Common-duct Stones of Liver Origin." *The British Journal of Surgery*, 17 (1930): 578–591.

———. "Nasopharyngeal Carcinoma." *The British Journal of Surgery*, 27 (1941): 517–537.

Digby, K. H., G. H. Thomas, and S. T. Hsiu, "Notes on Carcinoma of the Nasopharynx." *Caduceus*, 9 (2) (1930): 45–68.

Earle, H. G. "Basal Metabolism." *Caduceus*, 1 (1922): 81–85.

Editorial. "Woman as Doctor and Woman as Nurse." *The Lancet*, 17 August 1878: 226–227.

Fan, Ka-wai. "Pao-chang Hou, (1893–1967): Pathologist and Historian of Chinese Medicine." *Journal of Medical Biography*, 14(2) (2006), accessed on 11 February 2022. https://journals.sagepub.com/doi/abs/10.1177/096777200601400407.

Fan, T. W. "The Life and Works of Professor Pow-meng Yap." *Hong Kong Journal of Mental Health*, 28 (1999):16–20.

Fang, David. "Harry S. Y. Fang—The Legend Lives On." *Hong Kong Med J*, 16 (5) (2009): 402.

Fong, L. Y, J. H. Ho, and D. P. Huang, "Preserved Foods as Possible Cancer Hazards: WA Rats Fed Salted Fish Have Mutagenic Urine." *Int J Cancer*, 23 (1979): 542–546.

Foo, Stephen. "In Memory of Dr. Peter C. Y. Lee." In The Obituary of Dr. Peter CY Lee. Hong Kong College of Family Physicians, 2013, 14–15. https://www.hkcfp.org.hk/Upload/Commemorative/Obituary_and_Remembrances/obituary_Dr.PeterLee.pdf, accessed on 9/9/2022.

Fu, Louis. "The Contributions of Kenelm Hutchinson Digby to Orthopedics in Hong Kong Part 1." *Journal of Orthopedics, Trauma and Rehabilitation*, 19 (2015): 66–71.

George, J. "The Lady Doctor's 'Warm welcome,' Dr. Alice Sibree and the Early Years of Hong Kong's Maternity Service 1903–1909." *Journal of the Hong Kong Branch of the Royal Asiatic Society*, 33(1993): 81–109.

Haoran. "Huhuide yisheng xianggang haimian shi yi di yi ren" [Dr. Arthur Woo was the first to operate charity floating clinic in Hong Kong]. *Christian Weekly*, no. 2461, 23 October 2011.

Harrison, Mark. "Cantlie, Sir James." *Oxford Dictionary of National Biography*. Accessed on 24 January 2022, https://www.oxforddnb.com/view/10.1093/ref:odnb/9780198614128.001.0001/odnb-9780198614128-e-50530.

He, Gaojun. "Guangdong sheng zhengfu qudi yiwu zhi yuanyin" [Reasons for the Guangdong provincial government to ban certain medical services]. *Zhonghua yi bao*, 6 (1913): 1–10.

He, Gaojun. "Yu zhongguo kexue fada dang yi zhongguo wen shou ke bing yi kexue shu bao yijian shu" [If you want China to develop science, you should teach in Chinese and translate scientific publications—A proposal]. *Xinmin Bao*, 4 (6) (1917): 38–40; 4 (7) (1917): 38–41.

Ho, Faith C. S. "Hong Kong's First Professor of Pathology and the Laboratory of the Royal College of Physicians of Edinburgh." *J R Coll Physicians Edin*, 41 (2011): 67–72.

———. "Dr. Tseung Fat Im's Notebook of Professor Anderson's Lectures, 1924," *Hong Kong Med J*, 22 (2016): 298–99.

Ho, John H. C. "An Epidemiologic and Clinical Study of Nasopharyngeal Carcinoma." *Int. I Radiation Oncology, Biology, Physics*, 4(3–4) (1978): 193–198.

Hobson, Benjamin. "Report of the Medical Missionary Society's Hospital at Hongkong." *Chinese Repository*, 14 (1844): 380–381.

Hong, Chuang-Ye, and Fu-Mei Wang. "Chinese Translation of English Textbooks on Internal Medicine from the 1850s to the 1940s." *ScienceDirect, Journal of the Chinese Medical Association*, 77 (2014): 277–282.

Horder, M. "The Hard-Boiled Saint: Selwyn-Clarke in Hong Kong." *Brit Med J*, 311 (1995): 492–495.

Huang, C. T. "Prof Hou Pao-Chang." *Elixir*, 1, (1967), 15.

Huang, Rayson. "Eulogy: Professor James Blackburn Gibson." Hong Kong University Digital Repository at HKUL. *Interflow*, no. 71. March 1994.

Humphries, M. "Obituary: Sister Mary Gabriel O'Mahony." *Hong Kong Med J*, 12(5) (2006): 402.

Hussey, Kristin D. "Sir Patrick Manson at Home: 21 Queen Anne Street as a Hybrid Space." *J R Coll Physicians Edin*, 49 (2019): 84–91.

Jefferson, Laura, Karen Bloor, and Alan Maynard. "Women in Medicine: Historical Perspectives and Recent Trends." *British Medical Bulletin*, 114 (2015): 5–15.

Kelly, Fiona E, Kevin Fong, Nicholas Hirsch, and Jerry P. Nolan. "Intensive Care Medicine Is 60 years Old: The History and Future of the Intensive Care Unit." *Clin Med (Lond)*, 14(4) (2014): 376–379.

Khoo, U. S. "Handbook of Pathology." *Hong Kong Med J*, 24(5) (2018): 546–548.

King, Gordon. "The History of Tsan Yuk Hospital 1922–1955." *Bulletin of the Hong Kong Chinese Medical Association*, 8 (1956): 31–39.

King, Gordon and L. T. Ride. "The Relation of Vitamin B1 Deficiency to the Pregnancy Anemias—A Study of 371 Cases of Beri-beri Complicating Pregnancy." *J Obstetrics Gynecology British Empire*, LII(2) (1945): 1–18.

Lam, Cindy L. K. "Professor Sir David Todd, Honorary Fellow, Hong Kong College of Family Physicians." Accessed on 18 March 2022, https://www.hkcfp.org.hk/Upload/Commemorative/Obituary_and_Remembrances/obituary-Prof.%20DavidTodd.pdf.

Lam, Clarence C. K. "Journey Through Quantitative Hematology." *Hong Kong Med J*, 26 (6) (2020): 556–558.

Lam, S. K., and P. C. Lai. "Colonic Ether in Obstetrics and Gynecology." *Caduceus*, 7(4) (1928): 238–243.

Lau, C. S. "Professor Sir David Todd." *Hong Kong Med J*, 23(2017): 541.

Lau, Herbert K. "Dr. Arthur W. Woo. Rejuvenated the broken Hong Kong Rotary Club in 1945." Accessed on 24 April 2022, http://old.rotary3450.org/woo-a-w-dr/.

Lau, Herbert K. "Hong Kong Rotarian Dr. Tseung Fat Im, Instrumental in Forming the United College and the Establishment of the Chinese University of Hong Kong." Accessed on 18 March 2024, https://old.rotary3450.org/tseung-fat-im-hong-kong-dr/.

Lau, Herbert K. "Father of Rehabilitation in Asia, Sir Harry S. Y. Fang, M.B.B.S., M.Sc., J.P., Hon L.L.D. (HKU), D.S.Sc. D.Sc, Kt, G.B.M., C.B.E." Accessed on 26 February 2022, http://old.rotary3450.org/fang-harry-s-y/

Lee, A. W. M. "A tribute to the Emperor Extraordinaire: The Legend of Professor John HC Ho." *J HK Coll Radiol*, 8 (2005): 117–120.

Lee, S. H. "The 60-Year Battle against Tuberculosis in Hong Kong—A Review of the Past and a Projection into the 21st Century." *Respirology*, 13 (Suppl. 3) (2008): S49–S55.

Lett, Z. "Obituary." *Brit Med J* (Clin Res Ed) , 292 (1986): 208.

———. "Obituary, Dr. Kok Cheang Yeo, CMG, MD, DPH, DTM& H." *Hong Kong College of Anesthesiologists Newsletter*, September 2004.

Li, Shu Fan. "The Surgical Side of General Practice." *Caduceus*, 5(1) (1926): 14–19.

———. "Recent Development and Observations on Spinal Anesthesia under Novocaine Caffeine Compound." *Caduceus*, 6(3) (1927): 326.

———. "Reminiscence of 50 Years of Medical Work in Hong Kong and China." *Bull of the Hong Kong Chinese Medical Association*, 10 (1958):161–173.

Liu, S. "The New Life and I." *New Life Psychiatric Rehabilitation Association Annual Report*, 1990, 49–51.

Lo, Ronald. "Obituary- Dr. Zoltan (Lefty) Lett." Royal College of Anesthetists, accessed on 7 March 2022, https://rcoa.ac.uk/obituary-dr-zoltan-lefty-lett.

———. "'Dr. Zoltan Lett, MD, DA, FRCA, FFARCS, FANZCA, FHKCA, FHKAM (Anes)' on the Conferment of Honorary Fellowship of the Hong Kong College of Anesthesiologists at the 25th Congregation of the College," Accessed on 7 March 2022, https://www.hkca.edu.hk/archives/HKCAbulletin/E-news/doc/Citation-Zoltan_Lett.pdf.

Lo, W. H. "Development of Legislation for the Mentally Ill in Hong Kong." *Hong Kong Journal of Mental Health*, 43(1) (2017): 22–26.

Manson-Bahr, Philip. "Obituary. John Anderson MA, MD, BSc, MRCP, DTM and H." *Brit Med J*, April 11, 1931; 647–648.

———. "Sir Patrick Manson. The Founder of the Medical College of Hong Kong (October 1, 1887), and Its First Dean." *Elixir*, Spring (1956): 22–30.

Manson, Patrick. "Remarks on an Operation for Abscesses of the Liver." *Brit Med J*, 1 (1892):163–167.

Margetts, Edward L. "Pow Meng Yap (1921–1971)." *Canad Psychiat Ass J*, 17 (1972): 253–254.

Medical Research Council Working Party on Tuberculosis of the Spine. "A Controlled Trial of Anterior Spinal Fusion and Debridement in the Surgical Management of Tuberculosis of the Spine in Patients on Standard Chemotherapy: A Study in Hong Kong." *The British Journal of Surgery*, 61 (1974): 853–866.

Mo, Mimi. "Biographic Notes. The Legacy of Dr. Kok Cheang Yeo, the first Chinese Director of Medical and Health Services of Hong Kong." *JRASHKB*, 54 (2014): 181–194.

Moodie, A. S. "Tuberculosis in Hong Kong." *Tubercle, Lond.*, 44(1963): 334–345.

Nambiar, Raj M. "Obituary, Professor Tan Sri Guan Bee Ong PSM, OBE, MD, DS, FAMS (Hon) (1921–10 January 2004)." *Annals Academy of Medicine*, May 2004, accessed on 28 February 2022, https://annals.edu.sg/pdf200405/V33N3p398.pdf.

Ng, Jacob W. T., and John Y. H. Ho. "An Addendum to 'Doctor for Society'—Professor Lee Shiu Hung: 'Pass on Benevolence, Pass on the Legend'." *Hong Kong Med J*, 20 (2) (2014): 169.

Nixon, W. C. W. "J. Preston Maxwell, M.D., F.R.C.S., F.R.C.O.G." *British Medical Journal*, 2(5251) (1961): 590–591.

O'Mahony, M. Gabriel. "Doctor at Large-Hospice Care." *The Hong Kong Practitioner*, 10 (2) (1988): 3024–3027.

"Obituary, Benjamin Hobson, MB, MRCP." *Brit Med J* (29 March 1873): 355.

"Obituary, Philip Burnard Chenery Ayres. CMG, MRCS Eng. LRCP Edin, Late Colonial Surgeon and Inspector of Hospitals, Hong Kong." The Thames Database, taken from an obituary notice of 28 October 1899, printed in the *Lancet*. http://www.thamehistory.net/people/Ayres.htm.

"Obituary, Philip B.C. Ayres, CMG, MRCS." *Br Med J*, 2 (1899): 1140.

"Obituary, John Murray." *Brit Med J*, 8 August 1903, 339.

"Obituary, John Mitford Atkinson, M.B. (Lond.)." *Brit Med J*, 16 June 1917, 827.

"Obituary, Dr Alice Deborah Hickling." *Br Med J*, 6 October 1928, 635.

"Obituary, A. R. Wellington, CMG, MRCS, LRCP, DPH, DTM&H." *Brit Med J*, 25, November 1961, 1439.

"Obituary, A. W. Woo, OBE, MBBS, FRCS." *Br Med J*, 11 April 1964. Accessed on 23 April 2022, https://www.bmj.com/content/bmj/1/5388/988.full.pdf

"Obituary, Professor Hou Pao Chang." Nature 214 (1967): 539.

"Obituary, A. J. S. McFadzean, OBE, DSc, MD, FRCP, FRCP Ed, FACP." *Brit Med J*, 6 (1974): 723.

"Obituary, Sir Lindsay Ride C.B.E., Ed., M.A., D.M." *Br Med J*, 2 (6096) (1977): 1228.

"Obituary, Shiu-Hung Lee, b. 6 June 1933 d. 9 January 2014." *The Royal College of Physicians*, London. Accessed on 16 February 2022, https://history.rcplondon.ac.uk/inspiring-physicians/shiu-hung-lee.

Parry, Jane. "Obituary: John HC Ho." *Brit Med J*, 331 (2005): 578.

Paterson, Andrew. "Edward Hamilton Paterson." *Brit Med J*, 348 (2014): 1250.

Paterson, E. H. "Cleft Lip Surgery." *Bulletin of the Hong Kong Chinese Medical Association*, 11 (1960): 77–81.

———. "Cleft Lips and Palates in Hong Kong." *Hong Kong Nursing Journal*, 22 (1977): 45–50.

———. "The Kwun Tong Community Health Project." *Trop Doct*, 8 (1978): 85–89.

———. "Outside Europe. An Urban Community Health Project." *Brit Med J*, 280 (1980): 29–31.

Phoon, S. W. "Kenelm Hutchinson Digby, O.B.E., F.R.C.S. An Appreciation." *Bulletin of the Hong Kong Chinese Medical Association*, 7 (1955): 26–28.

Poynter, J. R. "Ride, Sir Lindsay Tasman (1898–1977)." *Australian Dictionary of Biography*, National Center of Biography, Australian National University, volume 16, Melbourne University Press, 2002. Accessed on 31 August 2022, https://adb.anu.edu.au/biography/ride-sir-lindsay-tasman-11524/text20557.

Prabook. "Herbert Earle." Accessed on 26 January 2022, https://prabook.com/web/herbert.earle/2347211.

Pryor, E. G. "A Historical Review of Housing Conditions in Hong Kong." *Journal of Hong Kong Branch of Royal Asiatic Society*, 12 (1972): 89–129.

Ride, Lindsay, K. D. Ling, E. Q. Lim, and S. F. Cheng. "Some Biochemical Aspects of Acute Cholera." *Caduceus*, 17(4) (1938): 175–201.

Ride, Lindsay. "Fifty Years of Medical Education in Hong Kong." *Caduceus*, 16(2) (1937): 45–61.

Roland, Charles. "Sir Albert Rodrigues, M. D., POW Experiences as a MO in Hong Kong 1941–1945." Interviewed in Hong Kong, China by Charles Roland 8 September 1987, *Oral History Archives*. Hannah Chair for the History of Medicine, McMaster University. Interview no HCM 8–87.

The Royal College of Surgeons of England. "Obituary: Guan Bee Ong." *BMJ*.,328 (2004): 771. Accessed on 28 February 2022, https://livesonline.rcseng.ac.uk/client/en_GB/lives/search/detailnonmodal/.

Saw, Swee-Hock, and Chiu Wing Kin. "Population Growth and Redistribution in Hong Kong, 1841–1975." *Southeast Asian Journal of Social Science*, 4(1) (1975): 126.

Senkoylu, Alpaslan. "Arthur Ralph Hodgson." *The Journal of Turkish Spinal Surgery*, 23 (3) (2012): 253–257.

Severn, A. G. M., and K. H. Digby. "Two Cases of Intrahepatic Stone Formation and Suppression of Bile." *Caduceus*, 3(3) (1924): 145–150.

Sim, Patrick P. "A Measure of Gold, Hong Kong Anesthesia at 50." *Anesthesiology*, 107(1) (2007): 153.

TAC. "Obituary, Sister Mary Aquinas, OBE, FRCPED." *Brit Med J* (Clin Res Ed), 292 (1986): 208.

To Kelvin K. W., and Kwok-Yung Yuen. "In Memory of Patrick Manson, Founding Father of Tropical Medicine and the Discovery of Vector-Borne Infections." *Emerging Microbes and Infections*, 1:1, 1–7, DOI: 10.1038/emi.2012.32.

Todd, David. "Obituary. Gerald Hugh Choa (b.21 March 1921 d.3 December 2001)." *Royal College of Physicians of Edinburgh*. Accessed on 17 February 2022, https://history.rcplondon.ac.uk/inspiring-physicians/gerald-hugh-choa.

———. "Professor A. J. S. McFadzean—An Appreciation." *Caduceus*, Special issue, the McFadzean Memorial Issue 1 (1975): 121–123.

Tottenham, R. E., and E. C. Crichton, "Clinical Report of the Rotunda Hospital for One Year. November 1st 1913 to October 31st 1914." *Transactions of the Royal Academy of Medicine in Ireland*, 3 (1) (1915) 287–325.

———. "Maternity Work in the Colony of Hong Kong." *Caduceus*, 5(2) (1926): 82–87.

———. "Strictures of the Vagina among the Chinese." *Caduceus*, 6(2) (1927): 150–154.

———. "Some Observations on the History and Treatment of Eclampsia." *Caduceus*, 7(1) (1928): 8–13.

Tseung, F. I. "Diabetes Mellitus. The Significance of Biochemical Tests in Its Diagnosis and Treatment." *Caduceus*, 5(3) (1926): 197–226.

University of Hong Kong. Herbert Gastineau Earle. Doctor of Laws honoris causa. Congregation 1936. Accessed on 28 January 2022, https://www4.hku.hk/hongrads/citations/m-a-m-b-herbert-gastineau-earle.

University of Hong Kong. Citation, Li Shu Fan, Doctor of Laws honoris causa. 55th Congregation (1961), The University of Hong Kong. Accessed on 3 February 2022, https://www4.hku.hk/hongrads/citations/mb-chb-frcs-shu-fan-li-li-shu-fan.

University of Hong Kong. Tseung Fat Im, Doctor of Laws honoris causa, 72nd Congregation, 1969, The University of Hong Kong. Accessed on 5 February, 2022. https://www4.hku.hk/hongrads/graduates/obe-mb-bs-jp-fat-im-tseung-tseung-fat-im

University Obstetric Department. "Clinical Report of the Department of Obstetrics and Gynecology of the University of Hong Kong 1937 and 1938." *Caduceus*, 18(2) (1939): 144.

Wang, C. Y. "Infantile Tetanus (Tetanus neonatorum) in Hong Kong: Its Prevalence and Sources of Infection." *Caduceus*, 6 (1927): 249.

Weil, M. H. "The Society of Critical Care Medicine, Its History and Its Destiny." *Crit Care Med*, 1 (1973):1–4.

Wellington, A. R. "Malaria in Its Relation to Man and Mosquitoes." *Caduceus*, 8, 3 (1929):117–129.

———. "The Life History of Mosquitoes," *Caduceus*, 9, 1, (1930): 15.

Woo, Sing Lim. "Dr. Tseung Fat Im, M.B.B.S. (Hong Kong)." *The Prominent Chinese in Hong Kong (1937)*. Hong Kong: Wuzhou shuju, 1937. Accessed on 4 February 2022,https://digitalrepository.lib.hku.hk/catalog/s7526c53d#?c=&m=&s=&cv=&xywh=-2095%2C-95%2C5389%2C1865.

World Health Organization. "History of the Development of the ICD." Accessed 2 July 2014, https://cdn.who.int/media/docs/default-source/classification/icd/historyoficd.pdf?sfvrsn=b9e617af_3.

Wu, Harry Y. J. "Triturator for Smallpox Vaccine Production." *Hong Kong Med J*, 25 (2019): 86–88.

Wylie, H. W. "Colonial Surgeon Extraordinary—The Era of Dr P. B. C. Ayres, CMG." *The Bulletin-Journal of the Society of Medical Officer of Health Hong Kong*, 1 (1969): 9–19.

Yap, P. M. "The Latah Reaction: Its Pathodynamics and Nosological Position." *Journal of Mental Science*, 98 (1952): 515–564.

———. "Suicide in Hong Kong." *Journal of Mental Science*, 194 (1958): 261–301.

———. "Koro- A Culture-Bound Depersonalization Syndrome." *British Journal of Psychiatry*, 111 (1965): 43–50.

Yeo, Dick. Excerpts from '*Glimpses of K.C.'s Life*' which was read by Dick Yeo at the Memorial Service held in Mountfield Church on 18th June 2004. Accessed on 14 February 2022, http://kcyeo.com/.

Yeung, C. Y. "Evolution of Child Health Care in Hong Kong." *HK J Paediatr* (New Series), 6 (2001): 66–71.

Young, Rosie. "Eulogy." In Memoriam: Professor Sir David Todd 1928–2017. Accessed on 17 March 2022, https://www.med.hku.hk/remembertodd/Eulogy.pdf.

Yu, W. K. "Palliative Care in Practice." *The Hong Kong Practitioner*, 9(6) (1987): 2531–44.

Yu, Y. L. "Reminiscence of Three Former Teachers: Prof. AJS McFadzean, Dr. Stephen Chang and Prof. Gerald Choa." *Hong Kong Med J*, 15(4) (2009) 315–319.

Websites

Biographic Dictionary of Medical Practitioners of Hong Kong, 1841 to 1941. http://hkmd1841-1941.blogspot.com

Department of Health. https://www.dh.gov.hk

Department of Pediatrics, HKU website. http://paed.hku.hk/

Gwulo Old Hong Kong. https://gwulo.com

Historical Laws of Hong Kong Online. https://oelawhk.lib.hku.hk/exhibits/show/oelawhk/home

History of Rotary International and District 3450. http://old.rotary3450.org/our_history/

Hong Kong Annual Digest of Statistics. https://www.censtatd.gov.hk/en/EIndexbySubject.html?pcode=B1010003&scode=460

Hong Kong Government Reports Online (1842–1941). https://sunzi.lib.hku.hk/hkgro/index.jsp

Honorary Degree Congregation, HKU. https://www4.hku.hk/hongrads/

Jockey Club School of Public Health and Primary Care. https://www.sphpc.cuhk.edu.hk/

Legislative Council, HKSAR. https://www.legco.gov.hk/

Royal Asiatic Society Hong Kong Website. http://www.royalasiaticsociety.org.hk

Royal College of Surgeons: Plarr's Lives of the Fellows Online. https://livesonline.rcseng.ac.uk/client/en_GB/lives/?

The Society for the Aid and Rehabilitation of Drug Addicts (SARDA), https://www.sarda.org.hk/eng/index.html

World Medical Association. https://www.wma.net/who-we-are/about-us/

Index

www.ingramcontent.com/pod-product-compliance
Ingram Content Group UK Ltd.
Pitfield, Milton Keynes, MK11 3LW, UK
UKHW022318230625
459998UK00004B/7/J

9 789882 37354